NUTRITION FOR THE GROWING YEARS

By Fredrick J. Stare and Margaret McWilliams:

Living Nutrition. John Wiley & Sons, Inc., New York, 1973.
Nutrition for Good Health. Plycon Press, Fullerton, CA., 1974.

By Margaret McWilliams:

Food Fundamentals. John Wiley & Sons, Inc., New York, 1966, 1974.
Illustrated Guide to Food Preparation. Plycon Press,
Fullerton, CA., 1969, 1971.

By Lendal Kotschevar and Margaret McWilliams:

Understanding Food. John Wiley & Sons, Inc., New York, 1969.

By Margaret McWilliams and Linda Davis:

Food and You. Ginn & Co., Boston, 1971.

NUTRITION
for the
GROWING YEARS

SECOND EDITION

By
Margaret McWilliams

Professor and Chairman
Department of Home Economics
California State University, Los Angeles

JOHN WILEY AND SONS, INC.
NEW YORK   LONDON   SYDNEY   TORONTO

Library of Congress Cataloging in Publication Data

McWilliams, Margaret
   Nutrition for the growing years.

   Includes bibliographies and index.
   1. Children--Nutrition. I. Title.
[DNLM: 1. Child nutrition. WS115 M177n]
RJ206.M26 1975   613.2   74-28180
ISBN 0-471-58738-9

Printed in the United States of America

10 9 8 7 6 5 4 3

Preface

The field of child nutrition is one which excites the researcher and stimulates the practitioner to make ever greater efforts to improve the nutritional status of the world's children. Although this has been an area of nutrition that has been of interest for many years, the programs centering around the implications of nutrition on child growth and development have been multiplying in the past decade. As a result, the significance of psychological, economic, and sociological influences in molding dietary patterns is being brought into focus.

World food problems are of particular concern; food shortages and nutritional ramifications have long been affecting some of the developing countries. Now these concerns are spreading to the United States, too. Children are particularly vulnerable to nutritional deficiencies, and an adequate diet is needed continuously if they are to achieve their potential, both physically and mentally. The interrelationship of nutrition and mental development is a particularly active research area at the present time.

Increasing importance is being attached to preventive dietary measures in childhood. Recently there has been attention on the possible causal relationship between overfeeding in the early years and obesity in adulthood. The potential of altering cholesterol levels in infant feeding to form the basis for a lifetime of sensible eating to minimize the risk of coronary heart disease also is being studied. Adequate diet of girls throughout the growing years is recognized as an important step toward optimizing the outcome of pregnancy. Such topics as these provide the framework for the review of child nutrition today which is the focus of this revision.

Nutrition for the Growing Years is designed to blend the theoretical basis of child nutrition with the practical realities of feeding infants and children. Developmental needs have been emphasized to clarify the reasons for dietary suggestions. Various ways of establishing good nutrition patterns for use throughout a lifetime have been discussed. Attention is given throughout this book to the practical problems faced by physicians, nutritionists, dietitians, nursery school teachers, educators, and parents as they strive to assist children in developing attitudes and dietary habits that will be an asset for a lifetime. The bibliographies at the ends of the chapters have been selected carefully to assist the reader who may desire additional information.

The tremendous amount of research in the field of child nutrition since the publication of the first edition of this book in 1967 has made this revision a stimulating and challenging task. It is my hope that this edition will help to promote interest in child nutrition and motivate professionals and parents to work toward better nutrition for all children.

I wish to express my appreciation to: Dr. Fredrick J. Stare, a constant inspiration as a nutritionist with a keen eye on human needs and behavior; Dr. Susan Calvert, a stimulating colleague in applied nutrition; Dr. Don McWilliams, my husband and encouraging reviewer; and Roger and Kathy McWilliams, our two children who have applied the theories in this book.

LOS ANGELES

1974

Margaret McWilliams

Contents

NUTRITION FOR THE GROWING YEARS

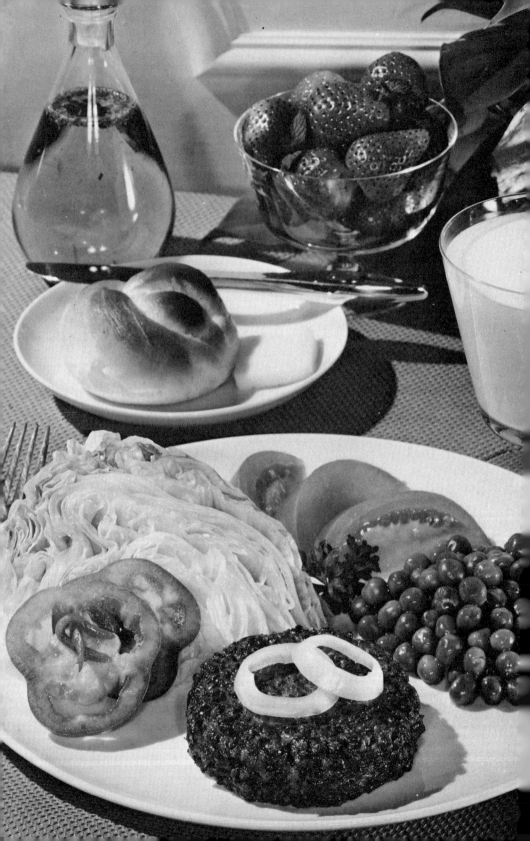

Chapter 1
Nutrition Basics

The achievement of good nutrition for all infants and children during the growing years is a goal of significance for the entire world. Adequate nutrition is one of the key factors in helping each person to achieve his full potential as an adult, and this state requires that a good diet be available and consumed throughout the early years. Each person is a summation of his total dietary history, a walking record of his nutritional status from conception. If the food supply is inadequate or the intake has been narrowed by economic factors, food prejudices, or other influences, an individual will be affected by his actual intake of foods.

Early life is recognized as being a particularly critical time for developing good dietary patterns and for providing the nutrients in the amounts required for optimum growth and development during this demanding period of rapid growth. This is a stage in the life cycle that has been the focus of extensive nutrition research in the past few years; in fact, the efforts in this realm of research have been intensifying as scientists begin to untangle and evaluate the multiple factors influencing total development of individuals.

The information presented in the subsequent chapters requires some knowledge of basic nutrition. The remainder of this chapter is an overview of nutrition. More extensive discussions of basic nutrition are available in the various nutrition texts listed at the end of this chapter.

THE NUTRIENTS

The nutrients needed by the body for growth and the maintenance of health may be divided into those contributing energy (namely, carbohydrates, fats, and protein), minerals, vitamins, and water. These essential nutrients are all available when one eats a varied and appropriately selected diet. However, a narrowly defined pattern of food preferences may lead to a deficiency of one or more of the nutrients needed for normal good health. The various nutrients and their roles are discussed below.

Carbohydrates

Carbohydrates are a class of nutrients that are maligned and misunderstood by many consumers because of misrepresentations and myths regarding their role. Starch, sugars, and cellulose are examples of carbohydrates which perform some important functions in the body and are required for good health.

Functions. The role of carbohydrates as sources of energy is vital to survival among many people in the world. Adequate starch and sugar help to spare protein for performing its unique functions in the body. Carbohydrates also provide glucose, a sugar required for the brain to function. Yet another role of carbohydrate is to aid in the utilization of fats in the body. With inadequate carbohydrate, ketosis develops because fats cannot be metabolized normally.

Cellulose is a unique carbohydrate in that it cannot be used by humans as a dietary source of energy. Unlike ruminants, humans are not able to break down cellulose to release energy. However, this inability to digest cellulose enables humans to use cellulose for bulk in the diet, thus promoting excretion of waste materials from the body.

On the negative side, carbohydrates (particularly sugars) that are allowed to remain in the mouth provide a favorable environment for the growth of caries-inducing microorganisms. This disadvantage can be eliminated by good dental hygiene and the avoidance of snacks when the mouth cannot be rinsed well.

Classification. Carbohydrates are all closely related chemical compounds made up of carbon, hydrogen, and oxygen. Some of these substances are simple in structure and small in size. These are called the monosaccharides and disaccharides; another designation for these compounds is sugars or simple sugars. Sucrose, the familiar granulated sugar, is an example of a disaccharide. Other examples of disaccharides are maltose and lactose (milk sugar); glucose and fructose (fruit sugar) are monosaccharides.

Starch (a polysaccharide) is very large compared with the sugars, but it is actually made up of units of glucose, linked together to make large molecules. Pectin is also a polysaccharide and is the carbohydrate used to gel jams and jellies. Cellulose is closely related to starch, yet its use in the body is very different. The glucose units of cellulose are joined together a little differently than are those of starch. This difference makes it impossible for cellulose to be digested by humans, but the material is a valued source of roughage.

Food sources. Carbohydrates are found in abundance in a wide range of foods. Granulated sugar is prepared from sugar beets and sugarcane. Syrups, including maple syrup and corn syrup as well as various fruit syrups, are also quite concentrated sources of carbohydrate. Starch is found in legumes and cereals. Of course, cereals are consumed frequently in modified forms, but much of the starch content still remains. Wheat is milled to make flour, and flour is utilized to make many foods commonly found in the diet. Breads of all types, cakes, pastries, cookies, pancakes, waffles, crackers, and doughnuts are familiar examples of foods containing starch. Fruits and vegetables are good sources of cellulose. Fruits also contribute sugars and pectin. Vegetables contain varying amounts of starch as well as cellulose.

Digestion and absorption. For carbohydrates to be utilized by the body, they must first be digested and absorbed. Digestion is the process of breaking down foods into the simple chemical molecules that can pass through the intestinal wall into the body proper. When sugars are eaten, the disaccharides are unchanged until they reach the stomach; here sucrose is broken into monosaccharides. Other disaccharides travel intact to the small intestine where they are broken into monosaccharides. Monosaccharides are then absorbed through the intestinal wall.

Starch digestion begins in the mouth with salivary amylase (a digestive enzyme that is also called ptyalin) beginning to split starch into smaller molecules. The action of salivary amylase continues while the food travels through the esophagus, but is halted when the food enters the acidic medium of the stomach. When the starch fragments (called dextrins) enter the small intestine, other enzymes (pancreatic amylase, maltase, sucrase, and lactase) continue the breakdown until monosaccharides are formed and absorbed.

Cellulose is made up of glucose units that are linked together in such a way that the enzymes in humans cannot split them apart. Because of this problem, cellulose remains as a very large molecule which cannot readily pass through the intestinal wall.

The intestinal wall in the small intestine is the site of the absorption of most nutrients. For absorption, each molecule must pass through the wall individually. A great deal of surface area is required for this process. The intestinal wall is of remarkable construction. Its surface is not smooth, but instead is made up of millions of tiny projections which sway and help to move the food bulk along through the intestine. These projections, called villi, increase the surface area significantly, thus facilitating absorption of nutrients. The surface area is increased even more by the microvilli that cover the surface of each of the villi.

When monosaccharides pass through this elaborate intestinal wall, they enter the blood stream, which transports them to the liver. In the liver, non-glucose monosaccharides are converted into glucose for utilization in the body. Glucose may be used for energy, converted to glycogen (the polysaccharide in animals that corresponds to starch in plants), or converted to fatty acids which will become fat in the adipose tissues of the body.

Metabolism. Energy is released from glucose by a complex process. During the numerous stages of this process, enzymes, coenzymes (containing various vitamins), and various chemical compounds are required. At various points along this complex metabolic pathway, energy is released to the body. In addition to energy, the other products resulting from the breakdown of carbohydrates are carbon dioxide and water. Carbon dioxide is carried from the cells where it is formed to the lungs where it is exhaled from the body. The water that is formed, sometimes referred to as metabolic water, ultimately is removed from the body via the lungs, skin, or urine.

Lipids

Classification. Lipids are another group of compounds found in foods. Within this category are found simple lipids (commonly referred to simply as fats and waxes), compound lipids, and derived lipids. The fats and oils in foods are made up of two components: fatty acids and glycerol. Glycerol, found in all common food fats, is a small molecular weight alcohol which is capable of combining with three fatty acids to form a molecule of fat. When three fatty acids are joined to glycerol, the molecule is said to be a triglyceride. Sometimes only two fatty acids or one may be combined with the glycerol. These are, respectively, diglycerides and monoglycerides. Triglycerides occur most commonly in foods, but mono- and diglycerides are used in some shortenings to improve the performance quality of the fat.

Fatty acids occur as free fatty acids in foods to only a limited extent. Ordinarily they are linked to glycerol. The characteristics of various fats are determined by the fatty acids that are attached to the glycerol. For example, butter has some rather small fatty acids included in the fat molecules. These contribute to the unique flavor and aroma of butter. Some of the fatty acids, particularly those in animal fats, are saturated with all of the hydrogen they can hold. These are called saturated fatty acids. A few fatty acids could hold only a little more hydrogen. These are the monounsaturated fatty acids. The polyunsaturated fatty acids have less hydrogen in them than the monounsaturated ones. In vegetable oils, the proportion of polyunsaturated fatty acids is relatively high in comparison with the quantities of polyunsaturates in animal fats.

Technologists can change the polyunsaturates into more saturated fatty acids by adding hydrogen, a process known as hydrogenation. When this is done, the fatty acids become firmer. An illustration of this process is the production of margarine or the hydrogenation of peanut butter. In these instances, vegetable oils are reacted with hydrogen, thus changing the starting material from a liquid into a solid that is spreadable at room temperature.

Sources. Some of the fats in the diet are quite conspicuous. The diner is well aware of the fact that margarine and butter are concentrated sources of fat. Salad oil, salad dressings, and fat surrounding meat cuts are also visible fats. Less obvious sources of fat are the marbling of fat within the muscle of meats, whipped cream, cheeses, chocolate, avocados, nuts, whole milk, and rich desserts. Fried foods make additional contributions of fat to the diet.

Digestion and absorption. The digestion of fat requires that fats be emulsified, that is, dispersed in the aqueous medium of the digestive tract in very small droplets. Emulsification is facilitated by increasing the fluidity of the fat. Thus, the fat that enters the mouth is warmed as it passes on through the esophagus and stomach. There is limited digestion in the stomach when the enzyme, gastric lipase, breaks down some fat that was in an emulsified form in the food that was eaten. Most fats proceed into the small intestine without being digested. In the small intestine, bile mixes with the fats to form an emulsion. This enables pancreatic lipase and intestinal lipase (enzymes in the small intestine) to split the fat molecules into glycerol and the component fatty acids. These fragments are now able to pass through the intestinal wall.

Upon absorption into the body, most of the fatty acids and glycerol recombine into mono-, di-, and triglycerides. These compounds are transported in the lymphatic system. During their voyage in the lymphatic system, the glycerides are combined with protein to form chylomicrons. These chylomicrons are sufficiently miscible with blood to be able to enter the blood stream just before the blood stream enters the heart.

Metabolism. When fats are utilized in the body, the fatty acids are first removed from the glycerol portion of the molecule. The glycerol then is metabolized in the same manner as the carbohydrates described above. The fatty acids are broken apart into fragments, each of which contains two carbon atoms. These fragments may be recombined to make different fatty acids or may serve as the building materials for sex hormones, cholesterol, and other complex compounds required in the body. Many of the two-carbon fragments are combined with the metabolic processes involved in carbohydrate utilization. These reactions result in the release of energy and the formation of carbon dioxide and water. For proper utilization of the fragments destined to be used for energy, sufficient carbohydrate must be available. Otherwise, these two-carbon fragments condense and form ketone bodies, which are toxic to the body when allowed to accumulate.

Functions of fats. Fat, gram for gram, is more than twice as good an energy source as either carbohydrate or protein. Pure fat provides nine kilocalories per gram; pure carbohydrates and proteins yield only four kilocalories per gram. Fats are recognized for their significant contribution to the energy needs of the body. Another important contribution of fats is their ability to provide a feeling of satisfaction as long as four hours after eating. This satiety value is due to the fact that fats leave the stomach much more slowly than carbohydrates and proteins.

The provision of energy is not the only role of fat in the diet. Some fats, particularly the vegetable oils, contain linoleic acid. This fatty acid is required for normal health of the skin. Since the body cannot manufacture this required nutrient, linoleic acid is called the "essential fatty acid". Fats also are needed in the diet because they serve as carriers of the fat-soluble vitamins (vitamins A, D, E, and K). Another important attribute of fats is that they are a distinct asset in making many foods more tempting and palatable.

Within the body, fat that is not used immediately is stored in fatty deposits or adipose tissues. These fatty deposits, because they reduce body angularity, are important as a beauty aid unless the depots become unattractively large. These stores are functional, too, for they serve as reserves of energy when food is unavailable. Epidermal fatty deposits are useful in helping to insulate the body and promote the maintenance of normal body temperature. Internal fatty deposits protect vital organs from physical impacts.

Dietary patterns. Interestingly, the percentage of the calories from fats is a rather sensitive indicator of the economic condition of a nation. As national income rises, the consumption of fat increases. In developing nations, the percentage of calories from fat in the diet occasionally drops as low as two to three percent. In contrast, Americans consume between 40 to 45 percent of their calories in the form of fat. Neither extreme is to be recommended. Higher levels frequently are accompanied by weight problems.

General dietary recommendations regarding fat consumption are:

1. Include approximately one percent of the day's calories from linoleic acid. For the person eating 2100

kilocalories per day, this recommendation could be met by using three tablespoons of corn, soya, or cotton-seed oil (in the form of salad dressings, margarines, or oil for frying).
2. Reduce the total amount of fat consumed by such measures as limiting the amount of fried foods and avoiding the use of large amounts of butter, margarine, sour cream, fatty meats, and salad dressings.

Proteins

Classification. Proteins are a unique class of compounds. Just as is true for carbohydrates and fats, proteins contain carbon, hydrogen, and oxygen. In addition, they contain nitrogen, an element which is unique to proteins in the living organism. All proteins are made up of building blocks called amino acids. There are 22 amino acids occurring in the proteins commonly found in foods. An individual protein may contain many of these amino acids, but will contain more of some than of others. The amino acid com-position (sequence and ratios) is different for each type of protein. Thus, one protein may be very high in its content of one amino acid, while another protein will contain larger amounts of another amino acid.

Some amino acids are essential amino acids. The term "essential" is used to designate the amino acids that are required by the body for growth and maintenance of tissues, but that cannot be manufactured in the body. In other words, essential amino acids must be contained in the proteins eaten in the diet. Adults require eight amino acids (methion-ine, threonine, tryptophan, isoleucine, leucine, lysine, valine, and phenylalanine) from dietary sources, and child-ren require these eight essential amino acids plus histidine.

The other amino acids are designated as nonessential, a term which actually is a bit misleading. Although the desig-nation of nonessential connotes that these are not necessary in the diet, just the opposite is true. Nonessential amino acids are important in helping to meet the body's total need for protein.

Proteins that contain all of the essential amino acids (plus many of the nonessential amino acids) are designated as complete proteins. These proteins are found in foods from animal sources (except gelatin). Incomplete proteins are proteins lacking one or more of the essential amino acids. These proteins are found in foods from plants. Animal proteins are generally more expensive than protein foods from plant sources. Both sources are important in the diet; plant proteins can be of great value in helping to reduce the amount of animal protein needed to meet the body's need for the essential amino acids.

Food sources. Animal protein sources include beef, veal, pork, lamb, fish, poultry (including ducks, chickens, turkey, goose, pheasant, and other fowl), eggs, milk, and cheese. Rich plant sources are provided by the legume family. Examples include kidney beans, lima beans, soybeans, navy beans, several other types of beans, and peas. Soybeans have been the subject of considerable research and are now used as the source of a protein that can be spun into fibers and used to fabricate plant "meats" or textured vegetable protein (TVP). The average protein content of legumes is approximately 20 percent. Cereals are other plant foods that contribute protein to the diet. Their protein content is much lower, (ranging from about seven percent in rice to as much as 12 percent in wheat) but cereals are used in sufficient quantities in many diets to make them qualify as a significant source of protein.

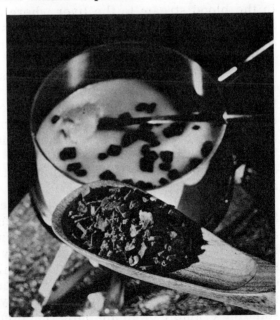

Textured soy protein products are increasing in their importance in the diet as an alternative or supplement to more costly meat proteins.

Digestion and absorption. Protein molecules are very large and must be digested so that the individual amino acids are released for absorption. This laborious process is begun in the stomach with pepsin (an enzyme acting on protein) attacking the molecule to split it into somewhat smaller fragments called polypeptides. These fragments then move into the small intestine.

In the small intestine the pancreatic juice contains trypsin (an enzyme) and the intestinal juice contributes carboxypeptidase, amino peptidase, and dipeptidase, which are the enzymes needed to complete the breakdown of the polypeptides that enter the intestine. The final products of protein digestion are the amino acids contained in the original protein molecule.

When individual amino acids are split off, they are absorbed through the intestinal wall into the blood stream. This is the normal process for absorbing the protein that is eaten. Occasionally, individuals may absorb a particular protein before it has been broken down to its component amino acids. When this happens, the body views the absorbed protein molecule as foreign protein and rallies its defenses. The result is an allergic response to the protein.

Metabolism. The absorbed amino acids are transported in the blood stream to the liver where an amino acid pool is formed. From there, the amino acids are carried to the tissues of the body for incorporation in proteins that are being synthesized by the body.

In the cell, various amino acids are assembled according to coded instructions provided for the specific protein to be formed. All of the amino acids required for the formation of this protein must be available if the protein is to be formed at all. Some of the nonessential amino acids can be formed to complete the requirements for the protein. However, all of the necessary essential amino acids must be available if the protein formation is to occur.

Protein synthesis is an essential process within the body. Since the intact protein molecules in foods are not available for the body's use, all of the proteins contained in the human body must be manufactured by appropriately assembling the amino acids that are available. The process of making larger molecules from smaller ones in the body is referred to as anabolism. Protein synthesis is an outstanding example of an anabolic reaction in the body.

Proteins in the body also undergo catabolic reactions, or the process of converting from a complex molecule into smaller compounds. In one such reaction, amino acids are changed to a related substance by breaking off the acid radical. Histamine is formed from histidine by this type of reaction. In other instances the amino group is removed, leaving a special type of acid. The amino group may be transferred to another compound to form an amino acid. Of course, amino acids formed in the body in this manner will always be nonessential amino acids.

When the amino group is broken off from an amino acid, two fragments remain. The amino group ultimately can be converted to urea and excreted in the urine. The non-nitrogenous fragment can be metabolized to provide energy, carbon dioxide, and water.

Some individuals are born with defects in their ability to metabolize amino acids in the normal manner. Phenylketonuria is the condition resulting when there is a defect in the metabolism of phenylalanine (an amino acid). This defect causes a buildup of phenylalanine and its derivatives and results in severe mental retardation unless special dietary precautions are initiated very early in life. Other inborn errors of metabolism have been observed, including defects in the utilization of histidine, leucine, and valine. As research efforts are expanded, there is some likelihood that other metabolic problems may be discovered. This direction in research is proving to be an aid in fighting the problems of mental retardation.

Functions. Protein can be used to provide energy, just as carbohydrates and fats do. However, protein performs some very unique functions, too. Protein is essential for the growth and maintenance of tissues throughout the body. Hormones, enzymes, and antibodies are all protein materials that must be present for normal body function. These are synthesized in the body from the amino acids provided by dietary proteins.

Within the body, there is need for regulating the fluids between the various compartments of the body. Plasma proteins are important for their role in helping to regulate the balance between the fluid levels in the cells and the blood stream. The relative neutrality of the body must be balanced very carefully and maintained within very narrow limits. Proteins are able to function as either acids or bases, hence are of considerable significance in maintaining the proper conditions within the body.

Protein in the diet. The need for protein is modified throughout life, ranging from 2.2 grams per kilogram of body weight for newborns to somewhat less than one gram per kilogram for adults. The very high level in infancy and childhood is dictated by the requirement for growth of tissues as well as maintenance of existing ones. Adults need protein for maintenance of tissues and the formation of some body compounds, but are not faced with the demands of growth.

Another way of interpreting this difference in requirements is from the standpoint of nitrogen balance. Growing children, persons recovering from surgery and burns, and pregnant and lactating women are in positive nitrogen balance, meaning that they are retaining nitrogen to supply the building material for new tissues. Adults maintain a neutral state; in other words, they excrete as much nitrogen as they consume. Persons with fevers are in a state of negative nitrogen balance because of the stress condition. This is an undesirable condition that requires an adequate intake of protein as soon as it can be tolerated.

Ideally, the protein intake will be scattered throughout the day in preference to providing it at only one or two meals a day. This pattern enables the protein to be utilized more efficiently in the body. One means of accomplishing this is to consume a glass of milk and some cereal or bread as a part of breakfast and to include a serving of animal protein or legumes at each of the other meals (plus at least one more glass of milk for adults). Numerous other variations of this pattern are available. The need for protein distributed throughout the day helps to emphasize the importance of eating a good breakfast. Without breakfast, most people will have practically all of their protein intake provided in a period of approximately six hours out of the 24 hour span of the day, a practice not consistent with optimum utilization of protein.

Protein needs can be met without eating meats, poultry, or fish, but the task is definitely more difficult than it is if at least one serving of these foods is included daily. The incomplete protein of a specific vegetable protein can be complemented by the addition of protein from another source. For example, refried beans provide incomplete protein by themselves, but the addition of some grated cheese provides the missing amino acids. The combination of several types of beans in a mixed bean salad is another way of complementing vegetable proteins. Nuts also can be added to provide still better variety. Some protein supplements have been developed using a mixture of vegetable proteins to make a complete protein food. Incaparina, developed by the Institute of Nutrition for Central America and Panama, is an example of just such a food product.

Kwashiorkor. When the intake of protein is restricted for a period of time, the physical condition deteriorates. The problem of an adequate intake of protein is particularly troublesome in some developing countries where children sometimes receive very restricted protein intake for the very important early years following weaning. Their poor diets reduce their resistance to various diseases and their unsanitary living conditions compound the problem, with the result that illnesses that normally are mild, may become threatening. Under these circumstances, kwashiorkor, the protein deficiency condition is likely to develop, particularly among the age group between one and four. The diarrhea and vomiting that accompany the illness compound the problems of a protein deficiency. These symptoms greatly impair the absorption of the amino acids that normally would be available to the body from the protein that is eaten. Children with kwashiorkor will be irritable and seemingly lazy. Their growth will be retarded and their muscle development will be very poor. Dark hair will sometimes develop a reddish-colored streak. The skin becomes scaly and blotchy. Anemia, diarrhea, vomiting, an enlarged liver, and very poor appetite also develop. Advanced cases often have a great amount of edema or bloating. Death results if the protein deficiency is great and treatment is not provided.

Protein-calorie malnutrition. In many instances where the protein intake is sharply curtailed, the total caloric intake is also distinctly low. This results in a problem very closely related to kwashiorkor – a condition referred to as PCM or protein-calorie malnutrition. When children have very severe limitations on all food intake, amounting to virtual starvation, they quickly develop marasmus. All of these conditions are the result of inadequate diets and may be corrected simply by providing appropriate dietary improvements, particularly more protein and an increase in total food.

ENERGY REQUIREMENTS

Energy becomes available to the body as carbohydrates, fats, and proteins are metabolized in the body. The body need for energy varies from individual to individual and day to day. There are three components which contribute to the daily need for energy: basal metabolism, activity, and specific dynamic action.

Basal Metabolism

The body requires energy to maintain its basic functions, including blood circulation, the functioning of vital organs and glands, breathing, maintenance of body temperature, and metabolism in the cells. The energy required for these essential life functions is known as basal metabolism. The actual amount of energy needed varies from one individual to another, for basal metabolic rate is influenced by several factors. Infants and young children have a high basal metabolic rate; in fact, almost twice as much energy per square meter of body surface is needed at age three as at age 75. Males typically have a higher basal metabolic rate than females. People with well developed muscles have a higher rate than those who are well endowed with fatty deposits.

The adrenal gland and the thyroid gland (endocrine glands) secrete hormones that influence basal metabolic needs. The effect of the adrenaline secreted by the adrenal gland is a temporary elevation of the basal metabolic rate for two or three hours. In contrast, the rate at which thyroxine is secreted by the thyroid gland has a continuing influence on basal metabolic rate. Too little thyroxine is reflected in a basal metabolic rate lower than normal; an excessively high basal metabolic rate can be caused by too much thyroxine. In the first instance, known as hypothyroidism, less energy than normal is needed to maintain the basal functions of the body. Conversely, hyperthyroidism requires more energy than normal because of the higher rate.

Physical Activity

Physical activity also requires energy, the amount varying with the activity patterns and body size of the individual. As expected, strenuous physical activities such as swimming require a relatively great amount of energy in comparison with reading, knitting, or other sedentary types of activities. Table 1.1 lists the energy requirement for a variety of activities. These figures are expressed as kilocalories per kilogram per hour. To apply these values to an actual situation, the value from the table must be multiplied by the weight of the individual (weight in pounds divided by 2.2 equals weight in kilograms) and by the fraction of an hour in which the activity was pursued.

Specific Dynamic Action

The body requires energy to utilize the food that is eaten. The energy required for converting and transporting food from the time it is eaten until its components have been utilized is termed the specific dynamic action of food. The amount of energy required for this purpose is dependent upon the amount of food consumed and is calculated roughly as ten percent of the energy required for basal metabolism and activity daily.

Energy Measurement

The body's need for energy is calculated and stated in units termed "kilocalories". A kilocalorie is the amount of energy required to raise the temperature of one kilogram of water one degree Celsius. The energy value of various foods (see Appendix) also is expressed in this terminology. Sometimes the terms "Calorie" or "calorie" are used to express the units of energy discussed in nutrition.

MINERALS

Minerals in nutrition are inorganic, crystalline chemical elements or compounds. The human body contains approximately four percent ash or mineral by weight, with the remainder being water, fat, carbohydrate, and protein. The

Table 1.1   Energy required for selected activities [a]

Activity	Kcal/kg/hr	Activity	Kcal/kg/hr
Bicycling (century run)	7.6	Piano playing (Beethoven's *Appasionata*)	1.4
Bicycling (moderate speed)	2.5	Piano playing (Liszt's *Tarantella*)	2.0
Boxing	11.4	Reading aloud	0.4
Carpentry (heavy)	2.3	Rowing in race	16.0
Cello playing	1.3	Running	7.0
Crocheting	0.4	Sawing wood	5.7
Dancing, foxtrot	3.8	Sewing, hand	0.4
Dancing, waltz	3.0	Sewing, motor driven machine	0.4
Dishwashing	1.0	Singing in loud voice	0.8
Dressing and undressing	0.7	Sitting quietly	0.4
Driving	0.9	Skating	3.5
Eating	0.4	Standing relaxed	0.5
Exercise		Sweeping with broom	1.4
Very light	0.9	Sweeping with vacuum cleaner	2.7
Light	1.4	Swimming (2 miles/hour)	7.9
Moderate	3.1	Tailoring	0.9
Severe	5.4	Typewriting rapidly	1.0
Very severe	7.6	Violin playing	0.6
Fencing	7.3	Walking (3 miles/hour)	2.0
Horseback riding		Walking (4 miles/hour)	3.4
Walk	1.4	Walking (5.3 miles/hour)	8.3
Trot	4.3	Walking downstairs	b
Gallop	6.7	Walking upstairs	c
Laundry, light	1.3	Washing floors	1.2
Playing ping pong	4.4	Writing	0.4

[a] Adapted from "Foundations of Nutrition" (5th edition) by Taylor, MacLeod, and Rose. Macmillan Co. 1956.

[b] Allow 0.012 kilocalories per kilogram for an ordinary staircase with 15 steps, without regard to time.

[c] Allow 0.036 kilocalories per kilogram for an ordinary staircase with 15 steps, without regard to time.

minerals comprising this small amount of ash in the body are designated as macronutrient and micronutrient (trace) minerals. The macronutrient minerals include calcium, phosphorus, potassium, sulfur, sodium, chloride, and magnesium; micronutrient minerals are iron, manganese, copper, iodide, chromium, cobalt, fluoride, molybdenum, selenium, and zinc.

Functions. The various minerals function in unique ways which will be cited below. As a group, however, minerals perform such vital roles as controlling water balance in the body, regulating acid-base balance, catalyzing various reactions in the body, performing structural roles, and providing key constituents in such compounds as enzymes, hormones, and certain other essential substances of the body. Inadequate intake of the various essential minerals will result in distinct physical malfunctions, depending upon the specific deficiency.

Water is found in cells, between cells, and in the bloodstream. The amount of water in each of these regions is determined, in part, by the concentration of minerals within and outside the cells. The distribution of minerals on either side of the cell walls influences osmotic pressure, thus partially determining the movement of water in and out of the cell.

The body generally is almost neutral in reaction, although the blood is slightly alkaline and the tissues less alkaline. Some of the minerals promote the formation of acids, while others form bases in the body. Organic phosphorus (phosphorus occurring in combination with organic compounds), chloride, and sulfur are the common minerals that promote acid formation. These are rather plentiful in meat, poultry, eggs, fish, and grain and cereal products. The minerals promoting the formation of alkaline products include calcium, iron, potassium, inorganic phosphate, magnesium, and sodium. Food sources of these minerals are abundant in the fruits and vegetables commonly contained in the diet. This may seem somewhat contradictory because fruits are acidic when they are eaten. However, they ultimately form bases in the body. Milk contains elements that contribute to an acidic reaction, but it also contributes inorganic phosphate and calcium, with the ultimate result that milk actually is a strong contributor to an alkaline reaction.

Some of the minerals, either as ions or as part of an enzyme system, catalyze reactions in the body. Magnesium, calcium, potassium, manganese, zinc, and iron are essential elements in a variety of metabolic reactions involving the utilization of carbohydrates, fats, and proteins. The absorption of some nutrients is facilitated by minerals; calcium aids in the absorption of the massive vitamin B_{12} molecule, and sodium and magnesium help in the absorption of simple sugars. Mineral ions (specifically calcium, potassium, magnesium, and sodium) are required for the transmission of nerve impulses and thus serve vital roles in muscle contraction and relaxation.

The function of calcium, phosphorus, and fluoride in the growth and maintenance of bones and teeth is of vital importance in childhood. However, minerals are required in adulthood, too, to maintain the integrity of the bones. Potassium is a mineral that is a necessary component of soft tissues. Sulfur is found in the proteins of hair.

Several minerals are components of essential body compounds. Two hormones include a mineral in their structures: insulin contains zinc, and thyroxine contains iodide. Among the vitamins, sulfur is a part of thiamin, and cobalt is contained in vitamin B_{12}. Hemoglobin requires an atom of iron. Hydrochloric acid in the stomach is a combination of chloride and hydrogen. Iron and copper are both contained in the cytochrome enzymes which are important in the release of energy. Zinc is a part of carbonic anhydrase (involved in the release of carbon dioxide from red blood cells) and carboxypeptidase (required in protein metabolism). Another enzyme with a mineral component is xanthine oxidase, which contains molybdenum.

Table 1.2 provides a summary of the functions and food sources of minerals. The following discussion also provides more detailed information about specific minerals and their roles in the body.

Calcium comprises approximately two percent of the body's total weight, making it by far the most abundant mineral in the body. The role of calcium in promoting growth is well-known and of considerable importance if growth potential is to be realized. The need for calcium is maintained throughout life to replace calcium that constantly is being removed from the bones. This dynamic nature of

Table 1.2 Minerals important in human nutrition – their principal food sources and body functions [a]

Mineral	Food Sources	Functions
Calcium	Milk, cheese, custards, puddings, cream soups, greens, small fish with bones in	Formation of bone, maintenance of bone, tooth formation, maintenance of teeth, clotting of blood, activation of pancreatic lipase, absorption of vitamin B_{12}, contraction of muscles (especially regulation of heart beat), transmission of nerve impulses
Chloride	Salt, meat, milk, eggs	Formation of hydrochloric acid in the stomach, maintenance of normal osmotic pressure, maintenance of acid-base balance
Cobalt	Animal sources	Synthesis of vitamin B_{12}, in intestine
Copper	Legumes, liver, cereals, nuts, shellfish	Catalyst for formation of hemoglobin, component of enzymes (cytochrome oxidase and catalase) required for release of energy, assistance in the formation of of elastin (connective tissue), formation of melanin (pigment in hair and skin), formation of phospholipids needed for myelin sheath of nerves
Fluoride	Fluoridated water, tea, sardines	Protection against dental caries, osteomalacia, and osteoporosis

Table 1.2 (Continued)

Mineral	Food Source	Functions
Iodide	Iodized salt, salt water fish, and shellfish	Formation of thyroxine to maintain normal rate of metabolism
Iron	Liver	Component of hemoglobin, component of myoglobin (protein pigment in muscle), component of enzymes (cytochromes, cytochrome oxidase, peroxidase, catalase)
Magnesium	Milk, green vegetables, nuts, bread and cereals	Catalyst for metabolic reactions involving change in energy state, conducting of nerve impulses, promoting calcium retention in teeth, release of thyroxine
Manganese	Cereals, legumes	Bone formation, component of arginase (enzyme required for formation of urea)
Molybdenum	Cereals, legumes, organ meats	Component of xanthine oxidase and aldehyde oxidase
Phosphorus	Meats (organic phosphorus); fruits, milk, and vegetables (inorganic phosphorus)	Component of bones and teeth, component of DNA (deoxyribonucleic acid), component of ATP and ADP (adenosine triphosphate and adenosine diphosphate), fatty acid transport in bloodstream
Potassium	Orange juice, bananas, dried fruits, potatoes, coffee	Maintenance of osmotic pressure, acid-base balance, transmission of nerve im-

Table 1.2 (Continued)

Mineral	Food Source	Functions
		pulses, catalyst in energy metabolism, protein formation
Selenium	Meats, seafood, grains from selenium-rich soil	Antioxidant *muscular dyst.*
Sodium	Salt, salt-preserved meats, milk	Maintenance of osmotic pressure, acid-base balance, relaxation of muscles, assistance in glucose absorption, transmission of nerve impulses
Sulfur	Meats, fish, poultry	Component of hair, fingernails, toenails, and skin, structural part of thiamin, pantothenic acid and biotin, component of amino acids (cystine, cysteine, and methionine)
Zinc	Whole grain cereal products, meats, legumes	Component of insulin, component of carbonic anhydrase, activation of enzymes involved in protein metabolism

[a]From Stare, F. and M. McWilliams. *Living Nutrition.* Wiley, New York. 1973.

calcium in bones is one of the primary reasons why calcium is considered so significant for adults as well as for children.

Teeth, although they are subject to some turnover in calcium, are much more stable in their structure than are bones. The most important need for calcium for deciduous tooth formation is from the middle of pregnancy until the deciduous teeth break through the gum. The important time for the permanent teeth is from the age of approximately three months until the teeth erupt.

Calcium functions in blood clotting in two places: to trigger the release of thromboplastin from the blood platelets and to convert fibrinogen to fibrin. Other significant roles of calcium include: activation of pancreatic lipase, the enzyme that digests fats in the small intestine; assistance with the absorption of vitamin B_{12}, a molecule that is difficult to absorb because of its bulkiness; and transmission of nerve impulses, including the contraction of muscles.

The absorption of calcium is influenced by a number of factors, varying widely from one individual to another and from one period of life to another. In general, calcium absorption is promoted by adequate vitamin D, the presence of ascorbic acid and amino acids, lactose, phosphorus, and a physical need for the mineral. When a diet is high in calcium, the body will absorb a much smaller percentage of the calcium in the food than it will if the diet regularly is very low in this mineral. However, the total amount absorbed will be greater when the dietary intake is high than when it is inadequate.

An inadequate intake of calcium (often complicated by an inadequate intake of vitamin D) may result in the stunting of growth in children or in teeth of poor quality. The lack of calcium may lead to malformed bones, such as bowed legs. Adults who have maintained an inadequate intake of calcium over a long period of time may develop osteoporosis or osteomalacia.

From a dietary standpoint, milk (or a calcium supplement if milk is not tolerated well) is an important component of the diet throughout life, not just in the growing years. The consumption of two glasses of milk daily by adults is recommended to insure adequate calcium in the diet. Various greens provide additional calcium to meet the body's need.

Iron is the mineral that perhaps is generating the greatest concern among nutritionists today. The population group wherein this concern is focused is women in the reproductive years, for iron is lost regularly through menstruation. Iron is a structural part of hemoglobin, the compound in blood that is capable of carrying oxygen to the tissues and carbon dioxide from the tissues to the lungs for excretion. When inadequate amounts of iron are available in the body, the hemoglobin level will drop, with a resultant drop

in the oxygen-carrying capacity of the blood. When hemoglobin levels are low, a person feels fatigued because of the
limited ability to carry oxygen to the tissues. This condition
is termed iron-deficiency anemia.

In addition to its role in hemoglobin formation, iron is
required for the formation of myoglobin, the pigment occurring in abundance in muscle tissue. Iron can be oxidized
and reduced. This ability makes it an important constituent
of oxidative enzymes such as the cytochromes, cytochrome
oxidase, peroxidase, and catalase. These enzymes are
essential for the release of energy from carbohydrates,
fats, and proteins.

Iron is absorbed from the intestinal tract with difficulty. Despite the fact that a number of people may have
a definite deficiency of iron, the absorption rate still is not
great. This is the reason that the recommended intake of
iron is so high. Fortunately, the body is very conservative
of iron once it has been absorbed; the mineral can be reused
when it is released from the red blood cells. The primary
mode of loss of iron that has actually been absorbed is
through bleeding.

For women, particularly those who are consuming less
than 2,000 kilocalories per day, there is need for constant
attention to including good sources of iron in the diet. Especially rich sources of iron are liver and heart. However,
meats are excellent sources, as are clams, oysters, spinach,
dried fruits, lima beans, and nuts. Enriched or whole grain
cereals are of significance in meeting the iron requirement
because of the frequency with which they generally are eaten.

The question of the level of iron enrichment in cereal
products has been a subject of rather heated discussions.
The prevalence of anemia in the United States supports
the arguments for increasing the level of supplementation
in flour and related products. However, there are some who
cite the toxic condition, hemosiderosis, which can result
when large amounts of iron supplements or extensive use
of iron cooking pots are a part of the living pattern. The
controversy is still unresolved at this writing, and the enrichment level has not yet been modified from the established level of 13 to 16.5 milligrams per pound of flour.

Copper is a mineral that functions in several ways in the
body. One of its important roles is as a catalyst in the formation of hemoglobin (although it is not incorporated in

the structure, as iron is). Melanin (a dark pigment in skin and hair) is formed from tyrosine in the presence of tyrosinase, a copper-containing enzyme. Copper also promotes the formation of phospholipids, which are important in the formation of the myelin sheath that coats nerve fibers.

The normal diet containing some cereals, nuts, legumes, or liver provides the amount of copper that seems to be essential for humans. No dietary recommendation for this nutrient has yet been established despite its importance in the body.

Fluoride is a mineral of nutritional significance because of its relation to dental health, one of the health concerns in America. Dental caries can be alleviated by nutritional measures. The ingestion of fluoride in drinking water (at the level of one part fluoride per million parts of water) is a preventive measure that is of demonstrated effectiveness in reducing the incidence of caries among young children. When fluoridated water is consumed throughout the period when teeth are forming, fluoride is deposited in the teeth in the form of fluorapatite, a hard crystalline material which is much more resistant to decay than is the hydroxyapatite which is normally present. This protection, when established in childhood, provides continuing resistance throughout the adult years, too. Fluoride is also deposited in bones, giving greater strength to mature bones.

The simplest way of providing fluoride is to fluoridate the city water supply, a measure that is both inexpensive and effective. Unfortunately, there has been considerable opposition to this procedure in some cities, and many children today do not have the opportunity to obtain fluoride at protective levels from the water they drink. In such instances, protection may be provided by topical application of stannous fluoride by dentists, by using fluoridated toothpastes, sodium fluoride tablets, or bottled fluoridated water. All of these alternatives are more expensive than fluoridating the water supply and are somewhat less effective.

Iodide is a key mineral element because of its role in the production of thyroxine. Thyroxine, the hormone secreted by the thyroid gland, is the material carrying the primary responsibility for regulating the basal metabolic rate. This hormone must have a supply of iodide available. When the iodide intake is inadequate, the thyroid gland will begin to enlarge in a futile attempt to produce more

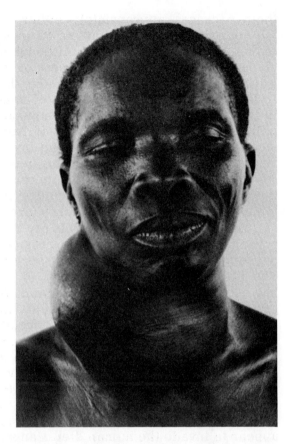

The large swelling on the throat is an obvious symptom of goiter caused by an iodine deficiency.

thyroxine. This swelling of the thyroid can be seen as a lump near the base of the throat. Persons with this problem have endemic goiter. At one time earlier in this century, goiter was a rather common problem in the region of the Great Lakes.

When iodide was found to be the key to preventing goiter, potassium iodide was added to table salt. This was the first nutritional food additive used in the United States and was implemented half a century ago. Iodization of salt was very effective in helping to reduce the incidence of goiter. However, the public gradually became complacent and began to ignore the need for iodized salt. With decreased use of iodized salt, the incidence of goiter once again began to increase. As a means of reminding people that iodized salt is an important health measure for many people, salt manufacturers were required in 1973 to begin labeling their packages appropriately either, "This salt supplies iodide, a necessary nutrient", or "This salt does not supply iodide, a necessary nutrient". Although not enough time has elapsed to assess the effectiveness of this labeling, such a warning presumably will help to stem the increase in goiter.

In general, appropriate levels of minerals are available in the normal, varied diet that emphasizes consumption of milk throughout life, a variety of fruits and vegetables, meat and other protein foods, and breads and cereals. No single food has all of the minerals needed for good health. However, all of the essential minerals are available from the foods that normally are included in the diet. The one mineral most likely to be in short supply is iron.

Toxicity. Some of the minerals are toxic to humans when consumed at levels greatly in excess of the quantities recommended; others may be toxic in very, very small amounts. The problem with large excesses of iron, hemosiderosis, has been cited earlier in this section. When fluoride is ingested during childhood at amounts approximately nine times greater than the amount recommended for fluoridation, the teeth will begin to discolor and assume a mottled appearance (although remarkably free of decay). Sodium and chloride in large excesses can cause elevated blood pressure when regularly consumed together as table salt. Livestock grazing on plants growing in cobalt-rich or molybdenum-rich soil have had some toxic effects, but such problems do not appear to invade the human diet. Manganese, when present over a long period of time in the air, will be breathed in and can cause a disruption of the nervous system. This also can be caused by extreme dietary modifications. However, the normal diet presents no possibility for manganese toxicity. Selenium is another mineral that can be toxic. When the intake of selenium is higher than five parts per million, the mineral is used in preference to sulfur. Again, the possibility of this kind of dosage being available in the normal diet is virtually nil.

Heavy metals, such as mercury and lead, are toxic. Although these materials have not been a problem in the diet in the past, recent developments in industry have resulted in the potential for high levels of these metals in foods on rare occasions. The accidental feeding of mercury-treated grain to hogs that subsequently were slaughtered and fed to humans resulted in a tragedy in New Mexico. Lead in paint has been the cause of lead poisoning among some children who have eaten flakes of this type of paint. The levels of mercury in swordfish were yet another area of concern. One of the principle reasons for the general concern, in fact the virtual public hysteria which the detection of heavy metals in some foods has created, is that analytical instruments are now much more sensitive than they used to be. The high levels of mercury that have been measured in some seafood may not be significantly higher than the content in the past. It may be that the analysis simply is more accurate. In any event, the increasing awareness of the potential for mineral contaminants in foods is of value in helping to prevent unsafe levels of consumption.

Vitamins

Carbohydrates, fats, and proteins are categories of organic compounds that can provide energy for the body. Minerals clearly are not organic in nature and they are not potential sources of energy themselves, although they do serve as catalysts for energy release in some cases. Vitamins represent yet another category of nutrients. Although they are organic compounds, they are unlike the other organic compounds considered previously because they are not, in themselves, sources of energy.

A working definition of a vitamin is that a vitamin is an organic compound which is essential for growth and the maintenance of life and is needed in the diet in very small quantities. This definition separates vitamins from minerals on the basis of the criterion of being an organic compound. The stipulation that the vitamins are needed in the diet in very small quantities differentiates these substances from carbohydrates, fats, and proteins, all of which are needed in far larger quantities. The requirement that the substance be essential for growth and maintenance of life separates vitamins from miscellaneous organic compounds lacking the essential character of the vitamins.

As a group, vitamins are somewhat diverse in their chemical characteristics and behavior. One common way of categorizing them is on the basis of solubility: water soluble and fat soluble. Using this classification, the fat soluble vitamins include vitamins A, D, E, and K; the water soluble vitamins are the B vitamins and ascorbic acid.

Fat soluble vitamins. Vitamin A was the first of the vitamins to be discovered. In 1912 two groups of investigators, Osborne and Mendel at Yale and McCollum and Davis at the University of Wisconsin, announced the discovery of this new substance. When these workers fed experimental animals a diet from which milk fat had been removed, the animals developed an eye ailment and subsequently died. Their experiments also showed that the symptoms could be reversed if butter fat or egg yolk was added to the diet. Green and yellow vegetables later were also shown to be of value in supplying the missing nutrient in the diets of these experimental animals. Finally the structure of the vitamin was clarified in the early 1930's, the vitamin was purified and crystallized in 1937, and the synthetic vitamin was first produced in 1946. This is the normal pattern for the study of vitamins.

Vitamin A actually has two active forms, vitamin A_1 (in the form of retinol, retinal, or retinoic acid) and vitamin A_2. Vitamin A_1 is by far the more important active form, for it occurs in such common foods as butter, liver, and egg yolk. In plants the carotenes are common pigments that can be modified in the body into active vitamin A. Therefore, green, leafy vegetables and orange vegetables are good potential sources of vitamin A. The carotenes include alpha-, beta-, and gamma-carotene. Vitamin A is rather stable during most food preparation procedures. However, its activity is lost when fats are oxidized.

Perhaps the best known function of vitamin A is in the prevention of night blindness. Vitamin A is needed to form a key compound (rhodopsin) in the visual cycle which functions in dim light. Unless sufficient vitamin A is available, the normal amount of rhodopsin cannot be formed, and the ability to see in dim light is impaired. With a normal dietary intake of vitamin A over a period of time, this vitamin will be stored in sufficient quantities to enable one to make the visual adjustment for several months. However, continued inadequate intake will result in permanent visual impairment.

Another function of vitamin A is the promotion of optimum growth. With inadequate vitamin A intake, growth will be retarded, with the bones being affected more than the soft tissue. The most serious problem on this score may be the retarded growth of the skull while the brain and central

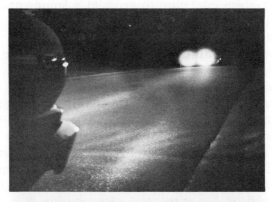

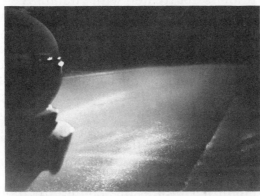

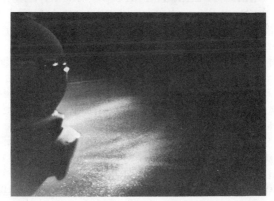

The bright lights of a car approaching at night (top) will not cause a normal person to have difficulty seeing a broad view after the car passes (middle); night blindness caused by a deficiency of vitamin A limits the ability to adapt to such changes and limits the visible field (bottom).

nervous system continue to grow at a somewhat more rapid rate. This situation can cause a pinching of nerves, and may result in permanent blindness.

The normal maintenance of the epithelial cells requires Vitamin A. When this vitamin is not supplied in sufficient quantities, keratin begins to form, and the outer layers of cells become very rough, like goose flesh. This condition also reduces resistance to infections. A similar problem develops in the eye in a vitamin A deficiency. The cornea becomes dry and then develops keratinized areas known as Bitot's spots. When this becomes severe, the condition is known as xerophthalmia. Blindness will be the ultimate outcome if the condition is not treated with vitamin A.

Sufficient vitamin A or its carotene precursors is available from the normal diet if a dark green, leafy or a yellow vegetable is eaten every other day. Spinach, carrots, winter squash, greens of all types, and broccoli are a few of the excellent vegetable sources of provitamin A (carotene). Cantaloupe and the various yellow fruits such as papayas and peaches are good fruit sources. Any milk or milk product containing milk fat contributes vitamin A, and liver is a particularly rich source of this vitamin.

When foods of this type are eaten frequently, there is absolutely no need for taking a vitamin A supplement. In fact, vitamin A capsules are potentially dangerous. This vitamin is stored in the body and may build up to toxic levels when excessive amounts of the vitamin are consumed for a long period of time. Hypervitaminosis A has been observed in adults who regularly consume 50,000 International Units daily. This amount is ten times the recommended dosage of 5,000 I.U. (1,000 retinol equivalents), daily for adult males. Symptoms in hypervitaminosis A include loss of appetite, blurred vision, excessive irritability, headaches, diarrhea, nausea, drying and cracking of the skin, and hair loss. These symptoms can be reversed by eliminating vitamin A from the diet until the condition is corrected. Such problems will not result when vitamin A is obtained only from food. The difficulty arises when large capsules of vitamin A are continued over a period of time.

Vitamin D is the fat soluble vitamin that promotes the absorption of calcium and phosphorus. As a result of its efficacy in enhancing the use of these minerals, vitamin D

is considered to be essential for optimum growth and calcification of the skeleton. It performs in a similar fashion
in the development of the teeth. When vitamin D levels are
inadequate, skeletal development of children will be poor.
The weak bones will not be strong enough to support the
child's weight and bowing of the legs results. This is the
typical problem noted in rickets, the vitamin D deficiency
condition.

Vitamin D commonly is provided in the diet by the fortification of milk at the rate of 400 International Units per
quart. This level of fortification was established because
a quart of milk then contains the levels of calcium, phosphorus, and vitamin D that are deemed to be desirable for
promoting optimum growth among children. Unless the
vitamin D content is stated on the container, milk will not
be a good source of this vitamin, for milk does not naturally
contain vitamin D.

One of the unusual aspects of vitamin D is that its status
as a vitamin is subject to a certain amount of questioning.
According to the definition of a vitamin, the designation of
vitamin D as a vitamin could be challenged. This unique
substance can be made in the human body in amounts sufficient to meet physical need (although this frequently is

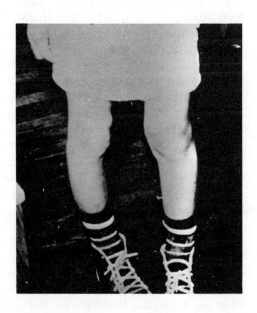

*Bowed legs are a symptom
of a vitamin D deficiency.*

not accomplished). The curious thing about vitamin D is that sunlight, when shining directly on the human skin, can convert cholesterol in the skin into active vitamin D. Of course, the problem is that many people have very little opportunity to expose their skin to the sun for a sufficient length of time. Furthermore, many climates are not conducive to good vitamin D production. The practical approach then becomes one of consuming the vitamin rather than producing it oneself. An interesting sidelight in this regard is that the increasing smog problem impairs vitamin D formation as well as causing respiratory problems.

The specification for vitamin D is deleted from the list of requirements for adults, with the exception of those who are pregnant or lactating. The recommendation for others is 400 International Units daily. The International Unit for vitamin D is the equivalent of 0.025 micrograms, a distinctly smaller value than the 0.3 micrograms of retinol which comprise an International Unit of vitamin A.

Vitamin D, like vitamin A, has the potential for creating a toxic condition when taken in excess for a period of time. Although the amount required to create hypervitaminosis D varies with the individual, a level of 10,000 International Units in children of school age and 100,000 International Units in adults usually will cause the problems to develop. Symptoms include excessive thirst, loss of appetite, vomiting, weight loss, irritability, high blood calcium levels, and finally calcium deposition in blood vessels, kidneys, and lungs, ultimately resulting in death. Such problems can only develop when massive supplements of vitamin D are being ingested. Food alone cannot create such problems.

Vitamin E has leaped into conversations with about as much fascination as weird reducing diets. This vitamin has been described as "a vitamin in search of an illness". The reason for this curious description is that a vitamin E deficiency has not been shown to result in an identifiable condition, such as is true for a vitamin D deficiency and rickets or a vitamin A deficiency and xerophthalmia. Perhaps it is because of this very vague aspect that vitamin E has been endowed with seemingly mythical qualities. For example, this vitamin is referred to as the anti-sterility vitamin. This is true when the vitamin is being considered in relation to white rats, but it has not proven to be the case in humans. In humans, the role of vitamin E is as an antioxidant. This means that the vitamin is oxidized readily in the body in preference to some other compound. In this manner, vitamin E helps to spare vitamin A, ascorbic acid, and polyunsaturated fatty acids. On the basis of such action, the value of vitamin E as a means of delaying the aging process has been suggested, but not proven.

The first time that a dietary recommendation for vitamin E was established was in the 1968 revision of the Food and Nutrition's Board's recommendations for the daily dietary allowances. The levels recommended in the 1974 revision range from 4 I.U. (one I.U. equals one milligram of synthetic dl-alpha-tocopherol) to 15 I.U. for male adults. Good food sources of vitamin E include green vegetables, meats, and vegetable oils.

Vitamin K, the last of the fat soluble vitamins, is of importance in normal clotting of blood. Because of this function, vitamin K frequently is referred to as the anti-hemorrhagic vitamin. Particularly good sources of vitamin K include egg yolks, liver, and dark green, leafy vegetables. Bacteria in the intestine are ready sources of the vitamin because the vitamin K they synthesize can be absorbed. Since such a ready source is always available after the first few days of life, a vitamin K deficiency is only a very remote possibility. Chronic diarrhea or poor absorption are the possible causes of a vitamin K deficiency. No recommended allowance has been established for this vitamin.

Water soluble vitamins. Ascorbic acid or vitamin C is a water soluble vitamin that has gained great popularity among armchair "nutritionists". This vitamin was recognized as being essential in the diet long before vitamins were known. Early explorers on long sea voyages frequently encountered a serious physical condition known as scurvy. In North America, Indians knew how to remedy the condition by brewing a beverage from spruce bark. The British Navy, under the guidance of Dr. James Lind, determined that citrus fruits could prevent scurvy on long journeys. Thus, as far back as the 18th century, the presence of an essential substance was noted. However, identification, isolation, and synthesis of this vitamin did not occur until two centuries later.

One of the important functions of ascorbic acid is the formation of collagen, an important type of connective tissue in the body. Cuts and scratches require the formation of collagen as a part of the healing process. This vitamin also facilitates the utilization of calcium in the body. A deficiency impairs calcification of bones and the formation of dentin, thus increasing the likelihood of weak and decaying teeth. In a deficiency of ascorbic acid, the fragility of blood vessels increases, a condition accompanied by minute hemorrhages under the skin. These are some of the primary functions of this important vitamin.

As is true with the other vitamins, regular ingestion of an adequate amount of this vitamin is a deterrent to infections, but colds and other types of infections still can arise when the level of ascorbic acid is adequate. The use of massive doses of this vitamin may be more effective in treating psychosomatic conditions than actual infections.

If ascorbic acid is not consumed regularly at recommended levels, a condition known as scurvy develops. This is the problem that killed so many sailors long ago. Symptoms of scurvy include tender calf muscles, muscular weakness, bleeding and swollen gums, subcutaneous hemorrhaging, poor wound healing, poor appetite, and occasionally sudden cardiac failure. Infants with scurvy tend to assume a frog-like position of the legs.

Adequate ascorbic acid is available from dietary sources such as oranges, grapefruit, strawberries, and tomatoes. Since this vitamin is not stored well in the body, a regular daily source of ascorbic acid is recommended. This is the reason for the recommendation of a citrus fruit daily.

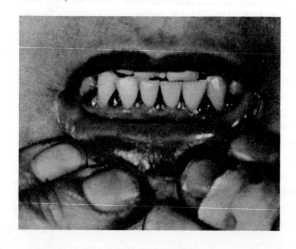

Symptoms of scurvy, a condition caused by an inadequate intake of ascorbic acid, include bleeding and swollen gums.

Ascorbic acid is very readily oxidized, and its vitamin activity is lost when oxidation occurs. Retention of ascorbic acid is aided by minimizing exposure of ascorbic acid-rich foods to oxygen. This means that oranges and other fruits should be cut shortly before being served, rather than being exposed to air for a long time.

Thiamin is the first of the group known as the B vitamins. This water soluble group of vitamins also includes riboflavin, niacin, pantothenic acid, pyridoxine, folacin, biotin, and vitamin B_{12}.

Thiamin (in the form of thiamin pyrophosphate or TPP) is a coenzyme that is important in carbohydrate metabolism. This role makes thiamin essential for the release of energy from carbohydrates and fats. This vitamin also functions in the formation of ribose, a sugar required for the production of DNA and RNA in the body.

A deficiency of thiamin results in a condition known as beriberi. Symptoms of this condition include depression, irritability, nausea, vomiting, and loss of appetite. People with this problem develop a very cautious and awkward

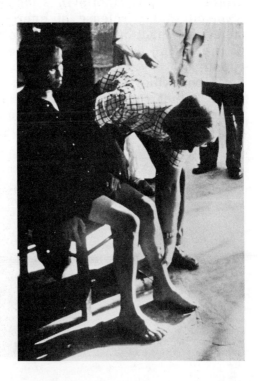

The impression of a finger remains after pressure is applied to the edematous legs of this thiamin-deficient patient who has developed wet beriberi.

walk. Young children may die rather quickly if beriberi develops; in adults the progress is considerably more leisurely, but still may be fatal. Death is triggered by malfunctioning of the heart. Sometimes beriberi takes the form of dry beriberi, in which the patient becomes very emaciated. This is in sharp contrast to wet beriberi with its accompanying edema or bloating.

Thiamin is available in useful amounts in whole grain and enriched breads and cereals, but not in refined, unenriched products. The vitamin also is available from meats, eggs, legumes, potatoes, asparagus, and milk. The primary concern with this vitamin in food preparation is to avoid an alkaline cooking medium and to minimize losses of this water-soluble material into cooking water.

Riboflavin is the vitamin that contributes a somewhat yellow-green color to milk whey. This vitamin is an essential component of flavoprotein enzyme systems (flavin mononucleotide and flavin adenine dinucleotide). These enzyme systems are essential for oxidation-reduction reactions that are a part of the metabolism of carbohydrates, fats, and proteins. In short, riboflavin is needed as a part of coenzymes involved in the release of energy from food. A specific metabolic reaction requiring riboflavin is the conversion of the amino acid tryptophan into niacin, one of the B vitamins.

Ariboflavinosis is the condition that develops when riboflavin is not consumed in adequate amounts in the diet. Symptoms of this problem include cracking at the corners of the mouth (angular stomatitis) and soreness of the lips

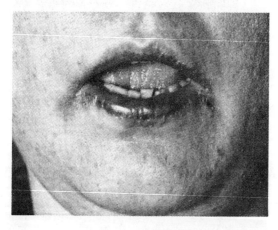

Ariboflavinosis, the condition caused by lack of riboflavin, is characterized by angular stomatitis and cheilosis.

(cheilosis). The tonue also undergoes a change to a magenta color and a smooth character. Young children with ariboflavinosis may become sensitive to light and their eyes may water readily.

A particularly good source of riboflavin is found in milk. Meats, eggs, fish, and green vegetables also contribute to the body's supply of this vitamin. One of the unique characteristics of riboflavin is its sensitivity to sunlight. This is the reason that milk should be marketed only in tinted glass or in plasticized cartons that block the sun's rays and protect the vitamin activity.

Niacin is a B vitamin that has been of particular interest in the United States, especially in the South. This vitamin is a key component of nicotinamide adenine dinucleotide (NAD) and nicotinamide adenine dinucleotide phosphate (NADP), compounds required to release energy from food. They also are of significance in the synthesis of fatty acids and the breakdown of glycogen.

When niacin is deficient in the diet, pellagra will result. The symptoms of this nutritional deficiency condition are sometimes referred to as the "three D's" – diarrhea, dermatitis, and dementia. Without treatment, a fourth D, death, also can result. The interesting aspect of the dermatitis of pellagra is its symmetrical nature, that is, the rashes will

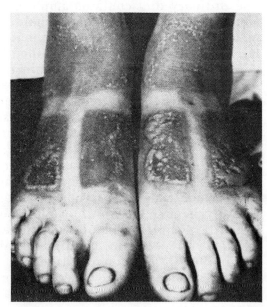

The dermatitis of pellagra, unique because of its occurrence on matching sides of the body, is the result of a niacin deficiency.

develop in approximately the same regions on both sides of the body in a symmetrical fashion. Pellagra can be remedied by increasing the intake of niacin.

Levels of niacin are high in meats of all types. Additional niacin is available from peanut butter, legumes, breads and cereals (whole grain and enriched), and some vegetables and fruits contribute small amounts. This vitamin is the most stable of the B vitamins, but it is water soluble and can be lost into the cooking water. Protein foods contain not only niacin itself, but also the amino acid tryptophan. Tryptophan can be converted into niacin in the body, thereby increasing the amount of niacin available from the diet.

Pyridoxine, also known as vitamin B6, is a B vitamin of particular importance in protein metabolism. This vitamin is involved in the transfer of amino groups to make new amino acids in the body, one important step in the formation of proteins in the body. Another function of pyridoxine is the breakdown of glycogen in the body to release energy. It also plays a role in the formation of antibodies. Vitamin B6 is required for the conversion of tryptophan to niacin.

A deficiency of pyridoxine is unusual, being far less common than beriberi, ariboflavinosis, or pellagra. However, irritability, loss of appetite, weight loss, and general weakness, are observed when a deficiency does develop. The ordinary diet contains ample pyridoxine, so a supplement is not necessary. Meats, whole grain cereals, spinach, potatoes, milk, and cabbage are the foods that contribute the largest fraction of pyridoxine to the diet.

Pantothenic acid is a B vitamin that is very prominent in the metabolism of carbohydrates, fats, and proteins. This vitamin is a component of coenzyme A (also called CoA). In addition to its role in releasing energy from food, coenzyme A is prominent in the formation of porphyrin for hemoglobin formation, for the synthesis of cholesterol, and for the production of some of the steroid hormones as well as for the synthesis of fatty acids in the body.

Although a deficiency of pantothenic acid is extremely unlikely in man, the problem has been produced experimentally. Symptoms include headaches, leg cramps, general fatigue with poor ability to sleep, abdominal discomfort, and limited production of antibodies.

A recommended allowance for pantothenic acid has not yet been set, but the average intake appears to be between

10 and 15 milligrams daily. This vitamin is available in many foods, with particularly high concentrations occurring in organ meats and whole grain cereals. There is little reason to be concerned with the intake of this vitamin if one is eating a reasonable quantity of food.

Biotin is another B vitamin that generally is present in adequate amounts in the normal diet. In fact, a deficiency is very difficult to produce. A deficiency of biotin was demonstrated finally by feeding a diet providing almost one-third of its calories from raw egg white, a diet that is not likely to be followed for long on a voluntary basis! The symptoms that developed included fatigue, nausea, loss of appetite, depression, dermatitis, and high cholesterol levels.

Biotin functions in the body in the release of energy from carbohydrates and fats, in the synthesis of fatty acids, and the removal of the amino group from amino acids. These are very important functions which can be carried on readily without supplementing the diet with additional biotin.

Folacin, also known as folic acid, is a B vitamin that is particularly important for its role in the maturation of red blood cells. Its ability to facilitate the transfer of single carbon units is utilized in the formation of such vital compounds as the purines in nucleic acids, thymine for nucleic acids, choline, and some of the amino acids. Because of these various synthetic functions, folacin is considered to be vital for cell growth and reproduction.

The need for folacin has been recognized rather recently, and it is now one of the vitamins stipulated in the Recommended Dietary Allowances. This vitamin is particularly abundant in spinach and other dark green, leafy vegetables, in mushrooms, liver, and kidney. Other fruits and vegetables are generally good sources. This vitamin is lost gradually during storage and during long periods of cooking.

A folacin deficiency is characterized by macrocytic anemia, diarrhea, and lesions of the alimentary canal. A limited intake of the vitamin or a physical condition which interferes with absorption can lead to this problem, although a folacin deficiency is not common.

Vitamin B_{12} is the B vitamin that finally provided the treatment for pernicious anemia, a condition that was fatal prior to the discovery of liver extract (containing vitamin B_{12}). Vitamin B_{12} is essential for the maturation of the red blood cells and also appears to play a role in the utilization of carbohydrates. With a deficiency of vitamin B_{12}, large and immature red blood cells are the typical pattern, and the functioning of the central nervous system is somewhat disturbed. This vitamin may function in the metabolism not only of carbohydrates, but also of protein and fats.

Vitamin B_{12} is a very large molecule which seemingly cannot be absorbed by some individuals. These people will develop a deficiency of the vitamin regardless of the level of the vitamin being ingested. For such individuals, injections of vitamin B_{12} circumvent the absorption problem and supply the physical need for the vitamin.

A vitamin B_{12} deficiency due to an inadequate diet can result when individuals follow a strict vegetarian diet with no animal food being consumed. Food sources of vitamin B_{12} are found in animal foods rather than in foods of vegetable origin. Thus, meat, milk, cheese, and eggs are all valuable sources of this vitamin. Vitamin B_{12} is synthesized in the intestinal tract by bacteria. However, the site of manufacture is too far down the tract to provide a practical source of this vitamin for humans.

The various vitamins function in unique, yet complementary ways in the body. They are essential for the metabolic reactions that result in the release of energy from food. Individual vitamins are of importance for the formation of a wide variety of essential compounds needed in the body. These vitamins are all available in the foods that can be purchased in any grocery store.

The key to adequate vitamin intake is a well balanced diet which includes a variety of fruits and vegetables, as well as meats, milk, and breads and cereals. Vitamin supplementation is an unnecessary expense for the individual who regularly eats a good diet. The vitamins that occur naturally in foods are the same compounds which may be added during the manufacture of food products. Either natural or synthetic vitamins are effective in the body; in fact, the body cannot distinguish between them. The functions and food sources of the various vitamins are summarized in Table 1.3.

Water

Many people do not even think of water as a nutrient, and yet death will occur in a matter of only a few days if water is not available. The importance of water is suggested

Table 1.3   Vitamins — their functions and food sources[a]

Vitamin	Food Sources	Functions
Vitamin A[b]	Margarine, butter, liver, egg yolk; milk; provitamin A sources include broccoli, carrots, greens, sweet potatoes	Vision in dim light, normal skin, optimum growth
Vitamin D[b]	Vitamin D-fortified milk, eggs, cheese	Absorption and utilization of calcium and phosphorus, optimum growth, calcification of bones and teeth
Vitamin E[b]	Vegetable oils, greens	Antioxidant to spare unsaturated fatty acids, vitamin A and ascorbic acid
Vitamin K[b]	Dark green, leafy vegetables, liver, egg yolks[c]	Blood clotting
Ascorbic acid[d]	Citrus fruits, strawberries, tomatoes, cantaloupe, broccoli, potatoes, cabbage, tropical fruits	Formation of collagen, normal strength of blood vessels, protection against infections, promotes calcification of teeth and bones, utilization of some amino acids
Thiamin[d]	Meats, eggs, legumes, enriched and whole grain cereals and breads	Coenzyme (TTP) to release energy from carbohydrates, fats, and proteins; aids in formation of ribose for DNA and RNA
Riboflavin[d]	Milk, meats, fish, poultry, asparagus, broccoli, legumes, whole grain and enriched breads	Flavoprotein (FMN and FAD) enzymes for cellular respiration and releasing energy, conversion of tryptophan to niacin

Table 1.3 (Continued)

Vitamin	Food Sources	Functions
Niacin[d]	Meats, poultry, peanut butter, whole grain and enriched cereals	Coenzyme needed to release energy from carbohydrates, fats, and protein; coenzyme involved in fatty acid synthesis
Pyridoxine[d]	Meats, bananas, beans, spinach, cabbage, potatoes	Metabolism of fats and carbohydrates; formation of non-essential amino acids; release of energy from protein; production of antibodies
Pantothenic acid[d]	Organ meats, whole grain cereals, and most foods	Component of coenzyme A; releases energy from carbohydrates, fats, and proteins; synthesis of cholesterol, fatty acids, and hemoglobin
Biotin[d]	Egg yolks, milk, organ meats, legumes, nuts	Deamination of proteins; release of energy from carbohydrates, fats, and amino acids; production of antibodies
Folacin[d]	Dark green, leafy vegetables, mushrooms, liver, kidney, fruits, vegetables	Transfer single carbon units to synthesize new non-essential amino acids, nucleic acids, and hemoglobin; cell growth; normal maturation of red blood cells
Vitamin B_{12}[d]	Meat, poultry, fish, milk, eggs	Maturation of red blood cells; maintain health of nervous tissues

[a]From Stare, F. and M. McWilliams. *Living Nutrition.* Wiley. New York. 1973

[b]Fat soluble vitamin.

[c]Much vitamin K is produced by bacteria in the intestine and absorbed through the intestinal wall.

[d]Water soluble vitamin.

by the fact that the normal body is approximately 55 to 65 percent water by weight.

Within the body, water is found in the cells, outside the cells, and in the bloodstream. This water is important partially because of its ability to serve as a universal solvent. This solvent capability makes it possible for water to transport nutrients to the cells and to remove waste products. Water serves as a lubricant, facilitating movement of joints. In its lubricant role, water helps food to move through the digestive tract. It also facilitates chemical reactions in the body. Another key function of water is to assist in regulating body temperature. Loss of water from the skin is an important mechanism for cooling the body. In a sense, water is a structural component of the body because its presence in cells helps to give the cell shape.

The normal intake of water recommended is about six glasses daily. Part of this can be provided by a variety of juices, soups, and beverages. In hot weather, the intake of water needs to be increased.

SUMMARY

Food contains carbohydrates, fats, proteins, minerals, and vitamins, all of which are important for growth and the maintenance of optimum health. Energy is derived from carbohydrates, fats, and protein. Protein also performs the unique role of providing the essential amino acids needed to manufacture the protein required by the body. Fats provide not only energy, but also serve as carriers of the fat soluble vitamins. Carbohydrates are required for the complete metabolism of fats.

Minerals are needed for a variety of reasons. They promote proper osmotic pressure and assist in maintaining the proper acid-base balance in the body. Various minerals are required for the body's structure, such as calcium in bones and teeth. Some are required for transmission of nerve impulses. Some minerals are structural components of various essential body compounds, such as iron in hemoglobin and iodine in thyroxine. Ions also act as catalysts in some metabolic reactions in the body.

The fat soluble and water soluble vitamins frequently serve as coenzymes to promote essential metabolic reactions in the body. Prime examples of these functions are provided by the roles that thiamin, riboflavin, and niacin perform in the release of energy from carbohydrates, fats, and proteins. Scurvy (ascorbic acid deficiency), xerophthalmia and night blindness (vitamin A deficiency), rickets (vitamin D deficiency), beriberi (thiamin deficiency), and pellagra (niacin deficiency) are vitamin deficiency conditions that have been particularly troublesome to man at various times in history and in various parts of the world.

BIBLIOGRAPHY

Bogert, J., et al., 1973. *Nutrition and Physical Fitness.* 9th ed. Saunders. Philadelphia.

Chaney, M.S. and M.L. Ross, 1972. *Nutrition.* 8th ed. Houghton Mifflin. Boston.

Fleck, H.C., 1971. *Introduction to Nutrition.* 2nd ed. Macmillan. New York.

Guthrie, H.A., 1971. *Introductory Nutrition.* 2nd ed. Mosby. St. Louis.

Mitchell, H.S., et al., 1968. *Cooper's Nutrition in Health and Disease.* 15th ed. Lippincott. Philadelphia.

Robinson, C.H., 1968. *Fundamentals of Normal Nutrition.* Macmillan. New York.

Stare, F. and M. McWilliams, 1973. *Living Nutrition.* Wiley. New York.

Williams, S.R., 1973. *Nutrition and Diet Therapy.* 2nd ed. St. Louis.

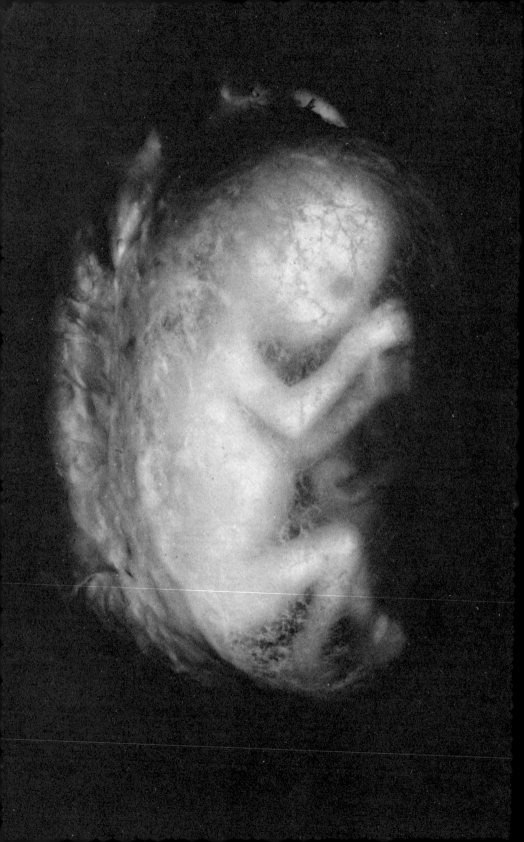

Chapter 2
Physical Development

The role of nutrition in growth and development is more readily understood when the study is based upon an overview of the changes that occur from conception through the achievement of physical maturity. Significant growth and differentiation occur throughout the antenatal period. Such changes necessitate an exploration of the placenta as well as the progressive development of the egg from fertilization until birth.

THE OVUM AND ITS DEVELOPMENT

During the period of approximately 14 days from fertilization of the ovum until implantation, there is little change in actual size, but tremendous changes in complexity are taking place. At the time of fertilization the egg, which is the largest cell in the body, begins to subdivide into smaller cells as the inactive ribosomes in the egg are triggered into activity. This period of free existence is the time of blastogenesis when cellular organization is initiated. Despite the significance of these developments, the ovum must rely on the nutrients present in the yolk sac until implantation, for other sources are not available during this period.

Blastogenesis proceeds as some cells (called trophoblastic cells) cover up other cells during cellular division and become the external cover of the embryo. At the end of blastogenesis, these external cells are separate from the inner cell mass. The cells which have been covered by the trophoblastic cells will become the embryo proper. Fluid separates the trophoblastic cells from the internal cells prior to the embryonic stage. The developmental sequences from conception to birth are outlined in Table 2.1.

Table 2.1   *Growth and development during antenatal period*

Stage	Age	Size	Development
Ovum	0–2 weeks	0.1–0.17 mm	
	0 week		Fertilization
	1 week		Penetration
	2 weeks		Subdivision:
			Trophoblastic cells (external cover)
			Embryo (internal cells)
			Implantation completed
Embryo	3–8 weeks	0.17 mm–3 cm 6 g	Three layers:
			Ectoderm (brain, nervous system, hair, skin)
			Mesoderm (voluntary muscles, excretory system, circulatory system, heart, bones, inner skin)
			Endoderm (inner lining of digestive system and respiratory tract, glands)
			Protein synthesis
	3 weeks	0.17 mm	Forebrain, midbrain, and hindbrain
	4 weeks	4 mm	Heart beats, neural fold for central nervous system. Digestive system forming. Beginning of budding of arms and legs
	5 weeks	5–6 mm	Central nervous system. Intestinal tract. Lungs, liver, skin

[handwritten annotations: "Blastogenesis" with bracket linking to Fertilization/Penetration/Subdivision; "Gastrulation / Formation / 3 layers (germ layer)" next to Embryo three layers; "Embryonic period" written in margin]

Table 2.1 (Continued)

Stage	Age	Size	Development
Embryo	6 weeks	11 mm	Umbilical cord and beginning of placenta. Arm buds. Bones
	7 weeks		Teeth germs. Lining of esophagus and intestine
	8 weeks	3 cm	Digits well formed. Tail-like process disappears. Face and features forming. Internal organs developing
Fetus	9–40 weeks	3 cm to 50 cm 6 g to 3500 g	Protein production. Continuing maturation in preparation for birth
	9 weeks	3–6 cm 7–27 g	Connective tissue, cartilage, and bone
	12 weeks	7–9 cm 28 g	Bone calcification, Sex readily determined. Nails developing. Eyes almost developed. Blood formation beginning in bone marrow. Adipose tissue
	16 weeks	10–17 cm 120 g	Maximum rate of growth. Strong heart beat. Hair on head. Muscles active. Myelination beginning
	20 weeks	18–27 cm 330 g	Brain is 13% of total weight. Enamel and dentine depositing in teeth. Creamy coating developing. Heart beat discernible
	24 weeks	28–34 cm 600 g	Eyebrows and eyelashes. Calcification of teeth. Lungs

Table 2.1 (Continued)

Stage	Age	Size	Development
Fetus			developing but not able to function. Eyelids separate
	28 weeks	35–38 cm 1000 g	Wrinkled skin. Lungs and intestines immature
	32 weeks	42–45 cm 1600 g	Subcutaneous fat deposits. Fair chance for survival
	36 weeks	47 cm 2500 g	Wrinkles smoothing. Vital organs developed. Good survival
	40 weeks	50 cm 3500 g	Fine hair disappearing. Skin still has creamy coating. Birth

EMBRYONIC PERIOD

The embryonic period, which is designated as the third through the eighth week of pregnancy, is the stage when rapid differentiation occurs. Gastrulation, the formation of the three germinal layers (ectoderm, mesoderm, and endoderm), marks the beginning of the embryonic period. At the beginning of this period, the embryo is disc-shaped and approximately 0.17 millimeters long. It is located between the amnion and yolk sac. The actual increase in size of the embryo is still quite small throughout the six weeks of this stage; the embryo assumes a three-dimensional aspect and attains a length of about four millimeters at the end of four weeks and continues to grow to a length of about three centimeters and a weight of six grams at the end of eight weeks.

The formation of the germinal layers is of interest because it is from these three layers that the total development will occur. From the ectoderm, the brain and nervous system and the outer skin (epidermis), hair, and nails will develop;

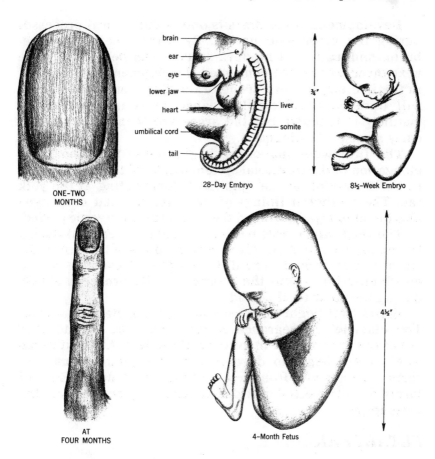

brain
ear
eye
lower jaw
heart
umbilical cord
tail
liver
somite
¾"

28-Day Embryo

8½-Week Embryo

ONE-TWO
MONTHS

4½"

AT
FOUR MONTHS

4-Month Fetus

Embryonic and fetal development during the first four months.

from the mesoderm come the voluntary muscles, the excretory system, the covering of internal organs, the inner skin layer (dermis), the circulatory system including the heart, and bones and cartilage; and from the endoderm develop the inner linings of the digestive and respiratory tracts and the glands, including the liver and pancreas.

During the fourth week, the neural folds fuse together to form the neural tube, the basis for the development of the central nervous system. The rest of the germ disk becomes the outer skin and associated structures. The lungs, liver, and digestive tract develop from the dorsal part of the yolk sac. By six weeks the main differentiation steps have been accomplished, and the arm buds appear.

Development of the brain is one of the critical processes during the embryonic period. By three weeks, the forebrain, midbrain, and hindbrain areas can be noted. In the next three weeks, the continued development has resulted in the five major areas of the brain. These areas, of course, will undergo considerable change in refinement before maturity is reached, but the areas are identifiable at this early stage of development.

The fifth week marks the beginning of the time when elongation of the intestinal system can be noted. This results in the formation of the umbilicus, terminating at the yolk sac. The epithelial linings of the intestine and esophagus also develop rapidly toward the end of the embryonic period.

The respiratory system has its initial development during the embryo stage. After six weeks the buds of the lungs, the trachea, and bronchi are differentiated. Movement of the developing lungs into the thoracic cavity proceeds slowly during the early fetal period.

Bones first begin to appear at approximately six weeks. The clavicle's appearance is followed soon by the long bones of the arms and then those of the legs. At about seven weeks teeth begin to develop from the teeth germs. The germs are derived from ectoderm and mesoderm. Enamel forms from the ectoderm; dentin and pulp derive from the mesoderm.

FETAL PERIOD

From the beginning of the third month of gestation through the approximately 40 weeks of age to delivery is designated as the fetal stage. This period is characterized by cell multiplication and an increase in the size of cells. Intercellular substances are formed and contribute to the growth characteristic of this period. Protein synthesis, an important development during the embryonic period, is a key part of the developmental process during the fetal period. In contrast to the synthesis of new types of proteins that marked the embryonic stage, the focus in the fetal stage is on continued production of the proteins developed in the embryonic stage. Both DNA (deoxyribonucleic acid) and protein content increase significantly during the fetal stage, resulting in gain in weight per nucleus.

myelitus: inflammation of spinal cord or of the
bone marrow —

Connective tissue, cartilage, and bones develop appreciably, beginning calcification with the third month. Adipose tissue appears usually during the fourth month, with increased deposition occurring during the last two months of pregnancy. These developments during the fetal period, in summary, represent an increase from 0.4 grams of protein to 362 grams at birth, and from a weight of six grams at the beginning of the third month to a fetal weight of approximately 3500 grams at delivery. The growth curve proceeds at a rather constant rate until the fetus reaches a gestation age of about 32 weeks. At this time the rate of gain is reduced, becoming sharply slower when the fetus weighs three kilograms.

Widdowson and Dickerson (1964) present interesting comparisons in the percentages of body weight contributed by various organs and tissues during the fetal period, at birth, and at adulthood. The brain develops extremely rapidly during the fetal period in relation to some other parts of the body. By 20 weeks of antenatal development, the brain represents 13 percent of the total weight, a value which persists through birth, but which becomes significantly lower (two percent) in adult man. Myelination is responsible for much of the weight gain of the brain after birth, with only limited myelination before delivery. By contrast, the heart changes only slightly in relative size, ranging from 0.6 percent of the body weight at 20-24 weeks fetal age to 0.4 percent in adulthood.

The heart will begin to beat at about the fourth week of fetal age and the chemical composition of the heart remains relatively constant. This early maturation of the heart is in contrast to the skin and skeletal muscles which assume their significant functions after birth. Some changes occur in fetal muscle from the fourth month until term. The relative proportion of water in muscle decreases appreciably as term is approached. Also, there is a drop in the sodium and chloride levels.

Calcification of the cartilaginous framework begins in approximately the eighth week. During calcification and development of the bones, there is a gradual and continuing loss of water, accompanied by an increase in both total nitrogen and collagen nitrogen, calcium, and phosphorus. The ratio of calcium to nitrogen shows an increase throughout the fetal period. The amount of calcium increases more

myelin - soft white somewhat fatty material
that forms a thick medullary sheath about
the protoplasmic core of a medullated nerve fiber

rapidly than does that of phosphorus, thus causing a higher calcium/phosphorus ratio at term than is found at the end of the first trimester.

PLACENTAL DEVELOPMENT

Development of the placenta is a critical part of the reproductive process. About the seventh day of gestation, the blastocyst penetrates the uterine mucosa. The trophoblast then begins to grow to make up a network containing small pits or spaces (lacunae). Maternal blood penetrates into these small lacunae by the 12th day, but does not circulate until approximately one week later. The reticulum (network) develops into a more regular form that resembles roots radiating from the chorion (outer membrane) of the placenta. Chorionic villi form and create intervillous spaces. The villi are penetrated by capillaries which ultimately are extensions of the two arteries from the embryo via the umbilical cord and the necessary return of fetal blood, also via the umbilical cord. Maternal blood circulates in the intervillous spaces, while the fetal supply remains in the villi. However, the large surface area created by the villi allows optimal exchange between maternal and fetal blood supplies despite the complete separation of the two.

The placenta is a highly complex structure and one which increases in size throughout the period of gestation. At the time of delivery the placenta usually will occupy a volume of approximately half a liter. Development of the placenta to this volume during gestation is generally considered to be important to the delivery of term babies of normal weight. Term babies (39 to 40 weeks of gestation) having a lighter than normal birth weight have been found by Aherne and Dunnill (1966) to have a mean placental volume approximately two-thirds of normal.

The value of the placenta in enhancing fetal development is related to vascularization and the adequacy of maternal blood circulation. Although evidence regarding this factor is somewhat limited in humans, there is an indication that smoking may limit circulation and constrict the uterine arteries (Gruenwald, 1966).

The placenta performs several functions in reproduction. Not only is the placenta charged with the responsibility of nutrient exchanges between maternal and fetal systems,

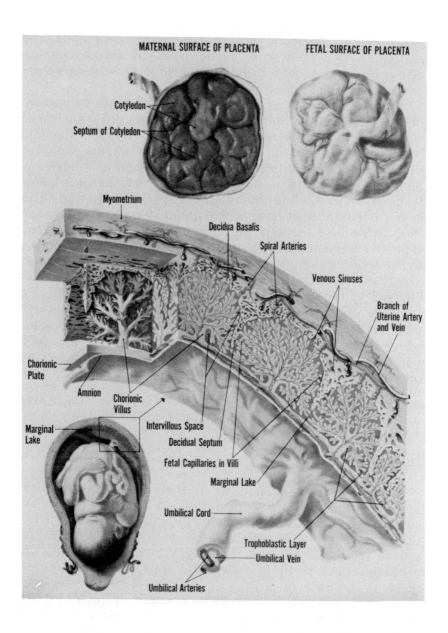

MATERNAL SURFACE OF PLACENTA   FETAL SURFACE OF PLACENTA

Cotyledon

Septum of Cotyledon

Myometrium

Decidua Basalis

Spiral Arteries

Venous Sinuses

Branch of Uterine Artery and Vein

Chorionic Plate

Amnion

Chorionic Villus

Marginal Lake

Intervillous Space

Decidual Septum

Fetal Capillaries in Villi

Marginal Lake

Umbilical Cord

Trophoblastic Layer

Umbilical Vein

Umbilical Arteries

Diagram of the placenta.

but it also has an endocrine function, namely synthesizing gonadotropic hormone at first and then estrogens and gestagens. The placenta participates in the exchanges of oxygen and carbon dioxide. It also serves in excretory exchange of urea, creatinine, and uric acid.

Nutrient exchanges are essential for the development of the fetus. Water, sodium, and potassium are transferred with ease through the placenta. Iodide crosses the placenta by active transfer, as does iron. Fetal plasma contains higher levels of iodide, calcium, magnesium, potassium, and phosphorus than does maternal plasma. Glucose is transferred to the fetal blood at a rate of more than 20 milligrams per minute at term, a rate about 10 times greater than that of fructose. Acetate and other precursors, used by the fetus to synthesize most of its lipids, are transferred readily to the fetus, while cholesterol penetrates slowly. Fatty acids are transferred with reasonable ease; phospholipids are cleaved by the chorionic tissue, and the free phosphate ion then becomes available to the fetus for synthesizing its own phospholipids. Amino acids are transferred to the fetus where they are used in protein synthesis. Hormonal polypeptides are transferred in limited amounts, and apparently only proteins of immunological significance are transferred from maternal to fetal supplies.

POSTNATAL DEVELOPMENT

Height

Although individuals do vary in their actual growth rates, an outline of typical growth patterns is of value when considering nutritional needs during the growing years. During the first year of life following birth, there will be an increase in length of approximately 50 per cent, making the average length of the year-old child approximately 75 centimeters. The rate of growth decelerates between the ages of one and two, with an average increase in height during this second year of between 12 and 13 centimeters. This growth is significantly less than the approximately 25 centimeters gained during the first year. After the second year, the growth rate levels off at the still slower rate of between five and six centimeters annually until the adolescent growth spurt is reached.

These values for growth rates are stated in rather general terms because much remains to be determined about the influence of a number of variables impacting growth rates. One variable that has been noted by a number of growth researchers is that of race. Negro infants have been shown to be more advanced in skeletal maturation than Caucasian infants from birth until approaching three years of age. Psychomotor development of Negro infants has been measured as being more advanced than Caucasian infants for a similar period of time, and dentition development follows a similar curve for most of the first three years. By the age of three, these differences generally have disappeared.

The rather regular slope of growth during the period preceding adolescence is altered at different ages, depending upon sex of the person as well as individual differences. Girls will enter a period of rapid growth between the ages of 10½ to 11. At approximately 12 years of age, the peak of the growth period will be reached. The period of rapid growth usually will last for about two to two and a half years and will add a total height increase of about 16 centimeters; most girls will return to a slower rate of growth between age 13 and 14. By about age 15, girls will have reached 99 percent of their adult height, with growth being completed for most girls by age 17-18 (see Table 2.2). The figure presents the graphs of height and weight for girls from ages 4 to 18. The impact of the adolescent growth spurt is not as evident in this presentation as it would be for an individual girl because the large numbers used in developing growth charts erase individual differences.

Boys reach the adolescent growth spurt at a somewhat older age than girls, although the duration of the spurt is about the same for both sexes. Boys usually begin the period of rapid growth at approximately 12½ to 13 years of age and reach the maximum velocity at age 14. The average gain in height during this period is about 20 centimeters, with much of this growth being the result of increasing length of the trunk. The differences in age of rapid adolescent growth because of sex difference result in a two to three year period between ages 11 and 14 when girls will be taller and heavier than their male peers. Growth in males generally continues at a slower rate following the adolescent spurt, until about

Table 2.2   Percentage of mature height attained at different ages[a]

Chronological Age (years)	Percentage of Eventual Height	
	Boys	Girls
1	42.2	44.7
2	49.5	52.8
3	53.8	57.0
4	58.0	61.8
5	61.8	66.2
6	65.2	70.3
7	69.0	74.0
8	72.0	77.5
9	75.0	80.7
10	78.0	84.4
11	81.1	88.4
12	84.2	92.9
13	87.3	96.5
14	91.5	98.3
15	96.1	99.1
16	98.3	99.6
17	99.3	100.0
18	99.8	100.0

[a]From Bayley's longitudinal study of 150 boys and girls in California. *J. Pediat.* 48: 187. 1956.

age 18 or older. The physical development of boys from ages 4 through 18 is described in the figure.

Weight

The changes in height that take place from conception to adulthood certainly are impressive. The development from an ovum just visible to the eye (approximately 0.1 millimeters long) to a newborn about 50 centimeters long is remarkable, and the increase in height of about three and a half times from birth to adulthood represents yet another milestone in growth. Despite these achievements in height, the growth changes as measured by weight are far more staggering in proportion. For example, the increase in weight from the ovum to delivery represents a factor of approximately 3 billion. In contrast to the maximum growth rate

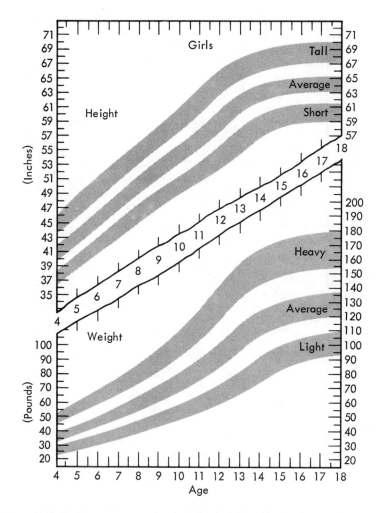

Height and weight tables for girls 4 to 18 in Iowa City, Iowa, schools (data collected in 1961). Prepared for the Joint Committee on Health Problems in Education of the NEA and AMA by Howard V. Meredith and Virginia B. Knott, State University of Iowa.

of height which occurs during the fourth month of fetal life, the maximum growth rate for weight takes place soon after birth. Weight generally increases approximately 20 times birth weight by the time adulthood is reached.

Weight is a far more variable measure of growth than is height, although some generalizations can be drawn. Female infants are approximately 140 grams lighter, on the

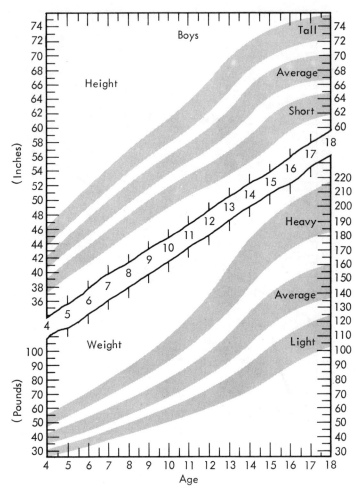

Height and weight tables for boys age 4 to 18 in Iowa City, Iowa, schools (data collected from 1961 to 1963). Prepared for the Joint Committee on Health Problems in Education of the NEA and AMA by Howard V. Meredith and Virginia B. Knott, State University of Iowa.

average, than are male infants at birth. Infants born of small mothers or of mothers of lower socioeconomic backgrounds tend to be lighter at birth than those born from more favorable backgrounds. First-born infants generally are lighter than those born later in the family sequence.

During the first year, infants usually about triple their birth weight. During the second year, the rate of increase in weight drops significantly, with the result that weight at the end of the second year is approximately four times birth weight. Weight gains then become fairly constant, averaging between 2.25 and 2.75 kilograms annually until the adolescent growth spurt is reached. The adolescent height spurt precedes the weight spurt by approximately three months, with girls adding an average of 16 kilograms and boys 20 kilograms during this period.

Skeletal Growth

The growth of the various systems of the body takes place at differing rates and periods of time. The head of the new-born is comparatively large in proportion to the development of the trunk and legs. At birth, the length of the head represents approximately ¼ the total length of the body, whereas in adults, the head length is approximately ⅛ the total height. At birth, the length of the legs represents about ⅓ of the total length of the body, a ratio which will change to about ½ in adulthood. This shift in the relative ratio of legs to total height means that there is an accompanying shift in the center of gravity. The young child learning to walk is more top heavy than an adult. Arms also are short at birth in comparison with their proportionately greater length in adulthood. The circumference of the head and chest are approximately equal at birth, and both of these measurements are smaller than the abdomen.

At birth, the measurements of the head are closer to maturity than are those of the remainder of the body, the trunk is next in its development, and the limbs are the least developed. The extremities of the limbs are more developed accordingly than are regions nearer the trunk. This means that the foot more nearly approaches adult proportions than does the calf, and the calf is ahead of the thigh. The final growth spurt in adolescence begins with accelerated growth of the hands and feet, followed by growth of the calf and forearm. The hips and chest then accelerate, with the shoulders coming next, and the trunk lengthening and the chest expanding last. The time required to progress through these various peaks of growth in adolescence is about a year.

The development of the skeleton occurs at different times at various points in the body, but following the maturational sequence: (1) development of bony centers (806 bony centers will be formed ultimately); (2) modification of the form or shape of the bony center; (3) fusion of groups of bony centers; and (4) orderly changes in the texture and composition of the bony centers. The jawbones and collarbones will appear as bony centers in the first six weeks of prenatal development, while a ridge at the top of the hipbone will not develop as a bony center until puberty. At the onset of ossification, the first hard bony tissue will be laid down in the bony center. The shape of the bony centers is modified as bones begin to touch each other. Some bony centers will fuse with others as a normal part of development. Some bony centers at the base of the skull will fuse before birth, while certain bones in the wrists and ankles will remain separate throughout life. Bones undergo changes in composition, ranging from the coarse and irregular bony tissues of early childhood to the more uniform secondary bone tissue of maturity.

The growth of bones may be studied by following the development of a long bone, such as is found in the arm or leg. Development begins with differentiation from the tissue into a white, rubbery substance known as cartilage. The cartilage becomes extended into the shape of a long bone, which then is encircled around the middle with a ring of actual bone tissue. This ring around the center of the long bone gradually extends toward both ends of the shaft, leaving only the ends of the bone cartilage extending beyond the bone sleeve. As the sleeve is developing, the cartilaginous tissue is replaced by spongy, osseous tissue. The length of the bone is increased by the extension of cartilage at both ends. Finally, the bony epiphysis appears in the cartilage at each end of the bone. From the center of the cartilage, the epiphysis replaces the cartilage, growing wider and wider. When the epiphysis becomes as wide as the bony sleeve on the shaft of the bone, only a thin disc of cartilage remains between the epiphysis and the shaft. Growth during childhood occurs as a result of active growth of this remaining cartilage. Eventually, when growth ceases, the cartilage is replaced on the outside by the hard bone of the sleeve and on the inside by spongy bone. Thus the bony epiphysis and shaft are fused together to terminate growth of the bone.

Bones grow in thickness as well as in length. The greater circumference of bone is achieved by laying down new layers of bone on the outside region of the bone. Concomitantly, older layers of bone are removed inside the bone. During the growing years, the inner region of the bone is filled with spongy bone tissue, but much of this spongy bone is gradually removed from the central region of the bone in adulthood, leaving the spongy bone only in the ends of the bone.

There has long been considerable interest in studying growth and maturation of children. The usual way of studying individual children is by the use of x-rays of the wrist and hand. Many of these x-rays have been evaluated very carefully and displayed in atlases that present typical rates of skeletal maturation. Skeletal age is evaluated in relation to chronological age because not all individuals grow and mature at the same rate. One child may be significantly smaller than average values for his age, but his skeletal maturity may also be somewhat retarded. In this instance, there will be a longer period of growth available for him, and the final height achieved may be predicted to be somewhat taller than a boy who was similarly short for his age, but who was more mature in skeletal age. Numerous discrepancies between skeletal and chronological age have been reviewed by growth specialists. In some individual instances, growth predictions may be of value in considering realistic future career goals in which size is of significant importance.

Teeth

Calcification. The growth and development of teeth must be considered in two different systems: the sequence of calcification and the sequence of eruption. Each of the 52 primary and permanent teeth undergoes a developmental phase in which a regular sequence is followed. In the case of the primary central incisor, calcification of the crown begins between the fetal age of four and four and a half months, with completion of calcification occurring after birth at the age of six to ten weeks, and eruption occurring at approximately six months. In contrast to the early formation of the central incisor, the third molar of the permanent teeth does not begin to calcify until between seven and ten years of age.

Development of teeth proceeds according to a template defined at the dentino-enamel junction. Deposition of the enamel matrix will proceed outward, layer upon layer, from this junction. Formation of the dentin proceeds in layers being deposited in an inward direction toward the pulp cavity. At the time the enamel has been deposited to its final size, the cells required for enamel deposition vanish and enamel formation cannot be resumed, even if the enamel of the tooth is injured. However, dentin can be formed along the surface of the pulp if the dentin is eroded due to the presence of dental caries. The rate of regeneration of dentin is quite slow, and thus is not adequate to combat developing caries in most instances.

Incremental lines in teeth indicate periods when calcification of teeth is interrupted. Rings or incremental lines normally develop at birth, three months, ten months, two and a half years, and five years. The ring occurring at birth is a reflection of the birth trauma and the adjustment to independence rather than a parasitic relationship. The line at three months is thought to indicate depletion of the fetal mineral stores. Massler, et al. (1941) have determined that the optimum conditions for calcification of primary and permanent teeth occur from the fourth month of gestation to delivery. The least favorable period was deemed by these researchers to be from birth to ten months; somewhat improved, but still poor circumstances were found between the ages of two and a half and five and between ages ten and thirteen. Calcification was more favorable at ages six to ten, and still more favorable between ten months and two and a half years.

Eruption. The eruption sequence for the primary teeth is somewhat different than for the permanent teeth, with the primary teeth eruption beginning with the central incisor at about six months of age. The first permanent tooth to erupt is the first molar or six-year molar. Until the loss of the first of his deciduous teeth, the child at about age six has the largest number of teeth that he will ever have. The eruption of the permanent teeth extends over a far longer period of time than the eruption of the primary teeth. The eruption process, which for the primary teeth requires only approximately a year and a half, continues usually for at least nine years for the complete eruption of the permanent teeth. Although the usual age for eruption of the first molar is six years, the third molar often does not erupt until after age 15.

Nervous System

The weight of many systems of the body will increase significantly from birth to maturity of an individual, with growth of the genital system, muscles, and pancreas representing the largest increase (approximately 30 to 40 times heavier at maturity than at birth). At the other end of the spectrum is the nervous system, which will increase its total weight less than five times during the maturation process. The brain doubles its birth weight during the first year after birth and the spinal cord will continue to mature, but the basic features of the nervous system are all present at birth. One of the important stages in maturation following birth is the development of the myelin sheath on many of the nerve fibers of the brain and spinal cord. The sensory tracts are reasonably well myelinated at birth, but the motor pathways need to develop this sheath. Nerve fibers will continue their growth in length and diameter even after myelination, but the formation of new nerve cells ceases at a fetal age of approximately six months.

Cardiovascular System

Considerable changes need to be made in the cardiovascular system at the time of birth, for the oxygenation of the blood in the placenta no longer is possible. During the fetal period, the lungs are by-passed, but oxygenation of the blood supply requires utilization of the lungs following birth. Thus, the by-pass of the fetal stage must be terminated. At birth the heart is somewhat larger in proportion to the rest of the body than it will be at maturity (0.75 percent at birth compared with about 0.4 percent mature weight). This relatively larger heart occupies some of the area that will later be required by the expanding lungs. During growth, the left ventricle walls will thicken considerably more than those of the right ventricle because of the difference in the work to be done. The arteries, veins, and heart will grow as the child grows, with a significant increase in the growth of the heart during adolescence. From birth to maturity the heart will increase in weight at a slightly slower rate than the overall increase in the body as a whole.

The white cells of the blood are numerous at birth and then drop to a somewhat lower level until the adolescent period. Red blood cells and hemoglobin counts decrease during the first three months of life; there is a rise at approximately three months, and a substantial increase in both values is normal during adolescence. Males experience a larger increase in red blood cells and hemoglobin in adolescence than do females.

Respiratory System

The respiratory system will increase its weight by 20 to 25 times from birth to maturity. This increase is comparable to the increase in the skeletal weight. As soon as breathing begins, the lungs increase rapidly in size and the air passages begin to change. The respiratory surface increases as additional alveoli and modifications of the respiratory bronchioles develop. The diameters of the tubes also increase. At puberty the larynx grows much more rapidly, a change that is particularly apparent in boys as their voices change.

Digestive System

Beginning with feeding after birth, the capacity of the small stomach increases rapidly. In fact, the capacity may triple in the first two weeks. Capacity is estimated at 30-90 cubic centimeters at birth, 90-150 cc at one month, 210-360 cc by one year, 500 cc at two, and up to 900 cc in later preadolescence. The stomach will gradually shift position as the infant grows, and by maturity the small intestine and sometimes at least part of the stomach will extend into the pelvic region. The small intestine (approximately 300-350 centimeters long at birth) grows throughout the early years and doubles in length by the beginning of adolescence. The liver, which has developed to approximately five percent of body weight at birth because of its role in blood formation during the antenatal period, will continue to grow. However, the liver represents only about two and a half percent of the weight of the adult. The gallbladder grows rapidly during the first two years.

The sucking response of the newborn develops very

quickly following birth, although premature infants require a few days for full development. Sucking triggers related contractions of the esophagus and peristalsis.

Excretory System

The newborn infant has a high percentage (43 percent) of its body weight as extracellular fluid compared with the 25 percent value found in adults. There is a decrease in the extracellular volume during early infancy and a somewhat smaller, yet significant decrease during adolescence. Infants exchange about half of their extracellular water daily, with considerable loss in fecal excretion. Dehydration can occur more readily in infants than in adults because of their limited ability to control water exchange.

The kidney weight increases slowly early in gestation and somewhat more rapidly in the later stages. The weight of the kidneys will increase 10 to 15 times before maturity is achieved. Weight gain is rapid during the first year and continues somewhat less rapidly into adolescence. Infants produce a relatively acidic urine. Disturbances such as diarrhea can quickly lead to acidosis and abnormal fluid balance, resulting in edema or dehydration.

Endocrine System

In males, the testes grow most rapidly during early infancy and again during adolescence, with growth continuing at a somewhat slower pace during the intervening period. In girls the ovaries double their birth weight by six months of age and double again during puberty. The uterus actually decreases its weight by half after birth, but regains its birth weight by age 11.

The pituitary gland is vital to normal growth processes. The anterior lobe of the pituitary gland produces a number of hormones including growth hormone, thyrotropin, corticotropin, two gonadotropins, and prolactin. Growth hormone aids in the synthesis of protein by promoting transport of amino acids across cell walls. It also aids in the breakdown of fatty acids and the formation of cartilage. Giantism or dwarfism can result if the anterior lobe of the pituitary gland fails to function properly.

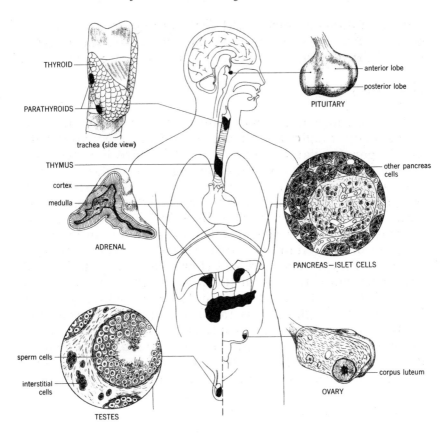

THYROID

PARATHYROIDS

trachea (side view)

anterior lobe

posterior lobe

PITUITARY

THYMUS

cortex

medulla

ADRENAL

other pancreas cells

PANCREAS—ISLET CELLS

sperm cells

interstitial cells

TESTES

corpus luteum

OVARY

Diagram of the endocrine system.

The thyroid gland is of significance because of its role in producing thyroxine and, ultimately, its role in influencing basal metabolism. When the thyroid gland is functioning normally, it promotes normal growth and development, including bone growth and sexual development, and maintains mental development. The thyroid gland is intimately related to the functioning of the gonads and the adrenals.

The adrenal glands lose about half of their birth weight by the age of three weeks, but they will slowly regain this weight and return to the original size by three years of age. The adrenal cortex produces steroid hormones: (1) aldosterone regulates water balance and sodium and potassium excretion; (2) corticoids influence growth and help to regulate carbohydrate-protein balance; and (3) androgens promote maleness and retention of nitrogen.

The parathyroid glands are significant for their role in regulating calcium and phosphorus metabolism. Parathyroid hormone is credited with freeing some calcium from depots in the bone to mobilize it as needed in the blood. This process is a normal part of bone formation, but hyperparathyroidism can lead to bone malformations.

SUMMARY

Growth and development proceed in a predictable and basically orderly sequence from fertilization of the ovum, through implantation and development of the embryo, the fetal stage, birth, childhood and adolescence. The stages prior to birth are parasitic, with nutrition being provided through the umbilical cord from the placenta as soon as this system is established. The newborn is able to draw upon his own body stores as well as the nutrients provided in his diet in the early stages of infancy.

The remarkable division, differentiation, and development of gestation have been reviewed. The factors that combine to determine the physical stature and the rate of development of the individual have also been examined. Genetic factors, diet, total environment and the functioning of the many complex parts of the human body combine to determine the growth achieved by an individual.

BIBLIOGRAPHY

Acheson, R.M., 1966. Maturation of the skeleton. In *Human Development*. Ed., F. Falkner. p. 465. Saunders. Philadelphia.

Aherne, W. and M.S. Dunnill, 1966. Morphometry of human placenta. *Brit. Med. Bull.* 22: 5.

Assali, N.S., ed., 1968. *Biology of Gestation.* Vol. I. Maternal Oranism. Academic Press. New York.

Assali, N.S., et al., 1968. *Biology of Gestation.* Vol. II. Fetus and Neonate. Academic Press. New York.

Assali, N.S., et al., 1968. Physiology of the placenta. In *Biology of Gestation.* Ed., N.S. Assali. Vol. I: 186.

Assali, N.S., et al., 1968. Fetal and neonatal circulation. In *Biology of Gestation.* Ed., N.S. Assali. Vol. II: 52.

Baer, M.J., 1973. *Growth and Maturation.* H.A. Doyle. Cambridge, Mass.

Donovan, B.T. and J.J. Van Der Werff Ten Bosch., 1965. *Physiology of Puberty.* Williams and Wilkins. Baltimore.

Falkner, F., ed., 1966. *Human Development.* Saunders. Philadelphia.

Falkner, F., 1966. General considerations in human development. In *Human Development.* Ed., F. Falkner. p. 10. Saunders. Philadelphia.

Giroud, A., 1970. *Nutrition of the Embryo.* C.C. Thomas. Springfield, Ill.

Gruenwald, P., 1966. Growth of human fetus. *Amer. J. Obstet. Gynec.* 94: 1112.

Lazzari, E.P., 1968. *Dental Biochemistry.* Lea and Febiger. London.

Massler, M., et al., 1941. Developmental pattern of the child as reflected in calcification pattern of teeth. *Amer. J. Dis. Child* 62, No. 1: 33.

Nesbitt, R.E.L., 1966. Perinatal development. In *Human Development.* Ed., F. Falkner. p. 123. Saunders. Philadelphia.

Rodahl, K., 1966. Bone development. In *Human Development.* Ed., F. Falkner. p. 503. Saunders. Philadelphia.

Ross Laboratories, 1973. *Premature Infant.* Columbus, Ohio.

Ross Laboratories, 1974. *Placental Development and Circulation.* Columbus, Ohio.

Shock, N.W., 1966. Physiological growth. In *Human Development.* Ed., F. Falkner. p. 150. Saunders. Philadelphia.

Sinclair, D., 1969. *Human Growth after Birth.* Oxford University Press. New York.

Tanner, J.M., 1969. Growth of children in industrialized countries with special reference to the secular trend. In *Nutrition in Preschool and School Age.* Ed., G. Blix, p. 9. Swedish Nutrition Foundation. Uppsala.

Waisman, H.A. and G.R. Kerr, 1970. *Fetal Growth and Development.* McGraw-Hill. New York.

Watson, E.H. and G.H. Lowrey, 1967. *Growth and Development of Children.* 5th ed. Year Book Medical Publishers. Chicago.

Widdowson, E.M., 1968. Growth and composition of the fetus and newborn. In *Biology of Gestation.* Vol. II: 1. Academic Press. New York.

Widdowson, E.M. and J.W.T. Dickerson, 1964. The elements. In *Mineral Metabolism* 2: 1. Academic Press.

Wynn, R.W., 1968. Morphology of the placenta. In *Biology of Gestation.* Ed., N. Assali. Vol. 1: 93. Academic Press. New York.

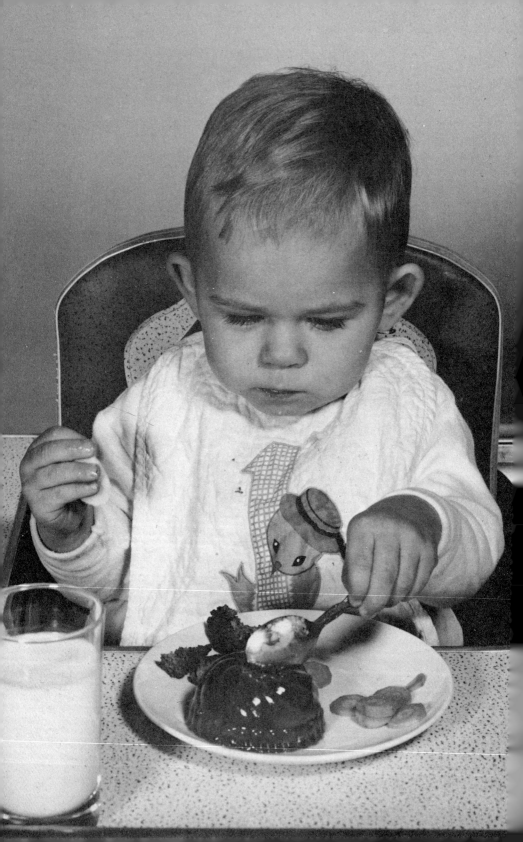

Chapter 3
Mental Development

A great deal of interest and research today centers around the interrelationship between nutritional status and mental development. Despite the high level of activity in this realm at the present time, much still remains to be demonstrated conclusively. There are still many areas where inferences are drawn because controlled studies have not been conducted. The conclusions are drawn presently from a combination of numerous observations over time, well controlled animal experiments, and limited human studies. There are many obvious reasons why controlled research in this area has not been conducted on humans. Nevertheless, information is beginning to emerge which strengthens the argument that nutritional status influences mental development.

PRENATAL CONSIDERATIONS

The nutritional status of the mother is of concern when considering the influence of nutrition-mental development interrelationships. A range of observations supports the conclusion that optimum nutrition of the mother throughout her early life and her pregnancy will promote optimal mental development in her offspring. Her nutritional status over the period when she was growing will influence her ultimate height and the dimensions of her pelvis, both of which have been shown to be related to prematurity, Caesarean sections, and infant mortality (Thomson, 1959; Baird and Illsley, 1953; U.S. Vital and Health Statistics, 1973). Concern for mental development goes back to the period of rapid brain growth between the sixth month of gestation to about the sixth to ninth month of life. At birth, division of the neuronal cells of the brain has practically stopped. Animals that have been deprived of sufficient protein during gestation have been shown to have fewer brain cells, a deficit which is apparently not overcome by feeding an adequate diet after birth. The birth of premature infants would reduce the time available for formation of new brain cells prior to birth. Controlled studies to validate this theory have not been conducted, but autopsies of children who died of malnutrition before the age of 2 (Winick, et al., 1970) revealed a small number of brain cells. Adequate nutrients for the cellular division to proceed normally would appear to be essential if the brain is to achieve its normal complement of cells before the age when cell division ceases. Autopsies of stillborn or infants who died within 48 hours of birth in the United States were reported by Naeye, et al. (1969). Again, smaller brains and other organs were reported, with the organs associated with poor families being smaller than those from more affluent backgrounds.

Chase, et al. (1971) noted that the cerebellum weight and the corresponding cellularity of that portion of the brain were the most affected part of the brain among small-for-gestational-age newborns. Biochemical differences such as low myelin lipids were also noted.

The brain, at birth, is already developed to about 25 percent of its mature weight, with growth during the first year of life bringing the size to approximately 70 percent of its expected adult weight. Differentiation as well as cell growth will be critical during this early developmental period. Although the most dramatic development of the brain is found during the gestational and very early postnatal period, there is a continuing process of myelination and dendrite branching which continues over a period of many years. The vulnerability of the brain to malnutrition definitely appears to be far greater during the cell division stage than it is later, but some vulnerability is considered to extend into the preschool period and beyond the infant stage.

Theories on the effects of malnutrition on brain development center around the developmental stage at which the nutritional insult occurs as well as upon the duration and severity. Brain development is categorized in 3 stages: (1) hyperplasia, (2) hyperplasia and hypertrophy, and (3) hypertrophy. Hyperplasia is described as cellular division, with increasing brain weight, increasing amounts of protein, and rise in DNA content of the brain. In the intermediate stage, this proliferation continues and the protein content and brain weight continue to rise, but the DNA level rises at a reduced rate. In other words, cell division and cell growth are occurring simultaneously. In hypertrophy, the DNA level does not rise, but the protein level and weight of the brain increase as a result of growth of existing cells. If severe nutritional deprivation occurs during the period of hyperplasia, the opportunity for cellular division may pass and the number of cells in the brain will be fewer than normal throughout life. The significance of a reduced number of cells is not known fully at this point.

Myelin formation is also important to the functioning of the brain and central nervous system. This substance, which acts as an insulator for the nerves, is a lipid complex that is a regulator in transmitting nerve impulses. Myelin formation begins approximately at birth and continues for about two years in humans. Prolonged malnutrition during this two-year period can result in decreased myelin formation, with less myelin being available per cell.

Wiener, et al. (1965) surveyed a matched group of premature and full-term infants at two intervals up to age seven to determine whether there was any difference in intellectual competence. When tested at age three to five, the children who had been born prematurely were rated as more retarded both intellectually and physically than the full term births. This same relative rating was observed in the subsequent tests between six and seven. Werner (1967) and others have reported a seemingly greater interrelationship between low birth weight and intellectual performance for children in the lowest social classes than among those born into higher social status. Thus, the lowest social classes have a greater likelihood of bearing infants of premature or low birth weight status, and these resulting infants are more likely to maintain their deficiency than are premature or low birth weight infants of higher social class.

POSTNATAL INFLUENCES

Malnutrition may take the form of suboptimal, but not acute malnutrition which can be maintained over a long period of time, or it may be a severe deprivation which will quickly result in hospitalization or lead to death. The effect of the nutritional insult will be determined by its severity, the duration, the stage in the life cycle at which it occurs, and the specific nutrient(s) missing or lacking in the diet. When considering the interrelationship of malnutrition and mental development, two deficiency conditions are of particular significance. These are marasmus and kwashiorkor. Although cases of either of these conditions are very limited in the United States, they are of broad concern and frequent occurrence in many of the developing nations of the world.

Marasmus

Marasmus may be described as chronic starvation. This overall lack of nutrients may be initiated during the prenatal period if the mother is living in very marginal or inadequate circumstances and is not receiving medical care and nutrient supplementation. If this situation is true for the mother, the infant will be brought into a similar environment and the condition will be perpetuated, often with fatal results. Marasmus is characterized particularly by a deficiency of both protein and calories. This condition may be noted during the first year of life.

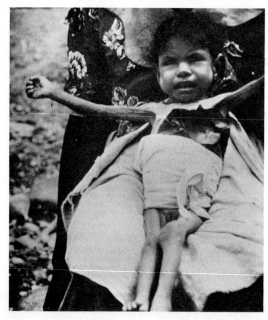

Marasmus is a nutritional deficiency condition due to severe deprivation of protein, calories, and other essential nutrients.

Kwashiorkor

Kwashiorkor is the condition that develops when protein is deficient in the diet over a period of time. Frequently this situation is triggered by the onset of a childhood illness which decreases the utilization of nutrients in the diet as a result of diarrhea and vomiting. Children from families with very limited incomes in developing countries are likely candidates for developing kwashiorkor. Usually this condition will not develop until after children are weaned; even though the mother may be receiving quite an inadequate diet, she usually will be able to produce sufficient milk for her infant to avoid kwashiorkor. The protein in her milk will safeguard against this illness despite the fact that the total protein available to the infant will not be sufficient in many instances to also promote optimal growth. The onset of kwashiorkor generally will occur somewhere between the ages of one and four, the period when mother's milk often is not provided and other sources of protein are perhaps severely restricted in the diet.

The individual role of malnutrition in influencing mental development is now extremely difficult to isolate from the other factors that also determine how effectively an individual interacts with his world. Young children who develop

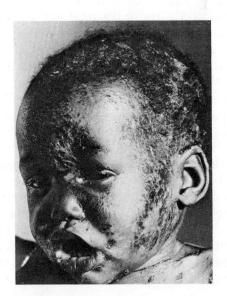

Protein intake may be reduced sharply following weaning, resulting in kwashiorkor.

marasmus or kwashiorkor often are hospitalized for treatment. This isolation provides different stimuli for learning as well as a different nutritional base.

Birch, et al. (1971) compared the intelligence of 37 Mexican children who had been hospitalized for kwashiorkor at some time between the ages of 6 and 30 months with their siblings who had not experienced malnutrition sufficient to hospitalize them. Verbal and performance tests on the formerly hospitalized children and their siblings revealed significantly higher levels of achievement for the siblings who had not been hospitalized than for those who had been hospitalized for kwashiorkor. Even more dramatic differences might be expected to be observed if pairings could be made with children from families of similar circumstances but without any diagnosis of malnutrition in the family. Presumably siblings in families with at least one child with kwashiorkor may be expected to also be experiencing suboptimal nutrition. Consequently, developmental differences between children in such deprived families could be predicted to be somewhat less than when comparing children experiencing optimal nutrition with those who have had kwashiorkor.

Other Significant Factors

Another aspect of nutritional deficiency and its relation to learning ability is illustrated by iron deficiency anemia. This type of a deficiency is not likely to result in hospitalization and isolation of a young child. However, iron deficiency anemia is a far more frequent problem in the United States than is either kwashiorkor or marasmus. The role of iron in the body is not suggestive of limiting brain growth significantly, as is true with a protein deficiency, and yet learning may be influenced by an iron deficiency.

In the instance of iron deficiency anemia, the hemoglobin level will be low and the oxygen-carrying capacity of the blood will be reduced. Hutcheson and Wright (1968) reported a survey taken in rural Tennessee which revealed that the highest incidence of anemia among the children (ranging up to six years of age) was in children one year old. Similar findings were noted by Gutelius (1969) in the Washington, D.C. area. Children with anemia will be more fatigued, be more irritable, and less motivated to explore their surroundings. This more limited interaction with environments for learning can promote a circumstance that again will inhibit or retard learning.

Inadequate levels of other nutrients, such as vitamin A or ascorbic acid, may contribute to the circumstance where learning is not optimal. When children have a decreased resistance to infections, they will be sick more frequently than when nutrition is optimal. Sickness means decreased attendance and participation in school and other settings for enriched experiences. Income levels do influence the adequacy of the diet that will be available to young children. Children from the low income areas are less likely to have an adequate diet than are children from more favorable circumstances. They also are likely to be living in more crowded and less sanitary housing, yet another factor that predisposes toward illness in the less advantaged group.

Yet another complicating factor in determining the role of nutrition in mental development is that children living in families which are less advantaged financially and socially are surrounded by an environment that is less stimulating and less directed toward learning. Their parents may have below average intelligence, their opportunities for learning may be quite restricted, and there may be little reinforcement and support for learning in the home. Added to this picture is the likelihood that the mother in the family has little knowledge of nutrition and, therefore, is handicapped in efforts to feed her family correctly with the limited amount of money available for food.

SUMMARY

The cyclic nature of impaired learning because of the combination of limited development of parents (particularly limited physical growth of the mother), possible impaired development of the fetus and infant, incidence of such nutritional deficiency conditions as kwashiorkor and anemia, limited benefits and attendance in school due to frequent illnesses and short attention span, and reduced earning potential due to the interaction of these factors all combine to perpetuate the problems of mental development and malnutrition. Some steps are being taken to interrupt this cycle and to attempt to promote better growth and greater achievement in school. These steps are an encouraging beginning, but much remains to be done before children will have an optimal opportunity for development from conception throughout life. Continuing research activities in the complex realm of malnutrition, learning, and behavior doubtless will be important in helping to achieve optimal development.

BIBLIOGRAPHY

Anonymous, 1973. Malnutrition, learning and behavior. *Dairy Council Digest* 44, No. 6: 1.

Baird, D. and R. Illsley, 1953. Environment and child-bearing. *Proc. Roy. Soc. Med.* 46: 53.

Birch, H.G., 1972. Malnutrition, learning, and intelligence. *Amer. J. Pub. Health* 62: 773.

Birch, H.G. and J. Cravioto, 1968. Infection, nutrition and environment in mental development. In *Prevention of Mental Retardation through Control of Infectious Disease.* Ed., H.F. Eichenwald. Health Service Publication 1962. Washington, D.C.

Birch, H.G. and J.D. Gussow, 1970. *Disadvantaged Children; Health, Nutrition, and School Failure.* Harcourt, Brace, and World. New York.

Birch, H.G., et al., 1971. Kwashiorkor in early childhood and intelligence at school age. *Pediat. Res.* 5: 579.

Champakam, S., et al., 1968. Kwashiorkor and mental development. *Amer. J. Clin. Nutr.* 21: 844.

Chase, H.P. and H.P. Martin, 1970. Undernutrition and child development. *New Eng. J. Med.* 282: 933.

Chase, H.P., et al., 1967. Effect of malnutrition on the synthesis of a myelin lipid. *Pediat.* 40: 551.

Chase, H.P., et al., 1971. Intra-uterine undernutrition and brain development. *Pediat.* 47: 491.

Committee on International Nutrition Programs, 1974. Relationship of nutrition to brain development and behavior. *Nutr. Today* 9, No. 4: 12.

Cravioto, J., et al., 1969. Mental performance of school children who suffered malnutrition in early age. In *Nutrition in Preschool and School Age.* Ed., G. Blix. p. 85. Swedish Nutrition Foundation. Uppsala.

Eichenwald, H.F. and P.C. Fry, 1969. Nutrition and learning. *Science* 163: 644.

Frisch, R.E., 1970. Present status of supposition that malnutrition causes permanent mental retardation. *Amer. J. Clin. Nutr.* 23: 189.

Gojulanathan, K. and K. Verghese, 1969. Socio-cultural malnutrition. *J. Trop. Pediat.* 15: 118.

Grifft, H.H., et al., 1972. *Nutrition, Behavior, and Change.* Prentice-Hall. Englewood Cliffs, N.J.

Gutelius, M.F., 1969. Problem of iron-deficiency anemia in preschool Negro children. *Amer. J. Pub. Health* 59: 290.

Hutcheson, H.A. and N.H. Wright, 1968. Georgia's family planning program. *Amer. J. Nurs.* 68: 332.

Johnston, P.V., 1974. Nutrition and neural development. *Food Nutr. News* 45, No. 3: 1.

Kallen, D.J., 1971. Nutrition and society. *J. Amer. Med. Assoc.* 215: 94.

Kaplan, B.J., 1973. Malnutrition and mental deficiency. In *Child Development and Behavior.* Ed., F. Rebelsky and L. Dorman. p. 99. Knopf. New York.

Martin, H.P., 1973. Nutrition: its relationship to children's physical, mental, and emotional development. *Amer. J. Clin. Nutr.* 26: 766.

Monckelberg, F., et al., 1972. Malnutrition and mental development. *Amer. J. Clin. Nutr.* 25: 766.

Naeye, R.L., et al., 1969. Urban poverty: effects on prenatal nutrition. *Science* 166: 1206.

Nutrition Foundation, 1973. Fetal malnutrition. *Nutr. Rev.* 31: 179.

Scrimshaw, N.S. and J.E. Gordon, 1968. *Malnutrition, Learning, and Behavior.* MIT Press. Boston.

Stein, Z.A. and H. Kassab, 1970. Nutrition. In *Mental Retardation.* Ed., J. Wortis. Vol. 2: 92. Grune and Stratton. New York.

Thomson, A.M., 1959. Diet in pregnancy. III. Diet in relation to the course and outcome of pregnancy. *Brit. J. Nutr.* 13: 509.

Werner, E., 1967. Cumulative effect of perinatal complications and deprived environment on physical, intellectual and social development of preschool children. *Pediat.* 39: 490.

Whitten, E.F., et al., 1969. Evidence that growth failure from maternal deprivation is secondary to undereating. *J. Amer. Med. Assoc.* 29: 1675.

Wiener, G., et al., 1965. Correlates of low birth weight: psychological status at 6–7 years of age. *Pediat.*, 35: 434.

Winick, M., 1972. *Nutrition and Development.* Wiley. New York.

Winick, M., et al., 1970. Cellular growth of cerebrum, cerebellum, and brain stem in normal and marasmic children. *Exper. Neurology*, 26: 393.

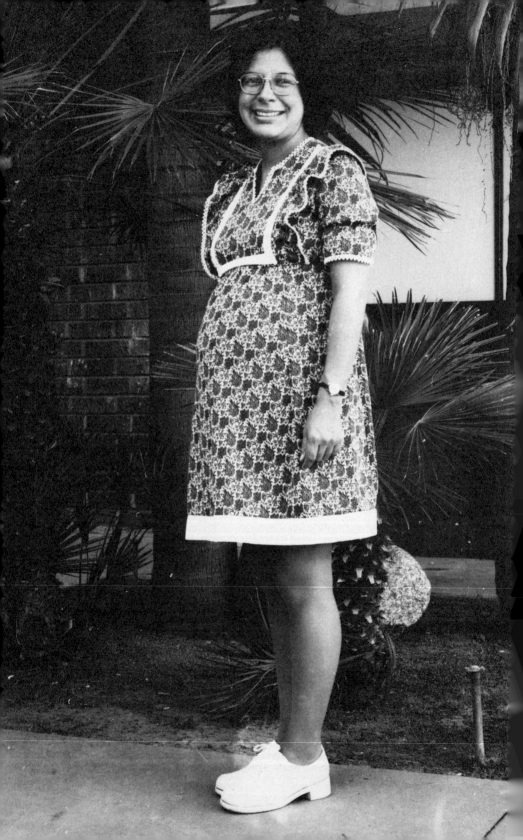

Chapter 4
Pregnancy and Lactation

Reproduction and the many ramifications of the quality of the product actually are influenced by several long term factors. Although nutrition and a range of social, psychological, and economic factors are of significance during the 40 weeks of gestation, the total picture must extend back in time. The physical condition of the woman who is to be pregnant will have an effect on the outcome of her pregnancy. This state of physical well being can be modified by appropriate dietary and activity modifications to enhance her physical condition, but not all facets can be modified after the reproductive age is reached.

PRE-CONCEPTION

Prognosis

A composite picture, based on world-wide data, could be sketched of the ideal physical situation for pregnancy. This picture of a woman who would have the best predictable chance for a successful outcome of pregnancy would be in her early twenties, more than five feet four inches tall, have a long oval pelvis, have had a successful prior pregnancy, live in an industrialized nation such as Sweden, be white, and of the professional or upper class.

The picture of the woman who might be predicted to have the best chances of a successful pregnancy is clearly not typical of the women who will be bearing children. In fact, one or more variations from this idealized pattern ordinarily will be found. Of course, even the woman with all of the above characteristics could have some other factor working against an optimum outcome, while many women with less than ideal circumstances will be successful in producing a healthy baby weighing more than 2500 grams. The figure of 2500 grams is generally the weight below which risks for the infant are found to be higher.

In 1971 Omran (Table 4.1) cited the consistent relationship of maternal age and stillbirth rate reflected in statistics from England and Wales. Revealed in these same statistics also was the reduced incidence of stillbirths among the upper social classes in comparison with the lower classes. These same data also indicate the higher stillbirth rate for firstborn and parities of four or more.

Birth weights of less than 2500 grams are considered to be a greater risk to the infant than if the birth weight exceeds this figure. Data of live birth weights in relation to the age and color of the mother are presented in Table 4.2. In the United States the data reveal a higher incidence of low birth weights before age 20, with the percentage being distinctly higher when the mother is less than 15 years old. There is a consistent difference between the data for whites and nonwhites, a difference which may be due to various social and economic factors. The data reported in Table 4.3 show similar patterns in relation to mortality of infants born to white and nonwhite mothers of various ages.

The above data support the need for good nutrition throughout life, for adequate quantities of nutrients are needed by girls throughout their growing years prior to the time that they mature and enter the reproductive period. During childhood the foundations for a healthy adult body are developed. Girls who have had inadequate dietary intakes during childhood, whether as a result of the various socioeconomic factors that limit food availability or because of poor dietary habits, will not achieve their optimum growth. Thomson (1959) noted that short mothers had a higher rate of prematurity and delivery complications at various income levels. These findings confirmed the report of Baird and Illsley (1953) that premature births occurred almost twice as frequently among women five feet one inch and under as among those who were at least five feet four inches tall.

The interrelationships of poor nutrition, suboptimal growth, increased risk of illness, impaired school performance, limited income, and greater risk in the outcome of pregnancy form a cycle that is very difficult to break. These

Table 4.1 Stillbirth, neonatal, and post-natal mortality rates in England and Wales, 1963 – 64 [a]

Mother's Parity	Social Class	Stillbirths/1000 Births			Neonatal Deaths[b]			Post-neonatal Deaths[b]		
		Under 25[c]	25-29	30 and Over	Under 25	25-29	30 and Over	Under 25	25-29	30 and Over
1	I, II[d]	10.5	12.3	18.0	9.6	9.4	12.6	3.9	2.6	2.4
	III	14.6	16.5	23.7	12.2	10.3	14.8	4.4	2.7	2.9
	IV, V	15.6	22.0	27.7	13.3	14.1	16.4	6.1	5.1	3.6
2, 3	I, II	8.6	8.8	12.6	8.8	7.3	8.8	4.3	3.9	2.9
	III	9.8	12.1	17.1	11.1	9.4	11.7	9.2	4.5	3.3
	IV, V	10.4	12.5	19.6	12.1	10.2	12.8	10.2	6.0	4.4
4 and Over	I, II	(5.1)	12.1	16.4	(12.8)	11.9	10.9	(10.3)	(4.7)	4.4
	III	11.4	17.3	25.9	16.5	14.5	15.0	17.3	10.2	6.2
	IV, V	13.2	20.5	28.1	16.3	15.6	15.8	15.4	12.5	8.1

[a]Adapted from Omran, A.R. 1971. *Health Theme in Family Planning.* Monograph No. 15, p. 19, 20, 23. Carolina Population Center. University of North Carolina. Chapel Hill, N.C. Data are from C.C. Spicer and L. Lipworth. 1966. "Regional and Social Factors in Infant Mortality," *Studies on Medical and Population Subjects,* No. 19, p. 13. Her Majesty's Stationery Office.

[b]Deaths are per 1000 live births.

[c]Mother's age in years.

[d]I represents the professional class; II, intermediate class; III, skilled; IV, partly skilled; and V, unskilled.

factors are all influential in the development of a baby. In truth, there is no clearly discernible starting point for discussing nutrition for pregnancy because the total picture starts far back in time.

Dietary Planning

Despite the complex factors that determine the outcome of a pregnancy, there is a great deal of work being done to help break the cycle and to promote optimum reproductive performance. Nutrition education programs and food distribution and production efforts are making inroads into the situation. However, successful reproduction is very much the personal concern and responsibility of the pregnant woman. Much is known today about the nutritional needs

Table 4.2   Percentage distribution of live births by birth weight under 2500 grams and by age of mother and color: United States, 1965 [a]

Age of Mother (years)	Birth Weight of 2500 Grams or Less (%)	Color	
		White (%)	Nonwhite (%)
Total	8.3	7.2	13.8
Under 15	18.7	13.0	21.3
15–19	10.5	8.5	16.4
20–24	7.9	6.9	13.3
25–29	7.3	6.5	12.2
30–34	7.9	7.0	12.8
35–39	8.9	8.0	13.4
40–44	9.0	8.3	12.5
45–49	8.7	8.5	9.8

[a]U.S. Department of Health, Education, and Welfare, Public Health Service. 1967. *Vital Statistics of the United States, 1965: Volume 1 – Natality.* U.S. Govt. Print. Office. Washington, D.C.

of pregnancy. This information can be applied effectively prior to and during gestation to aid in optimizing the pregnancy. Pregnancy evokes mixed feelings of excitement and satisfaction interspersed with some anxiety and concern, for this is the time when a woman is most intimately responsible for the well being of her offspring as well as for herself. Daily routines and habits assume new significance. Doctors quickly emphasize the importance of good nutrition during this period so that the daily food intake will meet the needs of both the mother and her unborn child with only moderate increases in caloric intake. Careful attention to diet throughout this period helps to provide the optimum circumstances for a successful pregnancy.

A discussion of nutrition for the pregnant woman actually should begin with a close look at the adequacy of her diet before conception. Ideally, body stores of nutrients such as calcium will be built up as she regularly consumes an adequate diet for several months, at least, before pregnancy is initiated. These reserves of the various nutrients are important assets in promoting and maintaining both optimum health of the expectant woman and normal development of the fetus. For women using contraceptive pills,

Table 4.3 Mortality of white and nonwhite infants by age of mother and age at death: United States, 1960 birth cohort [a]

Age of Mother (years)	Neonatal[b] (under 28 days)			Postneonatal[b] (28 days, 11 months)			Infant[b] (under 1 year)		
	Total	White	Non-white	Total	White	Non-white	Total	White	Non-white
Total	18.4	16.9	26.7	6.7	5.3	14.7	25.1	22.2	41.4
Under 15	41.2	32.1	46.5	17.6	15.5	18.8	58.7	47.5	65.3
15–19	22.7	20.4	30.9	10.1	7.7	18.6	32.8	28.1	49.5
20–24	17.3	15.9	25.3	6.9	5.5	14.8	24.2	21.4	40.2
25–29	16.6	15.3	24.2	5.8	4.6	13.1	22.4	20.0	37.3
30–34	18.3	17.0	26.4	5.3	4.2	12.0	23.7	21.2	38.4
35–39	19.7	18.4	27.3	5.8	4.5	13.9	25.5	22.9	41.2
40–44	23.1	22.0	29.4	7.5	6.1	15.4	30.6	28.1	44.7
45 and Over	31.3	31.8	28.9	9.8	7.1	21.6	41.1	38.9	50.5

[a]Source: U.S. Department of Health, Education, and Welfare, Public Health Service. 1967. *Vital Statistics of the United States, 1965: Volume 1 – Natality.* U.S. Govt. Print. Office, Wash., D.C.

[b]Rate per 1000 live births.

this means an increase in folacin and pyridoxine (and probably vitamin E) as well as eating a diet that supplies recommended levels of all nutrients.

Particular stress should be placed on proper dietary habits before pregnancy because studies have shown that adult women and teen-age girls in the United States frequently follow inadequate dietary patterns. It is a well-established fact that in the American population today teen-age girls compose the poorest-fed group; the young adult woman is only slightly better nourished than the teen-age female. Since the incidence of pregnancy during the teens is increasing, the nutritional problems of pregnancy are being imposed with increasing frequency upon the nutritional problems of the adolescent population. And since the teen-ager herself is still growing, she not only has the problem of meeting the nutritional needs of pregnancy, but also of meeting the needs for the growth of her body. Therefore it is imperative that good nutrition assume paramount importance so that both the pregnant teen-ager and her fetus may achieve the optimum levels of health and development.

The recommended daily dietary allowances, as revised in 1974 by the Food and Nutrition Board of the National Research Council, are given in Table 4.4.

Basic Four Food Plan. Wherever possible, the diet of the nonpregnant woman who is anticipating pregnancy should be given a careful check despite her age. The diet can well be evaluated on the basis of the Basic Four Food Plan, which is a simple food plan that any woman can use as a basis for planning meals for her entire family.

The Basic Four Food Plan is based on four food groups:
1. Milk and dairy products.
2. Meat and meat products.
3. Fruits and vegetables.
4. Bread and cereals.

In this plan the number of servings to be consumed in each group is specified to meet the nutritional needs of individuals of various ages.

The recommended number of servings in the milk and dairy products group is related to the age of the individual; for instance, two or more cups per day for the adult, four or more cups for teen-agers. The servings in this group may be glasses of milk; they may be milk used in cooking — for instance, milk used in cream soup or in custard; they also may be cheese or ice cream. The variety possible in this group is sufficient to provide appealing ways of consuming this group even for the person who does not regularly drink milk at each meal of the day. The value of the milk group should be stressed to the woman who is contemplating pregnancy, because the levels of calcium and phosphorus in milk provide important amounts of these minerals. An adequate intake of milk and milk products serves to increase the body stores of these minerals, should they be inadequate prior to pregnancy. In addition, milk and milk products are good sources of protein, which also should be stored in adequate quantities in the body before pregnancy.

Some people experience discomfort from drinking milk because of lactose intolerance. This condition is caused by a reduced level of lactase, the enzyme needed to digest lactose (the sugar in milk). Lactose intolerance occurs among some Blacks and Orientals. The consumption of small quantities of milk several times during the day may be a

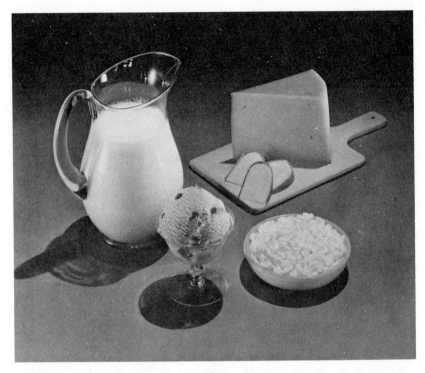

Milk, cheese, and ice cream are included as one group in the Basic Four Food Plan.

satisfactory solution to the problem. If milk cannot be consumed, a calcium supplement is recommended.

In the meat group two or more servings per day are recommended. The term "meat" in this group is used in a broad sense to include beef, veal, lamb, mutton, pork and porcine products such as bacon, as well as chicken, duck, turkey, and fish. Eggs are also suitable for inclusion in this category. These foods need to be included in the diet to provide the complete protein needed to build adequate stores of nitrogen in the body prior to pregnancy. Meats consumed in the recommended number of servings, in conjunction with the protein available from milk, will ensure adequate nitrogen storage for the woman anticipating pregnancy. All foods of animal origin, with the exception of gelatin, are classified as complete proteins; that is, they contain all of the amino acids needed by man for growth and development. Most protein foods from plants are incomplete proteins that lack one or more of the essential amino acids, but various vegetable proteins can be combined to provide all of the

Table 4.4   Food and Nutrition Board,
National Academy of Sciences – National Research Council
Recommended Daily Dietary Allowance, [a] Revised 1974

Designed for the maintenance of good nutrition of practically all healthy people in the U.S.A.

	Age	Weight		Height		Energy	Protein	Fat-Soluble Vitamins			
								Vita-min A Activity		Vita-min D	Vita-min E Activity[e]
	(years)	(kg)	(lbs)	(cm)	(in)	(kcal)[b]	(g)	(RE)[e]	(IU)	(IU)	(IU)
Infants	0.0–0.5	6	14	60	24	kg × 117	kg × 2.2	420[d]	1,400	400	4
	0.5–1.0	9	20	71	28	kg × 108	kg × 2.0	400	2,000	400	5
Children	1–3	13	28	86	34	1,300	23	400	2,000	400	7
	4–6	20	44	110	44	1,800	30	500	2,500	400	9
	7–10	30	66	135	54	2,400	36	700	3,300	400	10
Males	11–14	44	97	158	63	2,800	44	1,000	5,000	400	12
	15–18	61	134	172	69	3,000	54	1,000	5,000	400	15
	19–22	67	147	172	69	3,000	54	1,000	5,000	400	15
	23–50	70	154	172	69	2,700	56	1,000	5,000		15
	51+	70	154	172	69	2,400	56	1,000	5,000		15
Females	11–14	44	97	155	62	2,400	44	800	4,000	400	12
	15–18	54	119	162	65	2,100	48	800	4,000	400	12
	19–22	58	128	162	65	2,100	46	800	4,000	400	12
	23–50	58	128	162	65	2,000	46	800	4,000		12
	51+	58	128	162	65	1,800	46	800	4,000		12
Pregnant						+300	+30	1,000	5,000	400	15
Lactating						+500	+20	1,200	6,000	400	15

[a] The allowances are intended to provide for individual variations among most normal persons as they live in the United States under usual environmental stresses. Diets should be based on a variety of common foods in order to provide other nutrients for which human requirements have been less well defined. See text for more detailed discussion of allowances and of nutrients not tabulated. See Table I (p. 6) for weights and heights by individual year of age.
[b] Kilojoules (k J) = 4.2 × kcal.
[e] Retinol equivalents.
[d] Assumed to be all as retinol in milk during the first six months of life. All subsequent intakes are assumed to be half as retinol and half as β-carotene when calculated from international

Table 4.4 (Continued)

Water-Soluble Vitamins							Minerals					
Ascorbic acid (mg)	Folacin[f] (μg)	Niacin[g] (mg)	Riboflavin (mg)	Thiamin (mg)	Vitamin B$_6$ (mg)	Vitamin B$_{12}$ (μg)	Calcium (mg)	Phosphorus (mg)	Iodine (μg)	Iron (mg)	Magnesium (mg)	Zinc (mg)
	50	5	0.4	0.3	0.3	0.3	360	240	35	10	60	3
	50	8	0.6	0.5	0.4	0.3	540	400	45	15	70	5
	100	9	0.8	0.7	0.6	1.0	800	800	60	15	150	10
	200	12	1.1	0.9	0.9	1.5	800	800	80	10	200	10
	300	16	1.2	1.2	1.2	2.0	800	800	110	10	250	10
	400	18	1.5	1.4	1.6	3.0	1,200	1,200	130	18	350	15
	400	20	1.8	1.5	2.0	3.0	1,200	1,200	150	18	400	15
	400	20	1.8	1.5	2.0	3.0	800	800	140	10	350	15
	400	18	1.6	1.4	2.0	3.0	800	800	130	10	350	15
	400	16	1.5	1.2	2.0	3.0	800	800	110	10	350	15
	400	16	1.3	1.2	1.6	3.0	1,200	1,200	115	18	300	15
	400	14	1.4	1.1	2.0	3.0	1,200	1,200	115	18	300	15
	400	14	1.4	1.1	2.0	3.0	800	800	100	18	300	15
	400	13	1.2	1.0	2.0	3.0	800	800	100	18	300	15
	400	12	1.1	1.0	2.0	3.0	800	800	80	10	300	15
	800	+2	+0.3	+0.3	2.5	4.0	1,200	1,200	125	18+[h]	450	20
	600	+4	+0.5	+0.3	2.5	4.0	1,200	1,200	150	18	450	25

units. As retinol equivalents, three fourths are as retinol and one fourth as β-carotene.

[e] Total vitamin E activity, estimated to be 80 percent as α-tocopherol and 20 percent other tocopherols. See text for variation in allowances.

[f] The folacin allowances refer to dietary sources as determined by *Lactobacillus casei* assay. Pure forms of folacin may be effective in doses less than one fourth of the recommended dietary allowance.

[g] Although allowances are expressed as niacin, it is recognized that on the average 1 mg of niacin is derived from each 60 mg of dietary tryptophan.

[h] This increased requirement cannot be met by ordinary diets; therefore, the use of supplemental iron is recommended.

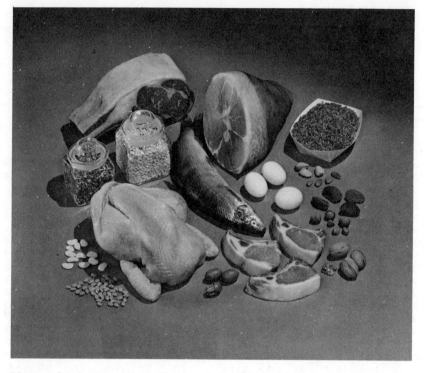

Plant and animal protein foods comprise a group in the Basic Four Food Plan.

essential amino acids. It is difficult, however, to ensure that all essential amino acids are being supplied when vegetable proteins are used exclusively. On this basis it is wise to be sure to include animal protein foods, too. Food costs may be eased by using animal and vegetable proteins in combinations, such as cereals with milk or refried beans with cheese.

The Basic Four Food Plan includes a total of four or more servings in the fruit and vegetable group. Within this group, one serving each day should be a citrus fruit or some other fruit high in ascorbic acid. A suitable substitute for citrus fruit in the diet is fresh strawberries. A second requirement in this group is that a serving of a dark green, leafy or a yellow vegetable should be consumed at least every other day. This requirement provides vitamin A in amounts adequate to permit normal functioning of the visual cycle in the eye and to promote healthy skin. The remainder of the four servings, above and beyond the serving of citrus fruit and green or yellow vegetables, can be met by any of the fruits and vegetables that might be used in the menus each day.

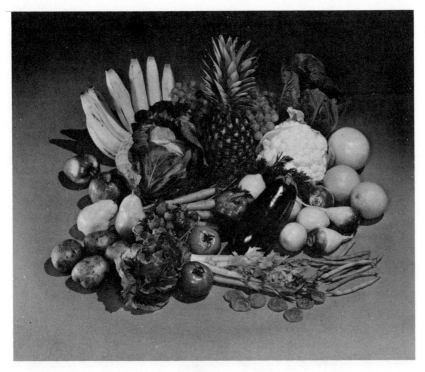

Special attention is given to citrus fruits and dark green, leafy or yellow vegetables in the fruit and vegetable group of the Basic Four Food Plan.

Fruits and vegetables are valuable sources of minerals in the diet and also contribute varying amounts of vitamins needed by humans.

The last group, the bread and cereal group, is of value because of its content of the necessary B vitamins. The recommendation is four or more servings of whole-grain or enriched breads and cereal products daily. Enriched cereals, flours, and related products will be labeled to indicate the nutrients that have been added.

Fats are not mentioned in the Basic Four Food Plan because it is assumed that butter or margarine will be consumed along with the breads and/or cereals in a meal. Since the average American consumes almost two times as much fat as he apparently needs for optimum nutrition, it seems unnecessary to add to the complexity of the food plan by adding a fifth group to spell out the need for fat.

Many people will not feel satisfied if they consume only the recommended numbers of servings in the four categories.

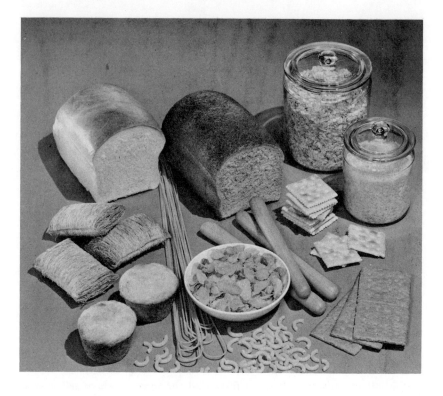

Whole grain or enriched breads and cereals are grouped together in the Basic Four Food Plan.

Actually this food plan is intended only as an outline of a food pattern that will provide adequate amounts of the vitamins, minerals, and protein needed by healthy persons. It is assumed that each individual will eat any additional servings of food necessary to provide adequate calories and a feeling of satisfaction throughout the day.

When planning a total diet for the day, it is not difficult to meet these various recommendations of the Basic Four Food Plan if the menus are varied and the food is consumed in reasonable quantities. Problems in meeting basic dietary needs often result from lack of knowledge of nutrition, carelessness in menu planning, limited acceptance of a wide variety of foods, or misconceptions about the value of foods with resulting emphasis on the narrow range of foods. The latter situation occurs in the diet of some food faddists. If attention is given to wise planning that includes adequate

amounts of the aforementioned food groups and if preparation and service of the food are done well, the average individual will not find it difficult to consume an adequate
diet. Adherence to this food plan for several months should
ensure that the normal woman will have adequate stores of
the various nutrients within her body before pregnancy.

Weight control. One additional nutritional problem should
be considered before discussing the diet of the pregnant
woman. For a more comfortable pregnancy with less likelihood of complications, it is advisable for a woman to attain
a weight within the normal range recommended for her
height before conception occurs (Table 4.5). In some instances this may mean that she will need to gain weight
before pregnancy. If so, this weight gain should be accomplished by following the Basic Four Food Pattern to ensure
not only that the necessary weight is gained, but also that
the body stores of the various nutrients are built up during
this period.

Perhaps the more common problem for the adolescent
as well as for the adult woman in the United States is that

Table 4.5   Desirable body weights for adult women prior to pregnancy

Height (without shoes)	Weight (without clothing – pounds)		
	Low	Average	High
5 feet	100	109	118
5 feet 1 inch	104	112	121
5 feet 2 inches	107	115	125
5 feet 3 inches	110	118	128
5 feet 4 inches	113	122	132
5 feet 5 inches	116	125	135
5 feet 6 inches	120	129	139
5 feet 7 inches	123	132	142
5 feet 8 inches	126	136	146
5 feet 9 inches	130	140	151
5 feet 10 inches	133	144	156
5 feet 11 inches	137	148	161
6 feet	141	152	166

[a]Adapted from Food and Your Weight. Home and Garden Bulletin No. 74. U.S.D.A.
Washington, D.C. 1973.

of overweight rather than underweight. It is important to be at an appropriate weight before starting a pregnancy in order to reduce the strain that pregnancy places on a woman.

When considerable weight reduction appears to be appropriate and desirable, it is wise to lose this weight under the guidance of a dietitian and physician. This team is able to provide the patient with (1) an appropriate diet for weight reduction, (2) medical supervision during the course of the dieting period, and (3) a feeling that someone else is interested in the outcome of the diet program. This latter contribution can be an extremely helpful psychological factor that will assist the patient in maintaining the discipline necessary for successful weight reduction.

Any reducing regimen should include the essential nutrients to ensure that a person will lose weight without depleting the body's stores of these nutrients, but this criterion becomes still more significant if the weight reduction takes place in preparation for pregnancy. The achievement of an appropriate weight before and during gestation not only will be an important morale booster to the pregnant woman, but also will make her pregnancy more comfortable.

Changing food habits. The period before and during pregnancy can be a very helpful period not only for building up the body's stores of nutrients, but also for retraining the dietary patterns of both the wife and husband. Because good dietary patterns in the home facilitate the development of good dietary patterns in the children during their formative years, it is valuable to the health and well-being of a family to have the parents apply good nutrition in their daily lives as well as in the lives of their children.

This period of nutritional concern prior to pregnancy can be viewed as a training period for both husband and wife if their dietary habits are less than adequate. Ideally the dietary pattern that emerges will be well balanced and appropriate for maintaining a desirable weight. The family will develop the pattern of eating not only lunch and dinner, but also breakfast. The acceptance and appreciation of a wide range of foods will be encouraged, and a general awareness of the importance of nutrition will develop during this period. This knowledge of good nutrition principles and their practical application will certainly be of benefit to the woman during both gestation and lactation, and, indeed, throughout her career as a wife and mother responsible for nourishing meals for her family.

It should also be mentioned that the foregoing discussion applies to any woman, whether she is contemplating her first or her tenth pregnancy. Certainly it is wise for her to replenish her body stores of nutrients after delivery before undergoing the stress of a subsequent pregnancy. Family planning, combined with adequate nutrition, can provide the time necessary for recuperation and replenishment. During this recuperative period the diet should be consciously controlled to ensure that all body stores have been replenished and that weight control is achieved before starting the next pregnancy.

NUTRITION DURING PREGNANCY

Early Adjustments

Nutrition assumes a role of added significance during pregnancy, for it is the mother's responsibility to consume a well-balanced diet of appropriate proportions to provide the nutrients necessary for the optimum development of her unborn child and for her own needs as well. She can best meet the challenge if she is given adequate information about the special nutritional demands of pregnancy and is shown practical ways of incorporating the recommendations into her daily dietary pattern. Physicians, dietitians, and nutritionists can be a very real help in assisting the pregnant woman to make the necessary adjustments.

One of the important nutrition concepts that should be pointed out to the pregnant woman is that the caloric needs are not greatly increased during pregnancy (Table 4.4). The National Research Council recommends an increase of 300 kilocalories per day for pregnant women to allow for the increasing growth and development of the fetus. The activity level of pregnant women, particularly in the latter part of pregnancy is generally low; however, the sedentary nature of many women's lives makes caloric needs for activities not a great deal different during pregnancy than it is during the nonpregnant state. Blackburn and Calloway (1974) estimated the caloric need of pregnant adolescents ages 14–19 to be 2400 kcal. These workers determined that their subjects were lying down or sitting 40 percent of the time.

Despite that fact that nutritional needs are not increased greatly during the first trimester, it is imperative that the recommended intakes be achieved daily to ensure that the body has the necessary nutrients available for the developing embryo during this critical period. It is apparent from an examination of Table 2.1 that important stages of cell differentiation are occurring during this three-month period. The dietary recommendations for this first three months of pregnancy can be met simply by following the Basic Four Food Plan, with an increase to a quart of milk daily (often in the form of skim milk) and larger servings of meat.

Academically this sounds so simple that there should not be any particular nutritional problem during the first three months of pregnancy. In actual practice, however, the achievement of the recommended intake and the utilization of food each day may be something less than optimum, depending on the condition of the woman. In some instances nausea can be an annoying, rather persistent problem that does influence the amount of food consumed and absorbed during the day. Nausea decreases the appetite of some women and also may interfere with the absorption of the nutrients provided by foods that are eaten. In such cases malnutrition may exist during this period even though the woman is conscientiously attempting to consume the recommended foods.

Today physicians can prescribe medications that help to combat the problem of nausea experienced by some women during the early stages of pregnancy. With such aids, achievement of adequate nutrition may cease to be a serious problem. Suggestions have also been made regarding diet plans to help minimize nausea. Perhaps the most practical of these suggestions is that of eating a couple of soda crackers before getting out of bed in the morning and then resting briefly after eating the crackers. This simple device is reasonably effective for the woman with mild problems. If nausea is a continuing problem in the early part of pregnancy, it certainly should be discussed with the physician so that the nausea can be relieved by use of the current medications designed for this purpose.

If nausea persists, nutrition can and should be bolstered through the use of a vitamin and mineral supplement to ensure that the woman is getting adequate amounts of the necessary nutrients during this period. These capsules, containing the appropriate levels of vitamins and such minerals as calcium, phosphorus, and iron, should be taken at a time during the day when nausea is not likely to be a problem. In this way the diet usually can be supplemented to avoid serious depletion of the maternal stores of these nutrients. Fortunately, during the second and third trimesters of pregnancy when the nutritional needs are somewhat higher, nausea usually ceases to be a problem, and therefore utilization of the nutrients is improved.

Weight Control During Pregnancy

The National Research Council's recommendation that caloric intake during pregnancy should be increased approximately 300 kilocalories for the average woman is intended merely as a guideline. A record of the actual weight gain will be kept by the physician, and his recommendations on caloric intake, based on the woman's needs, should be followed carefully. Weight gain should be monitored continuously by the pregnant woman.

Weight control may be a problem for some women who have worked outside the home before pregnancy and who have quit their jobs to remain home during the period of pregnancy. The transition from the business world to the environment at home may be difficult for some women, and they may find the constant availability of food to be a great temptation. To fight the tendency toward excessive weight gain in such situations, it is advisable for the pregnant woman to develop some new interests. She will thus occupy her mind with other thoughts and will be less inclined to snack during the day. In other cases it may be necessary for the physician or dietitian to assist the mother in developing a different dietary pattern.

The increased need for vitamins, minerals, and protein is out of proportion to the very small increase in energy requirements during gestation. To be adequately nourished during pregnancy, it is necessary to eat a diet that provides an optimum amount of nutrition with a minimum number of calories. In other words, rich foods and desserts should be eliminated from the diets of many women during pregnancy to prevent excessive weight gain. However, the daily caloric intake usually should not drop below 36 kilocalories per kilogram of body weight during pregnancy.

Excessive weight is a potential hazard for the unborn infant as well as for the mother. It has been shown that the likelihood of a stillborn child is increased appreciably when the mother is overweight during the period of pregnancy (Emerson, 1962). Toxemia also is more common among overweight pregnant women than among those of normal weight. This is a condition in which excessive amounts of water or fluid accumulate in the tissues (known as edema), accompanied by hypertension and perhaps albumin in the urine. If not checked, toxemia may result in convulsions.

Physiological Changes. Weight gain throughout the entire pregnancy generally should amount to a total of approximately 24 pounds for the woman who was within the recommended weight range prior to pregnancy. Pregnancy is not a period when tightly restricted diets are to be recommended because important mineral and vitamin intakes also will be restricted when caloric intake is too low. To accomplish this total weight gain for an optimum pregnancy, Jacobson (1972) recommends a steady gain, ranging from 0.5 to 0.8 pounds weekly, totaling 20 to 24 pounds for the entire 40 weeks. However, data by Hytten and Leitch (1964) suggest a gain of almost two pounds total by ten weeks, rising to a little less than one pound weekly in the last 20 weeks.

The weight gain of pregnancy is the result of numerous physiological changes in the mother as well as the development of the fetus. Maternal modifications involve the blood, respiratory system, metabolic, mammary, cardiac, and alimentary systems. Striking changes occur in blood volume and composition. The volume of plasma is constant until approximately the twelfth week, when the volume begins to increase to more than a liter above nonpregnant levels by the thirty-fourth week. A small drop in volume will occur during the remainder of the pregnancy.

Red cell volume increases, too, but at a rate distinctly less than plasma level, thus resulting in a reduced concentration of red cells and hemoglobin. This situation is termed the physiological anemia of pregnancy. There is still some debate about the significance of the usual drop in hemoglobin values to between 11 and 12 grams per 100 milliliters late in pregnancy (compared with average values of 13.5g/ 100 ml or more for nonpregnant women).

During the first half of pregnancy, there is an increase of one and a half liters in the cardiac output compared with the almost five liter output typical of the nonpregnant state. The heart rate is increased and the stroke volume is larger during pregnancy. Arterial blood pressure is essentially the same as it is in the nonpregnant woman. Venous blood pressure in the upper part of the body ordinarily will remain at normal levels during pregnancy, but high venous pressure may develop in the legs. This increased pressure in the legs contributes to the edema often observed in normal pregnancies. Yet another change of pregnancy is the enlargement and upward, forward shifting of the heart. The increased blood flow is focused in the placental region, although there is also an appreciable increase in the flow to the skin and kidney.

The respiratory rate does not change significantly during pregnancy, but the consumption of oxygen is increased at least 15 percent. This increased need is met by increased tidal volume, with the lung collapsing more than usual at the end of the breathing cycle.

The renal tract dilates by the tenth week of pregnancy and becomes more dilated on the right side than on the left during the latter stage of pregnancy. This dilation results in a larger urinary capacity and increases the tendency to develop infections in this region. Urine composition changes somewhat during pregnancy, too. Amino acids, iodide, sugar, and folacin are notably high in the urine of pregnant women. The loss of iodide may promote enlargement of the thyroid gland during pregnancy. Megaloblastic anemia may be the consequence of folacin loss. Urinary volume sometimes is very high during early pregnancy, a phenomenon that coincides with the unusual thirst that some women experience during this period.

Alimentary tract changes may include increased salivation in early pregnancy, a tendency toward heartburn because of relaxation of the cardiac sphincter, and reduced stomach acidity. The intestine relaxes a little during pregnancy, causing some tendency toward constipation. The gall bladder also may empty more slowly, with the result that bile becomes more concentrated.

Water retention in pregnancy is a matter of wide variation, although edema is noted in almost half of the women who are pregnant. In some instances, the edema will focus on the lower limbs, while in other cases it will be more generally distributed.

The components of weight gain during pregnancy have been studied throughout the reproductive cycle. The figure illustrates the components that constitute weight gain at various stages of a normal pregnancy. Most of the actual weight gain occurs during the last half of pregnancy; despite the significance of the changes of the first half, the total amount of matter involved is far less than in the latter half. In the middle of pregnancy, maternal stores of fat are deposited on the back, abdomen, and upper thighs. The average weight gained at term is constituted approximately by a fetal weight of 3.3 kilograms, 650 grams due to the placenta, 800 grams of amniotic fluid, for a total of almost 5 kilograms that will be lost at delivery. In addition, the uterus will have gained approximately 900 grams, mammary glands will weigh an additional 400 grams, and the increased volume of blood will weigh about 1250 grams. Additional weight gain represents retained water and fatty deposits.

Motivation for Weight Control. Control of weight within the guidelines outlined here is sufficient to assure optimal

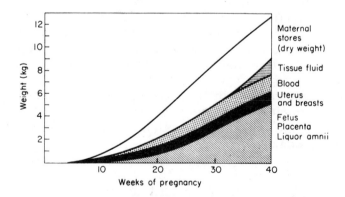

Components of weight gain in normal pregnancy. Reproduced by permission of the Committee on Maternal Nutrition, Food and Nutrition Board, National Research Council. In Maternal Nutrition and the Course of Pregnancy. *National Academy of Sciences. Washington, D.C. 1970. p.63.*

opportunity for development of a fetus of normal birth weight. Weight gain beyond this level will be excess stores of maternal fat, a change that may be very disheartening to new mothers.

The psychological lift that the new mother gets from being able to wear her regular street clothes after several months in maternity clothes should not be overlooked by the woman or her doctor during pregnancy. This goal, particularly in the latter stages of pregnancy, can provide considerable incentive for the expectant woman to control her food intake. Certainly it is hard on a woman's morale to find that her prepregnancy wardrobe is too tight on her after delivery. The motivation to quickly regain her former more shapely silhouette is sufficient to help many a woman curb what might otherwise be impulsive and excessive intakes of food.

This discussion has emphasized the problem of gaining too much weight, but in some instances inadequate weight gains are experienced. This situation is also undesirable because a distinctly underweight woman tends to produce a smaller baby, is more likely to have a premature baby, and is also somewhat less likely to be able to breast feed her infant satisfactorily (Bagchi and Bose, 1962).

Rationale for Dietary Recommendations

The nutritional needs of the pregnant woman, aside from the caloric needs previously considered, can be outlined by noting the contributions that the various food groups make toward meeting the nutritional needs of the pregnant woman.

Calcium and Phosphorus. Milk and milk products are valued during pregnancy because of their calcium and phosphorus content as well as their protein. These minerals are very important for the skeletal development of the fetus. In addition, they may be used to build the woman's stores of calcium so that she will be well prepared to nurse her baby. The need for calcium for the growth of the fetus is very limited at first, but it gradually increases during the first half of pregnancy. During the last three months the fetus requires an ever-increasing amount of calcium and, in order for the mother to supply this need, it is important not only that she has an excellent daily diet, but also that she has adequate stores of calcium in her own body to meet the demands of the fetus and of her body. The best way to ensure that adequate calcium will be available during this peak demand period is to form the habit of drinking a quart of milk a day during pregnancy. The addition of 2 extra glasses of whole milk to her regular diet represents the entire 300 kilocalories that are recommended to be added in pregnancy. If a woman needs to reduce her caloric intake, she can drink skim milk instead of whole milk. The reduction in calories is significant, but the calcium, phosphorus, B vitamins, and protein contents are not reduced when fat is removed.

Four 8-ounce glasses of milk (one quart) or their equivalent in other dairy products will supply the amounts of calcium and phosphorus (1200 mg each) that appear to be necessary during pregnancy. This intake in the early months supplies sufficient calcium and phosphorus to build up stores of these minerals in the pregnant woman and meet the needs of the developing embyro. Then, as pregnancy proceeds, the progressively greater needs of the fetus can be met with this intake without placing a stress on the calcium levels of the mother.

It is not necessary to consume all four servings of milk simply as glasses of milk. Sometimes other dairy products can be eaten to help meet this need. For example, one ounce of cheddar, Swiss, process, or other type of cheese is equivalent to approximately one-half glass of milk; one-half cup of cottage cheese may be substituted for one-half glass of milk; one cup of ice cream is comparable to one glass of milk. Many women might also prefer to prepare a part of the recommended intake of milk as baked custard, cornstarch pudding, or as milk drinks such as malted milks and eggnogs. Of course, the caloric content of these various alternatives cannot be ignored.

Protein. The need for protein for the growth of the fetus becomes particularly significant during the last six months of pregnancy. To meet this demand, the pregnant woman needs approximately 20 grams more protein daily than her husband. This, of course, is contrary to the usual consumption pattern in a family. It is extremely important, however, that a pregnant woman eat an adequate amount of animal or mixed vegetable protein to provide the protein needed by the fetus for tissue growth. The pregnant woman also needs protein for tissue growth that occurs in her own body during pregnancy. To be sure that this need is being met each day, it is wise for her to eat at least two 3-ounce servings of meat and an egg daily. The protein from these foods, combined with the protein available in milk, will meet her recommended allowance for protein during the last six months of pregnancy. Many women may wish to eat an additional egg or increase the size of the servings of meat slightly.

In planning the day's menu it is wise to have some protein served at each meal because the body can use this nutrient better when it is available frequently than it can if most of the protein is eaten in one meal. This suggestion can be implemented by serving an egg and a glass of milk for dinner, and a glass of milk before bedtime. This is only one means of offering protein at various intervals during the day. Other patterns may be more acceptable to certain women, but it is important to remember that:

1. Total protein intake should be increased approximately two-thirds above normal.
2. The protein foods should be consumed at intervals throughout the day rather than at one meal.

Some vegetable protein foods may be relied upon to furnish part of the day's protein need, but during pregnancy it is particularly useful to include animal foods generously in the diet. Vegetable products that may be used to provide some protein include baked navy beans, kidney beans, split peas, lentils, and other legumes. The wide range of textured soy products has done much to extend the potential for adequate protein from plant sources.

Iron. The need for iron is also increased in the pregnant woman to meet her own requirements and those of the developing fetus. Adequate iron stores in a woman's body when she becomes pregnant will be useful in meeting the increased need for iron during this period, but she will need to increase her consumption of iron. A woman with poor stores of iron prior to pregnancy will find it still more difficult to meet her needs and the needs of her fetus. The cases of iron-deficiency anemia in pregnant women are proof of the need for careful attention to meet the iron requirement during this period.

Liver is a particularly outstanding food to use in meeting the iron requirement, but other foods also make valuable contributions. Meats of all types, although not as high in iron as liver, are still excellent sources of the mineral. The yolk of eggs, whole-grain or enriched breads and cereal products, green and leafy vegetables such as spinach, and dried fruits are all appropriate foods to help provide iron in the diet in reasonable amounts. If the diet is very carefully selected, it is possible to meet the high need for iron during pregnancy without iron supplementation. However many women do not eat a diet containing the recommended level of more than 18 mg of iron daily. Therefore, a dietary supplement of ferrous sulfate often is needed during pregnancy.

Iodide. Iodide is important as a nutrient for the developing fetus as well as for the mother. Care should be taken to use iodized salt during pregnancy to ensure an adequate supply of this mineral. When iodide intake has been severely restricted during pregnancy, cretinism or severe mental retardation has occurred in the newborn. Other minerals needed in larger amounts during pregnancy include zinc and magnesium.

Vitamins. Vitamin needs are also greater during pregnancy. Vitamins A, E, thiamin, riboflavin, niacin, folacin, vitamin B_6, vitamin B_{12} and ascorbic acid all need to be included in the diet in larger amounts than they did prior to conception. In addition, vitamin D, which is not required for the adult woman, is once again considered to be essential in the diet. The increased need for vitamin D is doubtless the result of the need for bone-building materials for the fetus; the presence of vitamin D is essential for optimum absorption and utilization of calcium and phosphorus.

Ascorbic acid is necessary for collagen formation, that is, for the development of connective tissue in the body. Such tissue formation certainly must take place in the development of the fetus. In addition, ascorbic acid may have some influence on the utilization of calcium and phosphorus. The increased need for the B vitamins (thiamin, riboflavin, and niacin) is related to the developmental needs of the fetus, but is also necessitated by the slight increase in the amount of food that must be metabolized by the body. The increased need for folacin and vitamin B_{12} is to reduce the likelihood of developing megaloblastic anemia. Vitamin B_6 is needed for the tissue development associated with pregnancy. Vitamin A needs are increased during pregnancy to facilitate healthy development of skin and proper functioning of eyes.

By following these recommendations, a satisfactory intake of the main nutrients will be accomplished through normal dietary practices. Since the nutritional requirements are rather high in pregnancy and since absorption is likely to be somewhat hampered during the first trimester due to possible nausea, it is often the practice to supplement the food intake of a pregnant woman by the use of vitamin and mineral capsules. This practice, in general, appears to be perfectly appropriate and may be viewed as an insurance program to enable the mother to provide the necessary building materials for the fetus and for herself. It should be emphasized, however, that such supplements do not provide protein, which is an extremely important building material in the body; therefore the woman taking supplemental vitamin and mineral preparations should not be lulled into the feeling of security that she is consuming all the nutrients she needs simply by taking pills. Emphasis still needs to be given to consuming adequate amounts of protein through dietary sources.

Vitamin excesses. Excess amounts of most of the vitamins and minerals apparently are not a problem in humans. Excessive amounts of vitamins A and D, however, can present a hazard. Evidence is not extensive to date on this matter, but there is a distinct possibility than an excessive intake of vitamin D during pregnancy can cause mental retardation and possible physical deformities, including heart abnormalities, in the newborn. Therefore, intakes in excess of the 400 International Units of vitamin D recommended daily should be avoided. This amount of vitamin D is contained in a quart of irradiated milk and really should not be supplemented through the use of a pill containing the vitamin. Preferably, a vitamin supplement for the woman who is drinking a quart of irradiated milk daily should not include any vitamin D. Such capsules are difficult to find. Therapeutic (massive) doses of this vitamin ordinarily should be avoided.

The other vitamin that may possibly be toxic in excessively large doses is vitamin A. There is less evidence of definite harm to the fetus resulting from vitamin A intakes at very high levels, but again there appears to be no advantage in having unusually high levels of vitamin A. The recommended amount of vitamin A is 1000 retinol equivalents or 5000 International Units daily. Small supplements of vitamin A in a vitamin capsule apparently present no problem although levels above 2000 retinol units from supplements should be avoided. Unusually high levels, such as 20,000 to 25,000 I.U., are totally unnecessary and may be dangerous.

Common Misunderstandings

Some misconceptions and myths surround the dietary needs of the pregnant woman. One of the most common sayings is that the pregnant woman is eating for two. From the previous discussion it should be apparent that this statement cannot be taken literally, but rather it may be generalized that the total food intake for the pregnant woman should not exceed greatly the intake prior to pregnancy. The increased fetal need for calories for growth (especially in the last three months) is partially counterbalanced by some reduction of physical activity by the mother during the last trimester. This limited increase in the total need for calories requires that the diet be high in nutritive value in relation to the caloric content. Empty calories (foods high in calories, but low in vitamins, minerals, and protein) are luxuries that few women can afford weightwise during pregnancy.

Another misconception often expressed is that a pregnant woman's desire for a particular food indicates that she is lacking in some nutrient offered in the desired food. One of the foods sometimes mentioned in this regard is pickles. Pickles, of course, provide a pleasing contrast in texture and flavor in a meal, but they do not offer any unique substance in the food that cannot be gained by eating a variety of other foodstuffs. Other women may suddenly have a strong desire for fruits that are out of season or some other exotic and expensive food. Certainly it is fun to be humored and indulged in this manner, but it is unnecessary from a nutritional basis. Other seasonal and less expensive foods can well be substituted to meet the body's nutritional needs. The emphasis on food patterns for the pregnant woman should center on selection of a wide variety of foods in the proper amounts rather than on erratic consumption patterns that rely heavily on one particular type of food. Pregnancy is a particularly poor time in life to pursue food fads.

Some women pursue the practice of eating either clay or starch during pregnancy. Edwards et al. (1964) explored the motivation for pursuing this practice. Reasons for the practice varied from superstition that clay was needed if the baby was to be normal to indications that eating clay or starch was relaxing, pleasurable, and stimulating to the appetite. Assessment of infants born to clay or cornstarch-consumers versus those in the control group who did not consume these items indicated no difference in general size and weight, but the newborns of clay and cornstarch eaters were judged to be in poorer shape than those from the control group of mothers.

The high incidence of edema in pregnancy has led to the elimination or drastic reduction of salt in the diets of many women simply as a routine modification. This change may be needed in some instances, but the sodium, chloride, and iodide available in iodized salt generally are needed and should be eliminated only upon the recommendation of a physician.

Another fallacy often heard is that mothers will suffer during pregnancy if nutrients are not available for the fetus. The saying that a mother must lose one tooth for each child again reflects the idea that the fetus will develop normally at the expense of the mother's body. Actually, evidence indicates that both the mother and the fetus will suffer from inadequacies in the nutrients necessary for mother and fetus. The emphasis for nutrition during pregnancy, then, needs to be on ensuring an adequate intake to meet both the mother's needs and the needs of the developing fetus rather than depleting the body supplies of both individuals during the pregnancy period.

DIET FOR LACTATION

The period of lactation is often a time of great gustatory pleasure for the woman who has had to carefully control her caloric intake during pregnancy. This is the time when the food intake should be increased and certain degrees of latitude in the dessert department can be permitted.

Nutrition for the lactating mother is an important subject because the nutritional requirements are particularly high during this period. For example, the caloric intake of the lactating woman needs to be increased approximately 500 calories above the allowance recommended prior to conception. The nutrients that require emphasis (beyond the needs of pregnancy) during the period of lactation, in addition to the need for calories, are vitamin A, riboflavin, niacin, ascorbic acid, iodine, and zinc.

Recommended intake of folacin decreases, but is still well above the pre-gestation level. The recommended level of protein drops slightly from that for pregnancy, but still is much greater than before gestation. Iron intake once again returns to the level recommended for women in the reproductive years, that is 18 mg daily. Recommendations during lactation remain the same as in pregnancy for the following nutrients: vitamin D, vitamin E, thiamin, vitamin B₆, vitamin B₁₂, calcium, phosphorus, and magnesium.

The need for vitamin D is met by drinking a quart of milk daily. This amount of milk and dairy products is necessary to meet the calcium and phosphorus requirements as well as to supply protein for the lactating woman. The milk being secreted by the lactating woman represents much of the increased calcium need.

Emphasis not only should be given to the consumption of an adequate quantity of milk, but also should be directed toward providing enough protein. During lactation the need for protein is much greater than is the need for protein in the adult man. It is perhaps shocking or amazing to a husband to find that his meat needs take second place in priority to his lactating wife's need for protein; his needs will be approximately 56 grams of protein if he weighs 154 pounds, whereas his lactating wife (if she weighs 128 pounds) will need 66 grams of protein daily. A significant portion of the protein requirement can be met through the intake of milk. The remainder of the protein should be met by having a minimum of two large servings of meat per day to complement the protein in the milk.

Care should be taken to include an adequate amount of iron in the diet in order to help replenish the iron stores in the mother which may have been depleted during pregnancy and delivery. The iron that is absorbed during lactation will be used to rebuild the mother's stores of iron; even when the lactating woman has an adequate amount of iron in her diet, her milk will not contain a suitable amount of iron for the infant. However, some iron will be secreted in her milk if she is well fed.

The other needs for the lactating woman can be met by being certain that the recommended servings of the fruits and vegetables and of the bread and cereal group are being supplied in the diet. In order to meet the caloric needs for lactation, more than the recommended minimum numbers of servings in these two groups may be consumed.

The need for liquid in the diet of the lactating woman has been open to considerable discussion. The idea has often been expressed that lactation will be more successful if the woman has a large intake of fluids each day. It appears that the actual total amount of fluid intake each day is not significant in determining the amount of milk produced by the mother. The amount of milk consumed by the lactating woman, however, does appear to influence the amount of milk produced, and it is for this reason that milk is so important in the diet of the lactating mother.

The foods consumed by the mother who is nursing her child will influence to a limited extent the character of the milk she produces. For this reason it is often wise to limit the intake of strong-flavored or spicy foods during lactation to avoid the inclusion of materials in the milk secretion which might cause gastrointestinal distress in the infant.

SUMMARY

Consideration of nutritional needs during pregnancy actually should begin far in advance of conception, for nutritional adequacy throughout the growing years of the mother will influence the outcome of the pregnancy. When possible, a woman's diet ought to be evaluated for its adequacy prior to pregnancy and modified accordingly. Weight should be brought within the recommended range, also.

During pregnancy, the total weight gain recommended is approximately 24 pounds. This gain represents the summation of the mother's physical changes as well as those associated with fetal development. Since the increased need for nutrients must be provided by foods which increase caloric intake by only 300 kilocalories daily, a pregnant woman may need to drink skim milk (rather than whole milk), reduce her intake of fried foods and desserts, and increase the use of fruits and vegetables. If she has been eating limited amounts of protein-containing foods, she will need to increase serving sizes to provide the protein levels required for reproduction. An iron supplement probably will be needed, but large supplements of vitamins A and D should be avoided.

Caloric needs for lactation are increased by about 500 kilocalories above the recommendation for the non-pregnant woman. This increase should be provided by a diet containing a quart of fortified milk, two large servings of meat, four or more servings of breads and cereals, and ample servings of fruits and vegetables daily.

BIBLIOGRAPHY

Aznar, R. and A.E. Bennett, 1961. Pregnancy in the adolescent girl. *Amer. J. Obstet. Gynecol.* 81: 935.

Bagchi, K. and A.K. Bose, 1962. Effect of low nutrient intake during pregnancy on obstetrical performance and offspring. *Amer. J. Clin. Nutr.* 11: 586.

Baird, D. and R. Illsley, 1953. Environment and childbearing. *Proc. Roy. Soc. Med.* 46: 53.

Blackburn, M.L. and D.H. Calloway, 1974. Energy expenditure of pregnant adolescents. *J. Amer. Dietet. Assoc.* 64: 24.

Brewer, T.H., 1966. *Metabolic Toxemia of Late Pregnancy. A Disease of Malnutrition.* Thomas. Springfield, Ill.

Brown, R.E., 1973. Breast feeding in modern times. *Amer. J. Clin. Nutr.* 26: 556.

Brown, R.R., 1972. Normal and pathological conditions which may alter human requirements for vitamin B6. *J. Agri. Food Chem.* 20: 498.

Committee on Maternal Nutrition, 1970. *Maternal Nutrition and the Course of Pregnancy.* Food and Nutrition Board, National Research Council. National Academy of Sciences. Washington, D.C.

Edwards, C.H., et al., 1964. Effect of clay and cornstarch intake on women and their infants. *J. Amer. Dietet. Assoc.* 44: 109.

Emerson, R.G., 1962. Obesity and its association with complications in pregnancy. *Brit. Med. J.* 4: 516.

Erhardt, C.L. and H.C. Chase, 1973. Part 2. Ethnic group, education of mother and birth weight. In Study of Risks, Medical Care, and Infant Mortality. Ed., H.C. Chase. *Amer. J. Pub. Health Supplement* 63(Sept): 17.

Hodges, R.E., 1971. Nutrition and "The Pill". *J. Amer. Dietet. Assoc.* 59: 212.

Hurley, L.S., 1968. Consequences of fetal impoverishment. *Nutr. Today* 3, No. 4: 3.

Hytten, F.E. and I. Leitch, 1964. *Physiology of Human Pregnancy.* Blackwell. Oxford.

Hytten, F.E. and A.M. Thomson, 1968. Maternal physiological adjustments. In *Biology of Gestation.* Ed., N.S. Assali. Academic Press. New York.

Jacobson, H.N., 1972. Nutrition and pregnancy. *J. Amer. Dietet. Assoc.* 60: 26.

Metz, J., et al., 1965. Effect of folic acid and vitamin B_{12} supplementation on tests of folate in vitamin B_{12} nutrition in pregnancy. *Amer. J. Clin. Nutr.* 16: 472.

Milk, J.C., 1973. Adolescent parenthood. *J. Home Econ.* 65, No. 8: 31.

Nutrition Foundation, 1973. Etiology and implications of lactose intolerance. *Nutr. Review* 31: 82.

Nutrition Foundation, 1973. Fetal malnutrition. *Nutr. Review* 31: 179.

Nutrition Foundation, 1973. Maternal dietary supplementation and infant birth weight. *Nutr. Review* 31: 45.

Nutrition Foundation, 1973. Starvation in pregnancy: metabolic changes. *Nutr. Review* 31: 182.

Roe, D.A., 1973. Nutritional side effects of drugs. *Food and Nutrition News* 45, No. 1: 1.

Stare, F. and M. McWilliams, 1973. *Living Nutrition.* Wiley. New York.

Stearns, G., 1958. Nutritional status of the mother prior to conception. *J. Amer. Med. Assoc.* 168: 1655.

Sulman, F.G., 1970. *Hypothalamic Control of Lactation.* Springer-Verlag. New York.

Surgeon General, 1971. *Health Consequences of Smoking.* Public Health Service, Dept. Health, Education, and Welfare. Washington, D.C.

Thompson, M.F., et al., 1974. Nutrient intake of pregnant women receiving vitamin-mineral supplements. *J. Amer. Dietet. Assoc.* 64: 382.

Thomson, A.M., 1959. Diet in pregnancy. III. Diet in relation to course and outcome of pregnancy. *Brit. J. Nutr.* 13: 509.

White, P.L., 1966. Nutrition and genetic potential. *J. School Health* 36: 337.

Winick, M., ed., 1972. *Nutrition and Development.* Wiley. New York.

Winick, M., ed., 1974. *Nutrition and Fetal Development.* Wiley. New York.

World Health Organization, 1965. *Nutrition in Pregnancy and Lactation.* Tech. Rept. Series No. 302. Geneva, Switzerland.

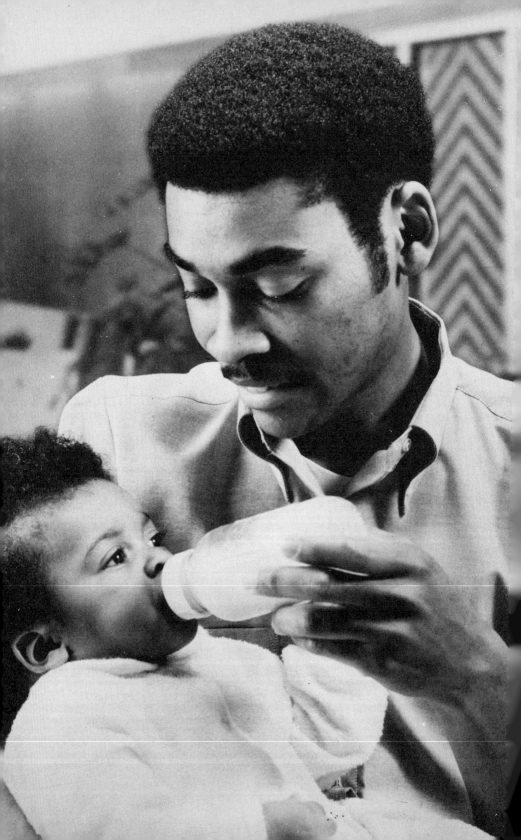

Chapter 5
Milk for the Infant

Once a baby is born, the questions regarding feeding of the infant focus not on whether milk is the most appropriate food for the baby, but rather on what type of milk is best for the newborn. Traditionally the milks used for feeding infants in the United States have been human milk or cow's milk, but this picture is quite different in some other countries of the world. For instance, in some countries remote from the United States, milk from the camel, water buffalo, or reindeer might be the most likely substitute for human milk when an alternative to breast feeding is required.

COMPOSITION OF MILK

Although studies have been made to determine the composition of the various types of milk, many mothers in the United States desire a clear-cut interpretation of these data in order to clarify the question of whether it is better to feed cow's milk or human milk to the infant. Mothers want to know which type of milk will promote the optimum rate of growth and which will most effectively aid in the development of a healthy baby. These questions require considerable discussion based, in part, on the difference in the composition of cow's milk and human milk (Table 5.1). However, tables indicating the percentage composition of fat, protein, and carbohydrate, as well as minerals and vitamins in human milk and cow's milk present only part of the picture that needs to be considered in comparing the types of milk.

Table 5.1   *Composition of colostrum, human milk, and cow's milk*

Nutrient	Colostrum[a] (1–5 days) (100 g)	Milk[b]	
		Human (100 g)	Cow's (100 g)
kcal	58	77	65
Protein (g)	2.7	1.1	3.5
Fat (g)	2.9	4.0	3.5
Carbohydrate (g)	5.3	9.5	4.9
Calcium (mg)	31	33	118
Phosphorus (mg)	14	14	93
Iron (mg)	0.09	0.1	Trace
Vitamin A (I.U.)	296	240	140
Thiamin (mg)	0.015	0.01	0.03
Riboflavin (mg)	0.029	0.04	0.17
Niacin (mg)	0.075	0.2	0.1
Ascorbic acid (mg)	4.4	5	1

[a]Data from Food and Nutrition Board, National Academy of Science. *The Composition of Milks.* National Research Council Publication No. 254. National Research Council. Washington, D.C. 1953.

[b]Data from *Composition of Foods,* Agriculture Handbook No. 8. Agricultural Research Service, U.S. Department of Agriculture. Washington, D.C. 1963.

Colostrum

Colostrum is the secretion from the human breast for the first few days after birth until mature human milk begins to be produced. Although the composition of colostrum will vary with the elapsed time from the birth, colostrum will be somewhat lower in energy value than mature milk; its protein content is higher, but its lactose and fat levels are lower. One of the important values of colostrum for newborns is its antibodies which provide valuable immunities to the infant. Breast feeding for even the first few days can be quite important because of the protection and nutrition provided by the colostrum.

Fat

The amount of fat in human and cow's milk is very similar, being just under 4 percent fat as an average figure. Fat from either type of milk can be utilized by most infants to meet their needs for this nutrient. The function of fat in the diet of infants is threefold.

First, fat is an important source of calories for the infant. It is true that energy can be obtained from protein and carbohydrate in the diet of the infant, but sufficient calories from fat make it unnecessary for the body to use protein for energy. It should also be recognized that fats contribute over twice as many calories per gram as do carbohydrates, which are another practical source of energy for the infant. Per gram, pure fat provides nine calories in contrast to approximately four calories for each gram of carbohydrate or protein. The caloric contribution of fat is significant because of the limited capacity of the small child and the need for calories for growth and physical activity during the early period. This possibility of providing sufficient caloric intake without an excessive volume by adding fat is of particular importance in the premature infant who has a limited capacity; in the ordinary full-term infant it is unnecessary to attempt to increase the amount of fat above the amount generally found in milk, that is, approximately four percent.

Second, the fat of both human and cow's milk is important not only for its caloric contribution to the diet, but also because vitamins A and D are carried in the fat portion of the milk. Because of this property, milk can be an important source of both of these vitamins.

Third, fats provide the body's only source of the essential fatty acid, linoleic acid. Both types of milk supply the small amounts of this unsaturated essential fatty acid needed by infants. Linoleic acid is necessary for optimum growth and also is an aid in maintaining healthy skin. Without adequate amounts of this essential fatty acid, the infant's skin will begin to be somewhat dry and scaly, and growth eventually may be stunted.

The fat found in human milk, of course, is not subjected to processing of any type before consumption. Cow's milk, however, does undergo pasteurization and also, in many instances, homogenization before being used in infant formulas. One particular value of homogenization is that the fat globules, by being forced through a very small aperture, are broken into much smaller fat particles which are easier to emulsify in the body than are the original fat globules.

The importance of emulsification is more easily understood by examining the process of digestion and absorption of fat in the body. In order for fat to be digested, it is necessary to have a great deal of surface area available for contact between fat molecules and enzymes. This extensive surface area becomes available when the fat is emulsified into extremely small particles, as can be done when the cow's milk is homogenized. Because of this greater ease of emulsification, the enzymes in the small intestine are able to break down the fat into its component fatty acids and glycerol. The fatty acids are then absorbed through the intestinal wall and become available to the body for energy, for transporting the fat-soluble vitamins, or as possible sources of linoleic acid.

Although there is only a limited difference in the total amount of fat in cow's milk versus human milk, there is a large difference in the amount of linoleic acid in the two. Human milk contains a total of 10.6 percent of its fatty acids as linoleic acid. In contrast, only 2.1 percent of the fatty acids of cow's milk are in the form of linoleic acid. The levels of various fatty acids in human milk vary a little as a result of individual dietary patterns. Cow's milk is rather high in its content of saturated fatty acids of moderately long chain length (16 and 18 carbons in length). Fats containing saturated fatty acid of these lengths are digested somewhat less readily by infants during the early weeks of life than are the shorter ones.

In bottle feeding not only is it possible to change the size of the fat globules by homogenization, but also it is feasible and sometimes desirable to modify the amount or the type of fat in the milk formula. The possibility of removing the animal fat from cow's milk and substituting vegetable fats has been explored. The vegetable oils or fats that are sometimes substituted in commercial milk preparations include the following: olive, soybean, cottonseed, coconut, corn, and safflower. These fats contain more linoleic acid and are more fluid than the original animal fat. They are therefore somewhat more easily emulsified and more readily digested and absorbed by the infant than the normal fats in cow's milk.

Modification of the type of fats in formulas may be of significance because of the influence of type of fat on cholesterol levels in infants. Formulas containing corn, coconut, or soybean oil resulted in lower serum cholesterol levels in infants than did the use of human or cow's milk. Although lower serum cholesterol levels are considered useful in reducing the likelihood of atherosclerosis in adulthood, the value in infancy is not yet known. Fomon (1971) suggests that there may be two possible hazards of a low serum cholesterol level in infancy: (1) normal cholesterol levels may be important as a challenge to develop the enzyme systems of metabolism that are needed to degrade cholesterol in the body, and (2) myelination of the brain may require dietary cholesterol to proceed at a normal rate, whereas polyunsaturated fats in the diet alter the type and quantity of fat circulating in the body. On the basis of these arguments, the necessity of feeding infants to achieve a low serum cholesterol value early in life is receiving critical questioning.

Protein

Protein is absolutely essential for proper growth and development of the child since this is the basic type of building material needed for tissue and muscle growth. Because of the significance of protein for the infant, protein differences in human and cow's milk are of particular interest; cow's milk contains 3.5 percent (by weight) protein and human milk contains 1.1 percent. Since cow's milk is obviously substantially higher in protein content than is human milk, the immediate assumption might be that cow's milk is definitely superior to human milk. This is not true, however, because of the difference in the type of protein in the two milks. Apparently the protein in cow's milk is easily digested by the young calf, but the enzymes in the human infant's digestive system appear to be slightly less effective in digesting this protein; the protein in cow's milk is not as well utilized by the human infant as might be desired.

The chief difficulty for infants digesting cow's milk seems to be related to the hardness of the curd formed from the protein in cow's milk. In technical literature this toughness of the curd is referred to as curd tension. When milk is consumed by the infant, the liquid passes into the stomach where a rather dramatic change takes place in the physical state of the milk. Rather than remaining in a smooth fluid form, the protein in the milk coagulates or forms curds such as are observed in cottage cheese. In order for the infant to actually use the protein in milk, it is necessary for the enzymes in the small intestine to break down the protein molecules contained in these curds into their component parts, the amino acids. These amino acids then can be absorbed through the intestinal wall and be used for the various body-building needs of the infant.

If the curd formed by the protein is a very soft, almost fluid substance, it is a comparatively simple matter for the enzymes to digest the protein and to isolate the amino acids for absorption into the body. But if the curds that are formed are rather hard and tight, the enzyme action is much less effective, fewer amino acids are isolated, and much less absorption takes place. This difference in rate of digestion can be demonstrated in a test tube by clotting whole cow's milk and clotting human milk and observing the digestion that takes place when a proteolytic enzyme is added to the substance. It can be seen that some digestion does take place in cow's milk, but the action is distinctly slower than it is in human milk. The value of the high protein content in cow's milk is reduced somewhat because of its slightly slower rate of digestion when compared to human milk; thus, the actual amount of available protein from the two milks is not as divergent as it would seem at first.

Raw cow's milk generally is not offered to infants because of the hazard of milk-borne contamination to the infant and also because of the digestive problems associated with the raw whole milk. Tuberculosis, undulant fever, and salmonellosis are sometimes transmitted by raw milk; such illnesses are serious at any age, but are particularly dangerous for infants.

The pasteurization of cow's milk is an essential step to safeguard the sanitation of the milk and this process also causes a change in the protein which helps to improve the digestibility of cow's milk. A still more significant difference in digestibility of protein is effected when pasteurized cow's milk is homogenized. Not only does the homogenization process break the fat globules down into the desired smaller particles, but also it causes changes in the nature of the protein which result ultimately in the formation of a softer curd in the infant's stomach. Because of the changes in the cow's milk protein due to pasteurization and homogenization, cow's milk is a suitable food for infants. Evaporated milk and dried milk have also undergone changes in the milk protein and consequently are suitable sources of protein for the infant when they have been reconstituted to the normal dilution.

The amount of protein in a child's diet is significant in determining the growth and development of the child. It has been suggested that about 1½ – 2 ounces of cow's milk per pound of infant weight will provide an appropriate amount of protein for growth; translated into practical terms, this means that the 10-pound infant should be consuming 15 – 20 ounces of cow's milk to obtain the amount of protein that is generally recognized as necessary for optimum growth.

The needs of the breast-fed infant are more difficult to measure since actual intake is more difficult to determine. Actually, the lack of visual evidence on how much milk a breast fed baby consumes is an advantage. With bottle feeding, there may be the temptation to urge the baby to drink all of the milk in the bottle, even when he does not need it. This may lead to excessive weight gain. Breast feeding removes this visual assessment of dietary needs and may prevent overfeeding.

When there is some indication that the baby is unusually hungry between breast feedings, it may be advisable to weigh the infant before and after each feeding to determine how much milk he is actually consuming. Usually good growth results on an intake of 2½ – 3 ounces of breast milk per day per pound. These weighings are usually unnecessary, however, because the growth rate and the satisfaction after feedings provide practical guides for the amount of milk needed by the breast-fed infant.

There are eight essential amino acids (methionine, threonine, tryptophan, isoleucine, leucine, lysine, valine, and phenylalanine) considered necessary for human adults and nine amino acids (the aforementioned eight plus histidine) that are essential for the growth and development of the young child. These amino acids occur in appropriate combinations in the proteins in both types of milk and at adequate levels to ensure good growth in infants (Table 5.2). From the standpoint of amino-acid composition, the two types of milk are appropriate foods for the young infant. It appears that it is unnecessary to supplement either of these types of milk with additional amino acids as long as the infant is consuming an adequate amount of milk.

Table 5.2　Comparison of the amino acid requirements of infants and children with the amino acid content of human and cow's milk (g./16 g. N)[a]

	Human Milk	Cow's Milk	Infant b	c	Children d
Arginine[e]	4.1	3.7	–	–	–
Histidine	2.2	2.7	2.4	–	–
Lysine	6.6	7.9	7.7	7.5	10.7
Leucine	9.1	10.0	10.9	10.9	8.0
Isoleucine	5.5	6.5	6.6	9.2	5.3
Methionine	2.3	2.5	4.8	3.3	–
Cystine[e]	2.0	0.9	–	–	–
Total sulfur amino acids	4.3	3.4	6.2[f]	–	4.8[f]
Phenylalanine	4.4	4.9	6.6	6.5	4.8
Tyrosine[e]	5.5	5.1	–	–	–
Total aromatic amino acids	9.9	10.0	–	–	–
Threonine	4.5	4.7	4.4	6.3	6.1
Tryptophan	1.6	1.4	1.6	1.6	1.6
Valine	6.3	7.0	6.7	7.6	5.9

[a]From *Evaluation of Protein Quality*, Publ. 1100, National Research Council of National Academy of Sciences, Washington, D.C., 1963.

[b]Recalculated from the data given in *Evaluation of Protein Nutrition*, Publ. 711, National Research Council of National Academy of Sciences, Washington, D.C.

[c]Recalculated from L.E. Holt, Jr., P. Gyorgi, E.L. Pratt, S.E. Snyderman, and W.M. Wallace, *Protein and Amino Acid Requirements in Early Life*, New York Univ. Press, New York, 1960.

[d]Recalculated from the data of I. Nakawa, T. Takahashi, and T. Suziki, *J. Nutr.*, 73:186 and 74:401, 1961.

[e]Nonessential amino acids.

[f]Methionine requirement in absence of cystine.

Carbohydrate

The question of carbohydrate in the infant's diet is primarily a question of the amount of energy (total number of calories) needed by the infant each day because the carbohydrate in milk is an important source of energy. Unlike proteins, which have a specific function in the growth of tissue, or fats, which are sources of the fat-soluble vitamins and the essential fatty acid, carbohydrates appear to serve primarily the function of providing energy for the various activities of the infant. By providing sufficient energy for this purpose, carbohydrate spares protein to perform its unique functions in the body rather than creating the need for the body to utilize protein for energy. A sufficient amount of carbohydrate also is necessary in the body to metabolize fats satisfactorily.

There is a significant difference in the amount of carbohydrate found in human milk and in cow's milk. The carbohydrate found in human milk is approximately twice as plentiful as the quantity in cow's milk (9.5 percent in human milk in comparison with 4.9 percent in cow's milk). This carbohydrate occurs in the form of lactose in both types of milk and is well utilized by most infants.

In order to compensate for the difference in the level of carbohydrate in the two types of milk, some form of carbohydrate customarily is added to infant formulas prepared with cow's milk. Although it is not the same sugar that is naturally found in milk, corn syrup is well utilized by infants and is frequently added to formulas. A less sweet substitute for lactose is dextrimaltose. This material provides energy for the baby without sweetening the milk formula quite so much. Pure lactose also is available for use in cow's milk formulas. The disadvantage of lactose is that it is fairly expensive; however, it does help to promote the absorption of calcium.

Minerals

Two minerals, calcium and phosphorus, may be singled out as being particularly vital to the growth and development of the young infant. Calcium is a very important mineral for the growth of the skeletal structure and teeth of the infant as well as for such functions as clotting of blood and response of nerves to stimulus. Phosphorus not only is a structural constituent of bones and teeth, but also plays a key role in metabolic processes. Both types of milk are outstanding sources of calcium and phosphorus; it has been noted that cow's milk contains more than three times as much calcium as human milk. On this basis one might expect that cow's milk would be clearly superior to human milk for the growth of the infant because of the greater quantity of both calcium and protein in cow's milk. (Adequate protein in the diet favors optimum absorption of calcium.) In growth studies of breast-fed and bottle-fed infants, at an age of 112 days breast-fed infants in the 90th percentile for length and weight were longer and heavier than their counterparts fed cow's milk (Aitken and Hytten, 1960). However, it was shown that there was no significant difference in size at the age of one year that could be attributed to the source of the milk. It appears that the young infant's need for these minerals will be met if he consumes 2½ ounces of human milk or 1½ ounces to two ounces of cow's milk per pound of body weight each day.

The other minerals needed by the infant occur in milk in reasonable quantities, with the possible exception of iodide and the definite exception of iron. Unless the nursing mother herself is receiving an inadequate amount of iodide, her milk will contain sufficient iodide to meet the infant's need; cow's milk used in formula feedings will supply the necessary iodide. Iron is decidedly inadequate in both human and cow's milk.

The question of a mineral supplement needs to be resolved in the minds of many women because there is much badgering of mothers by various companies promoting the sale of mineral and vitamin products. When milk is consumed in the recommended amount each day, it provides adequate amounts of the minerals needed for optimum growth and development, with the exception of iron and possibly fluoride. The use of multiple mineral supplements therefore really appears to be superfluous as long as the recommended amount of milk is being consumed each day. Until the age of approximately three months, an infant born from a well-nourished mother will have sufficient stores of body iron to meet his needs. By the age of three months the iron can be supplemented by adding various foods rather than by a mineral supplement.

Vitamins

The quantities of vitamins in milk also should be considered carefully. Vitamin A and the B vitamins (thiamin, riboflavin, and niacin) are present in adequate amounts in both types of milk.

Ascorbic acid, the vitamin needed for formation of connective tissue and other vital functions in the body is definitely inadequate in cow's milk and may be present in insufficient quantity in human milk unless the mother is consuming large amounts of ascorbic acid. The addition of orange juice within two weeks after birth is often done to compensate for this shortcoming of milk.

Vitamin D must be present in order to efficiently absorb and utilize the calcium and phosphorus that are present in milk. Without an adequate supply of vitamin D, it is possible for the infant actually to consume adequate amounts of calcium and phosphorus and yet develop deficiencies of these two minerals because of their poor absorption. If irradiated or vitamin-D enriched cow's milk is being fed to the infant, his vitamin D requirement will be met when he consumes a quart of milk each day. For the infant on human milk, vitamin D supplementation will be needed in order to have optimum absorption of the calcium and phosphorus needed by the infant.

The level of vitamin K in both human and cow's milk provides a comfortable margin of safety, since these milks provide more than 1 milligram daily in normal infant diets (actual need is estimated at approximately 5 micrograms daily). Despite this margin when feeding is well established, a parenteral dose of 1 milligram of vitamin K_1 is recommended to correct the vitamin K deficiency that is relatively common among newborns.

There is also a possibility that premature infants may have a vitamin E deficiency at birth. A vitamin E supplement of 0.5 milligrams per kilogram is recommended for premature infants. Breast-fed infants will receive somewhat more vitamin E in their diet than will infants consuming cow's milk.

From the preceding discussion it can be concluded that either human milk or cow's milk is a highly suitable food for human infants, but that milk alone does not provide adequate amounts of all the nutrients needed for optimum growth and development. To date there does not appear to be any significant difference in the growth rate of persons who were fed cow's milk or human milk as infants.

THE DECISION TO BREAST OR BOTTLE FEED

One of the important decisions to be made in considering the feeding of a baby is whether to breast feed or formula feed the baby. Since good nutrition of a normal infant can be achieved with either type of milk, this decision should be made individually after the advantages of both types of feeding have been considered carefully in relation to the needs of the family. Choice of feeding methods is an individual decision that should be acceptable to all members of the family. It is impossible, because of the many factors involved, to state flatly that one method of feeding is superior to the other for infants in the United States.

Safety of Milk Supply

One important advantage of breast feeding is that of sanitation of the milk supply; human milk, as it is fed to the infant, is certainly going to be as pure as it could possibly be. There is no possibility of spoilage such as might occur in an unrefrigerated milk formula, nor is there an environmental opportunity for the milk to be contaminated. Consistent with the sterile nature of the milk supply, infants who

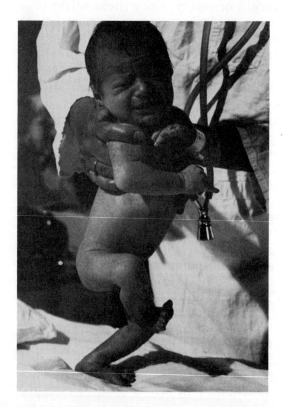

The newborn — to breast or bottle feed?

are breast fed have fewer respiratory ailments than do
infants fed by bottle. The problems associated with sanitation of bottle feeding, however, can be controlled satisfactorily if sterilization procedures are followed carefully and
if the bottles are handled with care during the feeding. It is
important to avoid handling the nipples or touching the milk
in the bottle during preparation and feeding. When the
mother understands the sterilization procedures and appreciates their importance, sanitation usually is not a serious
problem. If formula preparation is done carelessly, however,
bottle feeding can present a distinct hazard to the child.

The problems of sanitary formula preparation and refrigerated storage become more complex when one is traveling,
although commercial formulas in disposable containers are
now a practical means of meeting this contingency. Prompt
refrigeration of home prepared and opened containers of
commercial formulas is essential to safety. Milk is an excellent medium for microorganisms, and they will multiply
rapidly at room temperature.

In addition, there is the remote chance that a serious
error in formula preparation may occur. Perhaps the most
tragic case in recent years that might be cited to illustrate
this possibility was the episode in an Eastern hospital when
salt was accidentally substituted for sugar during preparation of a formula, a mistake that was fatal to the infants
drinking the formula. This type of error does not occur frequently in formula preparation, but it is still a possibility.
It may be concluded that, with ordinary precautions in the
home, formula errors are not likely to be a significant
problem.

On the other side of the coin is the fact that some medications will be transmitted in the milk supply of the lactating
woman. For example, breast feeding is not recommended for
infants if the mother is taking birth control pills. Arena
(1970) in discussing recommendations for lactating women
was opposed to the use of "any drug or chemical in excessive
amounts, diuretics, oral contraceptives, atropine, reserpine,
steroids, radioactive preparations, morphine and its derivatives, hallucinogens, anticoagulants, bromides, antithyroid
drugs, anthaquinones, dihydrotachysterol, and antimeta-
bolites". He pointed out that, on the basis of body size, a
drug is approximately 12 times more potent in an infant than
in his mother. Because of the transmission of nicotine in

cigarettes and marijuana, the use of these substances by lactating women definitely is not recommended. If a woman is smoking between 10 and 20 cigarettes or more daily, the milk supply will be affected and nicotine will be transmitted in harmful levels to the infant. Liquor, up to 2 cocktails daily, does not present a problem in the milk supply. Before taking any medication, a lactating woman should ascertain that the drug will not appear in her milk as a hazard to her baby.

Convenience

A reason that many mothers express for wishing to breast-feed their babies is that breast feeding is more convenient. There is no need to plan a time for formula preparation in the day's schedule; there is no problem involved in the refrigeration of formula, nor is there the problem of keeping the bottles clean and ready for formula preparation. The milk supply is constantly being produced while the mother is doing other things. This can be a particular advantage to the mother of a first child who will find herself extremely busy trying to reorganize her life and routine to encompass the responsibilities of caring for her expanded family. Time management to include time for formula preparation often is less difficult for a mother with several children than it is for the mother with her first-born infant, but the time saved by breast feeding is still valuable to the mother.

Allergies

Generally few allergy problems occur in the breast-fed infant, whereas there is somewhat more likelihood of development of an allergic response in infants fed cow's milk. This should not be construed to mean, however, that there is a great possibility for allergies if the infant is not breast fed. In actual practice this sensitivity becomes a factor for consideration only when it is suspected that there might be a problem because of a previous history of allergies in the family.

Mother-Child Relationship

Perhaps the foremost reason for breast feeding the infant in the United States is the psychological value that the mother and infant derive from this close relationship. Many mothers feel a sense of fulfillment by breast feeding their babies. They realize that they are helping to ensure that their children are well fed and adequately nourished by breast feeding. The infant responds well to the very warm close relationship between mother and infant. Therefore, for the psychological benefit to both mother and child, breast feeding is often a very appropriate choice of feeding methods.

Breast feeding, however, does not automatically effect a close psychological bond between all mothers and their infants. Some mothers may need to adjust to the total concept of motherhood more slowly and may find the adjustment easier if they are bottle feeding rather than breast feeding their offspring. The greater freedom accorded to the mother who is bottle feeding may be crucial to the new mother's adjustment to her new role. In such a case, breast feeding and its confining schedule would only accentuate the complications of her adjustment and would benefit neither mother nor child from the psychological viewpoint.

A mother with other young children in the family may find that breast feeding, rather than promoting the psychological bond between herself and the new addition, actually causes a feeling of antagonism or resentment because it may be very difficult to provide adequate care for her other young children during the nursing period. This problem is accentuated in nice weather when the mother is nursing her infant while the other children are playing outdoors. If a preschooler is playing outside and a difficulty arises or an accident happens while the newborn is nursing, the mother will not feel a comfortable relationship between herself and the infant; she will be distracted and will need to help the other child in the family. The anxiety the mother may feel while the other children are relatively unattended will certainly communicate itself to the newborn and interrupt the warm relationship that is so often depicted.

The desired closeness between mother and infant can be achieved during bottle feedings. A mother who always holds her baby when offering the bottle can develop a rewarding, warm relationship with her infant.

Feelings of Other Family Members

In some families there may be a possible advantage to bottle feeding because other children in the family may have a strong desire to help in caring for the infant. If there appears to be a strong feeling of jealousy developing in an older child, this feeling is amplified sometimes by the mother breast feeding the new arrival. In such a case it might be advisable to consider at least supplemental bottle feedings in order to let the older child assist with feeding the infant.

Acceptance of the newborn and the desire to help with the care of the newborn are adjustments that are not relegated uniquely to the older children in the family; the husband may face similar feelings as he adjusts to the newcomer in the family. If the mother is breast feeding the newborn, the father may feel that he is being prevented from becoming acquainted with his heir. The assistance that a father can

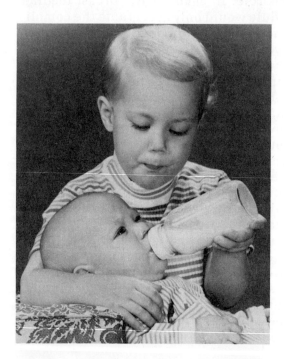

Other family members can share the pleasure of feeding the bottle-fed infant.

give is somewhat limited when the mother is breast feeding the infant, whereas the husband can participate with bottle feeding. If a father is strongly motivated to help care for his infant, it might be wise for the mother to consider either bottle feeding or supplemental bottle feedings from time to time so that the father can be included in the new experience.

On the other side of the ledger, it should be pointed out that some fathers prefer breast feeding because they cannot help with the feeding and are hence not called upon to do the feeding in the middle of the night.

Working Mothers

One of the major reasons emerging for bottle feeding in the United States today is the increasing number of working mothers. When the mother must return to work soon after the birth of her child, she really has no alternative to bottle feeding the infant. If possible it would be advisable for the mother to remain at home for perhaps the first month after the baby's birth in order to breast feed her infant during this period. She could then wean the infant to the bottle when she returns to work. This is one possibility that some working mothers might be able to consider seriously. In the event that the mother must return to work just as soon as possible, it is perfectly appropriate for her to plan to bottle feed from the beginning. The need for the mother to return to work is a decision that must be faced within the family, but the mother who needs to work should be reassured that it is certainly possible for her baby to be well fed on a formula rather than on human milk.

Physical Limitations

There may be several instances when, because of the mother's or the infant's physical condition, breast feeding is not the most desirable means of feeding the infant. If a mother has been sick during the period of pregnancy, lactation may place too great a physical strain on her and should not be undertaken. For instance, mothers with problems such as kidney disease usually should not undergo the additional physical strain of lactation. Also, mothers with tuberculosis present a distinct hazard to the child and should not attempt to nurse the infant.

Sometimes a premature baby must be bottle fed rather than breast fed in order to meet his specific nutritional needs. High-calorie formulas efficiently supply the necessary calories for the infant without overcrowding the child's small capacity for food.

In some cases the mother may have an inadequate milk supply for the infant and, in order to provide the necessary nutrients, breast feeding alone will not be adequate. It is possible in such cases to do supplemental breast and bottle feeding for a short time. Extended use of this supplemental method, however, is time consuming and often frustrating to both mother and child and hence is not usually continued for longer than a period of two to four weeks.

Economic Aspects

One of the reasons that is often given for breast feeding is that it is more economical. On the surface this might appear to be true, for breast feeding requires no purchase of equipment and ingredients or formula. Therefore it would appear that the feeding of the breast-fed infant is virtually without cost. This is not true, however, because the nutritional needs of the lactating woman are considerably greater than are her needs prior to pregnancy. Actually the economic decision is based on whether one wishes to spend money directly on milk for formula or indirectly on the additional food needed for the mother to produce milk; in either case, milk will cost money.

Personal Considerations

It should be pointed out that perhaps one of the most enticing reasons for some women to breast feed their babies is that the nutritional requirements for the lactating woman are high, and this then can provide one time in a woman's life when she can eat larger quantities of food without being quite so concerned with the effect of this large intake on her physical shape. The high number of calories required for lactation (500 kilocalories more than before pregnancy, most of which will be contained in the daily milk secretion) affords considerable choice of foods in the diet. This opportunity is particularly appealing to the woman who has had to be extremely careful about curbing her food intake to control her weight gain during pregnancy.

The anxiety that some women have for their figures may influence their attitude toward breast feeding. It is an obvious fact that a woman's breasts will become enlarged and somewhat heavy during lactation. Whether lactation causes any permanent change in the figure depends largely on the woman herself. During the period of lactation there will be little stretching of breast tissue if the mother is careful to wear properly fitted brassieres at all times – not just during the day, but also when she goes to bed at night. If this is done there should be little change in the woman's figure after breast feeding is discontinued.

Breast feeding is a normal part of the total reproductive cycle and may be of benefit to the mother in two very tangible ways. The nursing process aids in returning the uterus to its normal size more quickly. This role can be noted by the uterine contractions often felt during nursing. In addition, the risk of breast cancer is somewhat lower among the population which has nursed infants compared with those who have not. For some women, the delay in subsequent conception as a result of lactation and its tendency to deter ovulation is yet another benefit. A survey of women in Nigeria (Gioiosa, 1955) showed that the average time for the first menstrual period was 16 months after delivery for women who breast fed in the study; this was in contrast to an average of between 55 and 59 days for non-lactating women in the study.

Immunities

One of the compelling reasons for breast feeding for at least a limited period is to transmit antibodies from the mother to her infant. In this manner, some immunity to the viruses of mumps, influenza, and poliomyelitis may be developed in the newborn. Thus some protection is provided against antibodies that may be traversing the gastrointestinal tract. These antibodies afford some local immunity.

Social Aspects

Perhaps one of the biggest reasons for bottle feeding in the United States is related more closely to a social rather than a nutritional question. Many women feel that it is not socially acceptable to breast feed their infants. They may sense that it is best for the child to be breast fed, but they are not able to accept this as being an acceptable means of caring for their babies.

A transition in incidence of breast feeding has been occurring in different social classes in the United States over the past few years. Less breast feeding is being done in the lower social classes. In these population groups it appears to be a matter of prestige if one can bottle feed rather than breast feed. Some of this change may be due also to the greater number of working mothers in the lower social classes and to the economic need for these mothers to return to work soon after the birth of the baby. In these cases breast feeding would not be possible.

In contrast, there is an increasing acceptance of breast feeding in the upper social classes. The increase in the upper classes is of considerable interest for it reflects increasing appreciation of the value of breast feeding.

There has been considerable interest generating by the LaLeche League to encourage mothers to breast feed. Their efforts have received widespread publicity in the United States. However, the incidence of breast feeding in the nation still is not large. Fomon (1971) reported that 80 percent of the infants were fed commercial formulas at the time of discharge from the hospital in 1970, with 27 percent being at least partially breast fed. By two months of age, breast feeding was occurring for only 15 percent of the infants studied, a level which dropped to less than 10 percent by four months of age. At the age of four months, 40 percent of the infants were receiving commercial formula and 40 percent were fed whole cow's milk. By six months of age, 70 percent were drinking whole cow's milk.

The Actual Decision

The final decision as to which type of feeding to follow should be made by the individuals involved with the care of the child. If a woman has strong feelings that she will not be able to accept breast feeding from the social viewpoint, this might be a compelling reason for not attempting to breast feed. If a mother must go back to work as soon as possible, then bottle feeding is the obvious answer for her. In many instances the mother may have some question as to which she feels would be best for her to do with her infant. This decision should then be talked over with her doctor during pregnancy in order to make an intelligent decision before the birth of the baby.

The mother and father also should discuss this question in order to arrive at an answer that is acceptable to both of them, for this does need to be a mutually acceptable arrangement. It is very difficult for a mother to successfully breast feed her baby if her husband does not wish to have her do this. The opposite situation may also arise; the father may have strong feelings on the desirability of breast feeding and the mother may not wish to nurse her baby. In such a case, breast feeding would not be an acceptable answer.

In the United States, where standards of sanitation are high and supplies of milk are plentiful and wholesome, it is possible to meet the nutritional needs of most infants by bottle feeding. In some countries the sanitation problems or the limited supplies of milk make it almost mandatory for a mother to breast feed her infant. But in this country it appears that the question of breast or bottle feeding should be answered by the true feelings of both the mother and the father as well as by the total picture within the home. Once the decision has been made, the American mother should be fully satisfied that either breast or bottle feeding can be a highly successful method of feeding most infants.

It is extremely important that a mother not feel guilty about bottle feeding her infant. There can be a very warm relationship between a mother and her bottle-fed infant. This can readily be achieved to the satisfaction of both mother and baby as long as the mother feels confident that bottle feeding is a wise decision. The problem arises when the mother feels guilty about not breast feeding her infant.

In some cases there may not be a clear-cut decision about the advisability of breast versus bottle feeding, or there may be the problem of an only partially adequate human milk supply for the infant. In many such instances the mother may wish to supplement breast feedings with a bottle until the age of approximately one month, at which time it is appropriate to change over exclusively to bottle feeding.

BREAST FEEDING

Success with breast feeding usually can be traced to the mother's treatment in the hospital. When the mother is in a hospital where the doctors and personnel are sympathetic with her desire to breast feed her infant, the likelihood of successful breast feeding is greatly increased. New mothers often need encouragement and kindly interest in their success in this new endeavor. If nurses will take the time to assist the mother in feeding the breast-fed infant and will make the effort to get the babies to the mothers at the appropriate time, success in breast feeding can be greatly increased. Several studies in this country have shown that helpful attitudes on the part of all those associated with the mother during her stay in the hospital will increase the success of breast feeding. The practices of a rigid 4-hour feeding schedule, giving supplementary bottles, and keeping babies from nursing for the first 24 hours after birth are contrary to establishing successful breast feeding.

If the milk supply is to be adequate, there usually should be a rise in mammary skin temperature and uterine contrac-

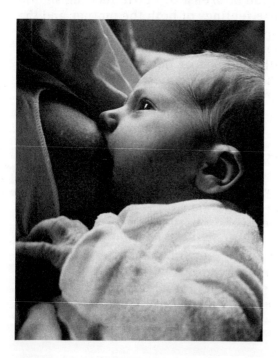

Success in breast feeding is promoted by supportive hospital personnel and a relaxed atmosphere.

tions during nursing on the second day after delivery. Another good indicator of the adequacy of the human milk supply is the amount of fat in the milk at seven days.

For a variety of reasons, some mothers cannot successfully breast feed. One of the possible explanations for inability to breast feed the infant is that the mother actually has a genetically poor milk-producing capability. This is the real reason for some mothers, but apparently is not the leading cause for failure to produce adequate milk for breast feeding. Failure to breast feed successfully often results from a multiplicity of psychological factors.

Perhaps one common reason for failure in breast feeding is that the mother actually does not wish to breast feed her infant. She may have verbally expressed the desire to breast feed her infant because other people expect her to do this, but subconsciously she may not wish to and therefore may have an inadequate supply of milk for her child. Some mothers are apprehensive and worried about the care of their babies and may become so anxious that their milk production is impeded. Then it often develops that the more concerned they become about the success of their breast-feeding efforts, the greater is their failure. In such cases it would be far better to encourage the mother to bottle feed her baby in order to relieve her anxiety as much as possible and to increase her pleasure in her baby. It seems probable that many mothers in this group will be able to nurse subsequent children satisfactorily.

Changes in the mother's routine also may cause a reduction in the supply of breast milk. It is not uncommon for a mother to have an adequate supply of milk when she leaves the hospital, only to have this supply diminish when she is at home. The additional strain of attempting to organize her household and to work the baby into the usual routine may cause the mother considerable anxiety and fatigue, thus resulting in failure to produce an adequate supply of milk.

With the short stay in a hospital that is now common after the birth of an infant, establishing satisfactory lactation becomes a problem. The mother's milk usually will begin to flow on approximately the third day. In some hospitals she might be released at this time. In others she might stay an additional day or two, but even after five days in the hospital many women do not feel really relaxed and comfortable with the new baby. These anxieties can create serious obstacles to successful lactation. It appears that, for the mother who desires to breast feed and who indeed has these feelings of anxiety, a somewhat longer stay in the hospital would enhance her possibility of success in lactation.

Technique

Probably most women will have more success with breast feeding if they feel they understand the fundamentals of the technique for breast feeding. The time for the first nursing varies from one physician to another and from one hospital to another. Therefore no flat rule can be stated. Some hospitals have the baby nurse briefly four hours after delivery. Others may wait as long as three days to begin breast feeding. The most common time interval, however, is somewhere between twelve and twenty-four hours after delivery. The reason for having the baby nurse this soon after delivery is not one of nutrition, but rather is one of acquainting the baby and the mother and helping the mother to gradually become accustomed to nursing the baby. This early period of nursing actually might be looked upon primarily as a practice period when both the mother and the infant are learning the techniques involved in the nursing operation. However, less weight loss occurs in infants when breast feeding is initiated early rather than waiting 24 hours to begin.

Nursing will be facilitated when both mother and baby are comfortable. The mother may wish to lie on her side facing the baby or she may prefer to sit up with the baby's head resting in the bend of her arm as she holds him. When the baby's cheek is touched with the nipple, he will instinctively turn toward the nipple. Most of the areolar (pigmented) portion of the breast should be in the baby's mouth in order to most effectively stimulate milk flow without causing soreness or cracking of the nipples.

The length of time for nursing the baby should be controlled more carefully in breast feeding than in bottle feeding in order to keep the mother's nipples from becoming cracked and sore. It appears that the majority of the milk will be obtained during the first 5 to 7 minutes of nursing. Therefore nursing time reasonably may be limited to approximately ten minutes the first few days. This time may be extended gradually to 15 to 20 minutes, but certainly should not exceed one-half hour.

The milk supply is stimulated when the infant empties the breast at each feeding, but there is some controversy regarding offering one or both breasts at each feeding. There presently appears to be no clear-cut answer as to whether both breasts should be offered at each feeding or only one breast each time. The doctor is the one best qualified to answer this question for the individual woman.

Duration

The most appropriate period of time for nursing the baby cannot be clearly delineated, but actually should be worked out between the mother and her doctor. Where possible, it appears advantageous to continue breast feeding until the baby is approximately five to seven months old. Should it be necessary to stop breast feeding sooner, however, there is usually no particular problem as long as the individual lives where a clean supply of milk is available. In the United States it is often inconvenient for the mother to continue lactation for such long periods of time, and there appears to be little benefit to the child from this prolonged lactation.

The importance of nursing for an extended length of time cannot be overemphasized in areas where milk supplies are not adequate and sanitation is a problem. In such conditions the nursing of infants to the age of at least one year, and preferably longer, in some of the underdeveloped countries is extremely important and should be encouraged.

It is wise occasionally for the mother to give a bottle of formula to the infant rather than to exclusively breast feed the infant. This practice serves a dual function; the mother has an opportunity during the supplemental feeding to go out and do something to entertain herself and break the routine of the constant care that is involved after the birth of the baby. This break in the routine will be a great psychological lift for the mother which actually may serve to increase the flow of breast milk. Not only is the offering of an occasional bottle good from the mother's viewpoint, but also it is helpful from the child's standpoint because it introduces the child to a new flavor and a new feeling, thus expanding his knowledge. This practice facilitates the transition from breast to exclusively bottle feeding, a fact that is sometimes particularly appreciated when a sudden change from breast to bottle feeding becomes necessary.

Ordinarily, weaning is best achieved by gradually reducing the nursing time and supplementing the feeding with milk from a bottle or a cup. If weaning is delayed until the age of about ten months, it is possible to wean directly to the cup rather than to the bottle.

BOTTLE FEEDING

Formula Selection

Commercially prepared formulas.   The bottle-fed infant may be fed a variety of formulas; one may choose to use either a formula prepared in the home or a prepared product purchased from a drug or grocery store (in a dried form, in a concentrated fluid preparation, or a ready-to-feed fluid form). Selection of a particular commercial product should be made with the guidance of the pediatrician. Examples of commercial formulas are presented in Table 5.3.

Among the commercial formulas available, there are many choices to be made. A review of the ingredients listed on the label shows choices between lactose, dextrins, maltose, sucrose, and glucose as the source of carbohydrates

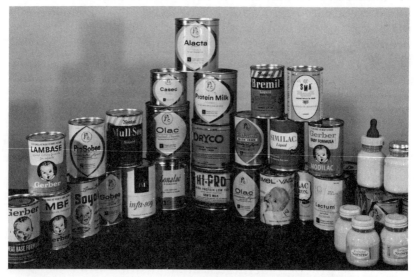

Many products currently are available for bottle-fed infants. Products specifically for infants with allergy problems are on the left; powdered milk products are in the center; and concentrated liquid and ready-to-feed formulas are on the right.

Table 5.3   *Examples of formulas suitable for commercial production* [a]

Formula	Milk, oz.	Water, oz.	Carbohydrate	Approximate Caloric Value	
				per oz.	per 100 ml
Evaporated milk					
1	6	18	1 tbsp. dextrimaltose, or ½ tbsp. light corn syrup, or 1 tbsp. dextrose	12	41
2	7	17	2 tbsp. dextrimaltose, or 1 tbsp. light corn syrup, or 2 tbsp. dextrose	15	51
3	8	16	2 tbsp. dextrimaltose, or 1 tbsp. light corn syrup, or 2 tbsp. dextrose	17	57
4	11	19	4 tbsp. dextrimaltose, or 2 tbsp. corn syrup, or 4 tbsp. dextrose	20	67
Prepared milk (liquid)					
1	1	3	—	10	34
2	1	2	—	13	44
3	2	3	—	16	54
4	1	1	—	20	67
5	3	2	—	24	81
6	3	1	—	30	101

Table 5.3 *(Continued)*

Formula	Milk, oz.	Water, oz.	Carbohydrate	Approximate Caloric Value per oz.	per 100 ml
Prepared milk (powder)					
1	1	4	—	10	34
2	1	3	—	13	44
3	2	5	—	16	54
4	1	2	—	20	67
5	3	5	—	24	81
6	3	4	—	30	101

[a]Prepared by Baby Formulas, Inc., of Southern California, 6115 Manchester Blvd., Buena Park, Calif.

in the products. The various sources of fat range from the natural fat content of cow's milk through others from plant sources, such as soybean, coconut, safflower, and corn. There is a choice between products with iron added and those without this enrichment. Protein levels also may be varied between commercial products. The nutrient labeling is an important guide to selection of a specific product if a commercial formula is to be used.

Yet another choice is available between concentrated products, dried or powdered products, and ready-to-feed or full strength formulas. The concentrated products are designed to be prepared by adding an equal volume of sterile water to dilute the formula to the correct concentration. This type of formula is easier to transport because of the reduced volume and weight of water contained in it. However, the formula does require that sterile water be available and that the entire contents of the can be prepared and refrigerated until it is used. In contrast, the ready-to-feed formulas may be available in feeding-size portions, thus eliminating the need for refrigerator storage since the unopened bottles are processed to not require refrigeration until opened. The cost of the ready-to-feed formulas may be slightly higher than the concentrated product.

Powdered formulas are particularly useful for supplemental feedings for breast fed infants. Although they are slightly less convenient to prepare than the concentrated liquid formulas, their preparation basically is quick and easy. The storage life of an opened container of powdered formula is significantly greater than is an opened can of liquid formula.

The formulas available for normal infants are based on a caloric value of 20 kilocalories per fluid ounce (67 kilocalories per 100 milliliters). Some formulas are prepared for infants with a need for calorically concentrated mixtures and a low renal solute load. For normal infants the renal solute load need not be considered in selecting a formula if the total volume of formula consumed is at least 100 milliliters per kilogram of body weight per day.

For infants with special dietary needs, commercial formulas of special design may be the most appropriate answer to meeting nutritional needs. For example, there is a commercial product designed for infants with steatorrhea and other chronic diarrheas. This product is formulated so that fat contributes less than 30 percent of the calories, as contrasted with the 50 percent contribution in cow's milk.

A formula with carbohydrate other than lactose may be

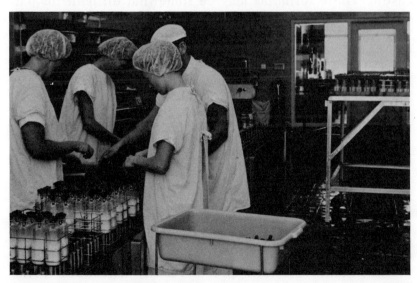

In some cities, commercial firms prepare formulas for distribution to hospitals in the area.

the answer for an infant with a lactase deficiency. Milk-free formulas are more expensive than those with a milk base, but they are of great value when feeding an infant with galactosemia or a congenital or acquired lactase deficiency.

Allergies may be found among some infants. The most common causes of these allergies have been noted to be due to milk, wheat, and egg. In such instances, soy formulas provide a suitable alternative. The oil in these formulas may be from the soy itself or from coconut. Soy formulas should be reviewed for total nutritional content, with appropriate supplementation being provided if the formula itself is not complete for meeting nutritional needs. Soy formulas are effective for many infants who do not tolerate cow's milk or goat's milk formulas. The soy formulas ordinarily are more expensive than cow's milk.

Meat-based formulas provide yet another alternative for feeding infants with special dietary problems. When cow's milk, goat's milk, and soy formulas do not enable the baby to thrive, a meat-based formula may be required. These formulas may be made commercially from beef or lamb hearts, usually with sesame or corn oil added. The protein efficiency ratio of these formulas is about 80 percent that of casein. These formulas may be somewhat difficult for parents to accept at first because their color and odor are so very different from milk formulas. However, infants who do not have a preconceived notion that their food should be white and taste like milk generally will accept these formulas. The cost, as might be anticipated, is significantly higher than other types of formulas.

Formulas prepared in the home. Formulas prepared in the home are less expensive than commercial formulas. The choice of milk for such formulas includes evaporated, homogenized, pasteurized, or dried milk.

Evaporated milk is a very useful product for a formula base because it is easily obtained in the store, can be stored without refrigeration until being opened, and is relatively inexpensive. In addition, the fat in evaporated milk is in very small particles, and the protein has been modified by the evaporation process so that it forms a rather fine, soft curd in the infant's stomach and is readily digestible in the intestine.

Probably the least expensive milk to use in preparing an

infant formula is dried milk. The milk can be either dried whole milk or dried skim milk. Dried skim milk has the advantage of having a longer potential storage life, but either type can be kept a long period of time, particularly if the unused portion is kept in a tightly covered can and stored in a cool place.

If skim milk is used in formula preparation, an oil should be added to provide the needed linoleic acid and the calories. Infant diets ordinarily should consist of between 7 and 15 percent of the calories from protein, 35 to 55 percent from fat, with the balance being provided by carbohydrates. Skim milk formulas will have only about 3 percent of their calories from fat and 40 percent from protein unless they are modified by the addition of an oil. The added fat is needed if an infant is to receive sufficient calories in a day without ingesting an unreasonably large volume of food. The use of skim milk in infant diets is likely to require such a large total volume of food that the infant will establish a pattern of overeating, a pattern that can lead to obesity as the calorie content of the diet is modified later in childhood. Estimates of total caloric needs for growth and activity vary, but range above 90 kilocalories per kilogram of body weight per day. If skim milk is used for feeding infants without the addition of an oil, the infant usually will be ingesting less than the amount (90 kcal/kg/day) needed for optimum growth and activity. This pattern will lead to depletion of body stores of fat.

Occasionally the question arises as to whether sweetened condensed milk is an appropriate food for infants. The use of sweetened condensed milk as an infant formula definitely is not wise because of the high number of calories contributed by added sugar. Not only does this milk provide a high number of calories, but also it accustoms the infant to sweet flavors and may cause him to show a decided preference for sweet foods at the expense of less sweet foods that provide more nourishment in the diet.

The need for energy obviously varies with the infant, with infants at age four months generally consuming between 100 and 105 kcal/kg/day on ad libitum feeding and the amount dropping to less than 100 by eight months of age. Excessive weight gains usually accrue if infants between the ages of four and eight months consume more than 100 kcal/kg/day. Sweetened condensed milk formulas or formulas high in fat will promote ingestion of excess calories and lead to the development of excess numbers of adipose cells in the body.

Formula Preparation

In order to make cow's milk more easily digestible by the human infant, modifications are made in the milk when it is prepared for infant feeding. Water is added to dilute the milk; the resulting reduced concentration of protein is more easily digested. Some form of sugar often is added to the formula to increase the caloric value of the diluted formula to approximately that of an equal volume of human milk.

The formula chosen should meet the needs of the individual infant. As the infant begins to consume close to a quart of formula each day, the formula usually is altered to contain less water. Such changes are best made at the doctor's suggestion.

Equipment. The equipment necessary for bottle feeding depends on the type of milk to be used in the preparation. It is convenient, however, to have enough bottles to provide one bottle for each feeding during a 24-hour period (usually six are required). These bottles may be made of glass or a boilable plastic. Plastic, of course, has the advantage of being unbreakable. Nipples and plastic covers are available in various designs. The choice of type is an individual matter.

Other items are of value when preparing formula. A bottle brush with bristles that extend across the end of the brush is required for cleaning the bottles. Although it is not essential, it is helpful to have a funnel for filling the bottles. Also, if canned milk is used, a punch-type can opener is necessary. A pair of tongs makes the handling of the equipment much more sanitary.

Terminal method of sterilization. With the wide availability of canned commercial formulas the terminal method of sterilizing formula has been diminishing in popularity. Basically, the terminal method consists of sterilization of the formula in the bottles. The steps actually involved can be outlined as follows:

1. Bottles, caps, and nipples should all be carefully washed; water should be forced through each nipple

to make certain that the holes are not clogged with formula from previous feedings. Careful rinsing ensures complete removal of the detergent used for cleaning the bottles.

2. If the formula is to contain evaporated or homogenized milk plus sugar, the correct amounts of these ingredients should be added to the appropriate quantity of water in a pan or mixing pitcher.

3. When the total amount of formula is ready, it is then divided into the number of bottles needed for the day's feedings.

4. Nipples are then placed in an inverted position on the bottles and the caps are screwed on to the tight position and then loosened about three-fourths of a turn. The loosening of the caps is necessary to prevent excessive pressure from building up in the bottles.

5. Place the bottles, in their rack, in the sterilizer and add water to the half-way point on the bottles. Put the lid on the steamer and heat the water to boiling.

6. Maintain the water at an active boil for 20 to 25 minutes.

7. If the short boiling time of 20 minutes is used, the formula should be cooled in the covered sterilizer for two hours and then refrigerated. For a 25-minute sterilization period, it is appropriate to remove the bottles from the sterilizer and, after letting them cool briefly at room temperature, store them in the refrigerator. Tighten caps before storing.

Sterile field method. The sterile field method employs separate sterilization of the formula and the bottles, followed by careful combination of the two. The preparation of equipment and formula is as follows:

1. All equipment should be carefully washed and rinsed, as explained in the terminal method.

2. The clean equipment is then placed in the sterilizer with the bottles either inverted or laid on their sides.

3. One to two inches of water are added. When the water comes to a boil, the sterilization period begins and is continued for five minutes. These items are ready for use when they are cooled sufficiently so that the tongs can be handled comfortably.

4. Cans to be opened in formula preparation should be rinsed first. Then sufficient formula is mixed for the day according to the physician's directions. To allow for evaporation during preparation, it is wise to prepare an extra ounce or two of formula.
5. The formula is then gently boiled in a pan for five minutes.
6. After the formula has cooled, it is poured through a funnel equipped with a strainer into the desired number of sterile bottles. Nipples are added, in an inverted position using sterile tongs. Caps are added and the completed formula is stored in the refrigerator.

Preparation of commercial formulas. The procedure outlined in the preceding section on the sterile field method is appropriate when a commercially prepared formula is used. If the formula selected is in a concentrated rather than a ready-to-feed form, the water used for diluting the product to the desired concentration can be boiled and then combined with the formula. Boiling the formula itself, however, is unnecessary.

Bottle-Feeding Technique

Only a short time ago, it was quite generally agreed that formula should be warmed until it just barely felt warm when tested on the inside of the arm. It is now a fairly common practice, however, to feed cool or sometimes even cold formula. Most infants do not object to the cool liquid unless they have been preconditioned to warm milk. In today's mobile society, it can be a real convenience to not be burdened with the problem of finding a place to warm a baby's bottle.

To achieve a satisfying parent-child relationship during bottle feeding, it is imperative that the child be held during feedings; bottle propping is definitely undesirable. The traditional way of holding the baby in one's lap and resting his head in the bend of the arm provides support for the baby's head and is comfortable for both parent and infant.

The nipple should be equipped with holes that permit the milk to drop from the inverted bottle at a regular pace rather than to flow in a stream. If the holes are too small, they can easily be enlarged with the aid of a sterile needle. When nipples begin to let the milk run out too rapidly, they should be discarded. It should be necessary for the baby to suck on the nipple to order to get his milk.

When the baby is drinking, small air bubbles will pass up the side of the bottle. Occasionally a nipple may collapse, resulting in a partial vacuum which impedes milk flow. This is easily corrected by loosening the cap to let air into the bottle, and then tightening the cap to resume the feeding. Care should be taken to prevent the baby from sucking in air during a feeding since this may cause gas discomfort in his stomach. The use of a well-designed nipple which does not collapse will aid in controlling this problem.

Sanitation should be kept in mind with regard to all aspects of infant feeding. Breast feeding is basically a very sanitary procedure, but bottle feeding requires awareness of good sanitation. The preparation of the formula should be handled as just described. The nipples should not be touched when preparing a bottle for feeding or during the feeding process. The amount of milk that will be used in one feeding should be placed in the individual container. If a little milk or formula is left in the bottle, this can be discarded. Milk is an excellent medium for growth of microorganisms and infants are very susceptible to infections. To reduce the risk to infants, formulas should be kept carefully refrigerated until ready for use. Periods of standing at room temperature or in even warmer places are to be avoided to reduce the possibility of contamination. Of course, all materials for formulas should be scrubbed well, and one's hands should be freshly washed when preparing to feed infants.

DIARRHEA AND DIETARY MANAGEMENT

Infants with diarrhea are very susceptible to dehydration. To minimize this hazard, infants can be fed either dilute skim or dilute whole milk or dilute formula. This diet aids in replacing some of the fluid that is lost without adding to the renal solute load. The practice of boiling milk to feed to infants with diarrhea is not as satisfactory as the above procedure because the loss of some water during boiling will increase the mineral concentration in the remaining boiled milk and add to the renal solute load. Of course, as soon as the diarrhea has been controlled, the formula should be returned to regular strength rather than continuing on the dilute ratio.

FEEDING THE PREMATURE INFANT

Premature infants (gestational age of 270 days or less or weighing less than 2.5 kilograms) have special requirements because of their higher proportion of water to body weight and their less developed systems. They will not be able to nurse as vigorously, and their enzyme systems are less well prepared to handle food. Despite these limitations, nutritional needs of these infants are high. The routine suggested for feeding newborn premature infants is discussed in Chapter 12.

SUMMARY

Cow's milk and human milk are the nutrient sources most frequently used in feeding infants in this country. For the normal infant, either of these milks may be a very appropriate food to provide his early nutritional needs. The choice of milk source is one that needs to be considered by the parents, with the decision being made in relation to their total situation. Either type of milk has been shown to be effective in promoting excellent growth and development. Although their nutritional composition is not the same, there are some advantages to each type of milk. The advantages have been reviewed in the chapter.

BIBLIOGRAPHY

Aitken, F.C. and F.E. Hytten, 1960. Infant feeding: comparison of breast and artificial feeding. *Nutr. Abstr. Rev.* 30: 341.

Applebaum, R.M., 1970. Modern management of breast feeding. *Pediat. Clin. N. Amer.* 17: 1.

Arena, J.M., 1970. Contamination of the ideal food. *Nutr. Today* 5, No. 4: 2.

Barness, L.A., 1972. *Milk and Milk Products in Human Nutrition: Fat.* Ross Laboratories. Columbus, Ohio.

Czajka-Narins, D.M. and W.B. Weil, Jr., 1972. *Developmental Nutrition: Calories.* Ross Laboratories. Columbus, Ohio.

Fomon, S.J., 1971. Pediatrician looks at early nutrition. *N.Y. Acad. Med.* 47: 569.

Fomon, S.J., 1973. *Skim Milk in Infant Feeding.* Maternal and Child Health Service. HEW.

Fomon, S.J., 1974. *Infant Nutrition.* 2nd ed. Saunders. Philadelphia.

Gioiosa, R., 1955. Incidence of pregnancy during lactation in 500 cases. *J. Obstet. Gynec.* 70: 162.

Gyorgyi, P., 1962. Protective effects of human milk in experimental staphylococcal infections. *Science* 137: 338.

Jelliffe, D.B., 1962. Culture, social changes and infant feeding: Current trends in tropical regions. *Amer. J. Clin. Nutr.* 10: 19.

Jelliffe, D.B. and E.F.P. Jelliffe, 1974. Confidence and the science of lactation. *J. Pediat.* 84: 462.

Knowles, J.A., 1965. Excretion of drugs in milk - a review. *J. Pediat.* 66: 1068.

Kon, S.K., 1972. *Milk and Milk Products in Human Nutrition.* UNIPUB, Inc. New York.

Ladas, A.K., 1970. How to help mothers breastfeed. *Clin. Pediat.* 9: 702.

LaLeche League International, 1958. *Womanly Art of Breastfeeding.* Franklin Park, Ill.

Macy, I.G., et al., 1953. *The Composition of Milks,* Publ. 254. National Research Council of National Academy of Sciences, Washington, D.C.

McRedmond, A., 1970. *Mammary Glands and Breast Feeding.* Ross Laboratories. Columbus, Ohio.

McRedmond, A., 1973. *Premature Infant.* Ross Laboratories. Columbus, Ohio.

Meyer, H.F., 1960. *Infant Foods and Feeding Practice.* Thomas, Springfield, Ill.

Meyer, H., 1968. Breast feeding in the United States. *Clin. Pediat.* 7: 708.

National Research Council, 1953. *Meeting Protein Needs of Infants and Children.* Publ. 843. National Academy of Sciences, Washington, D.C.

Newton, N., 1971. Psychologic differences between breast and bottle feeding. *Amer. J. Clin. Nutr.* 24: 993.

Newton, N., and M. Newton, 1967. Psychologic aspects of lactation. *New England J. Med.* 277: 1179.

Nutrition Foundation, 1973. Feeding baby of low birth weight. *Nutr. Reviews* 31: 14.

Nutrition Foundation, 1973. Fresh cow's milk and iron deficiency in infants. *Nutr. Reviews* 31: 318.

Nutrition Foundation, 1973. Overfeeding in first year of life. *Nutr. Reviews* 31: 116.

Nutrition Foundation, 1973. Postnatal growth of small-for-date babies. *Nutr. Reviews* 31: 51.

Pearson, H.A., 1972. *Developmental Nutrition: Iron.* Ross Laboratories. Columbus, Ohio.

Pyramid Rubber Co., 1961. *Modern Methods of Preparing Baby's Formula.* Ravenna, Ohio.

Reinken, L. and B. Mangold, 1973. Pyridoxal phosphate values in premature infants. *Internat. J. Vit. and Nutr. Res.* 43: 472.

Schaefer, O., 1969. Cancer of breast and lactation. *Can. Med. Assoc. J.* 100: 625.

Shank, R.E., 1970. Chink in our armor. *Nutr. Today* 5, No. 2: 2.

Smith, N.J., 1972. *Developmental Nutrition: Challenge of Obesity.* Ross Laboratories. Columbus, Ohio.

Williams, H.H., 1959. Differences between cow's and human milk. *Symposium 7: Infant Nutrition.* Council on Foods and Nutrition. Amer. Med. Assoc., Chicago.

Ziegler, E.E. and S.J. Fomon, 1971. Fluid intake, renal solute load and water balance in infancy. *J. Pediat.* 78: 561.

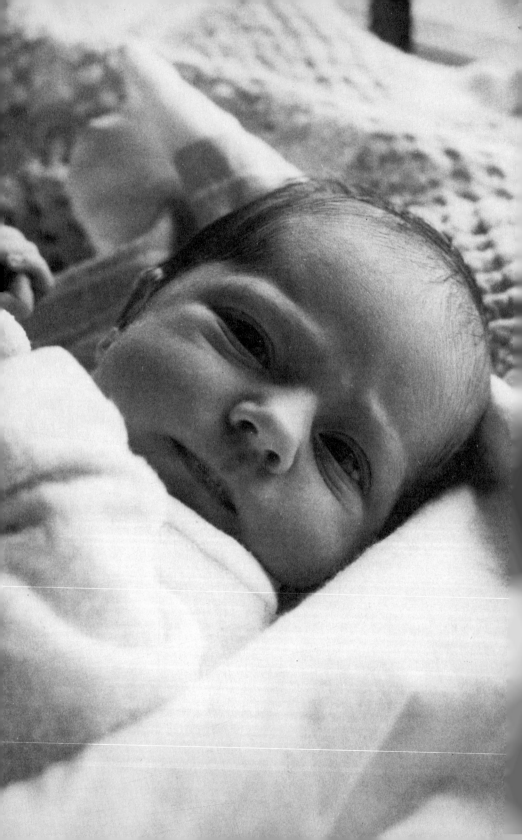

Chapter 6
The First Year

Probably the biggest single responsibility a mother feels when she brings her baby home from the hospital is that of feeding her new-born infant. Since the basic food for infants usually is milk, feeding sounds very simple until one is confronted with the practical aspects of the problem. Most hospitals have routines established which place little responsibility on the mothers. Therefore the home situation, where she is in sole charge, may suddenly seem quite different to the new mother.

ESTABLISHING A SCHEDULE

One very practical question that many mothers ask is, "How often should a baby be fed?" Two schools of thought exist as to the means of determining the time that should elapse between feedings. At one extreme is the school that feels babies should be fed by the clock, that is, at carefully regulated intervals. Mothers who are insecure in their new role may like clock feedings because rigid guidelines are provided and they are not required to make decisions. The second school, that of demand feeding, recommends feeding whenever the infant wakens and demands to be fed. This latter philosophy, on the surface, might appear to be the more logical way of determining when to feed the baby. To an inexperienced mother, however, this method may prove to be a little more complicated in practice than it sounds in theory, for she may be confused as to what a particular cry means. Does it mean that the baby is hungry and needs to eat, or does it simply mean that the baby is uncomfortable and needs some assistance and reassurance?

It would appear that, for the average baby and mother, the simplest way of establishing a baby's routine would be to integrate the two schools of thought, using the demand feeding system combined with the clock technique; that is, encouraging the baby toward a somewhat systematic feeding schedule, but allowing some variation according to the particular needs indicated by the crying of the baby. It certainly seems foolish to awaken a sleeping child when the clock says it is time for a meal, but on the other hand, it also is a bit ludicrous to feed a baby who has just finished a meal an hour earlier. Therefore, a mother probably will be most comfortable with a baby if she encourages him toward a schedule of approximately four-hour intervals between feedings. However, premature or very small babies will need to eat as often as every two or three hours for a few days.

In many instances the baby will already be established on a time interval of four hours between feedings since this is the approximate schedule of most hospitals. Some babies, however, may need to be gradually encouraged in this direction. Most mothers of first babies find some comfort in an approximate schedule such as this, rather than using completely demand feeding.

Establishment of a schedule is most easily accomplished by being certain that the baby has had an adequate meal at each feeding. This may mean, for some sleepyheads, that the mother might need to rouse the baby rather than putting him back in bed when he drowses off after consuming only an ounce or two of milk.

In general it is unwise to get in the practice of giving more food soon after the baby finishes a meal. If a well-fed baby rouses after approximately one hour, it is much more likely to be a gas pain upsetting him than a hunger pain. Therefore feeding is not appropriate at such a time and, after relief of a gas pain by burping, the baby probably will go back to sleep until close to the time for the next feeding.

It is extremely wearing on both mother and baby if frequent feedings become the pattern. Should this situation develop, mothers can gradually extend the time between feedings so that they begin to work back toward the desired schedule. A four-hour schedule (six feedings per day for the young infant) seems to work well for both breast- or bottle-fed babies. It permits the baby time to rest before it is time to commence the next feeding, and it also gives the mother time to do other jobs. Small infants probably will not be able to achieve a four-hour schedule until a weight of approximately eight pounds is achieved.

As the baby matures, it will gradually be possible to eliminate the middle of the night feeding. This, from the parental viewpoint, is extremely desirable. One can work toward this routine by having a good feeding at approximately ten o'clock at night and then encouraging the baby at the usual middle of the night feeding to gradually wait just a little longer. With the average size baby, sleeping through the night will occur at three to six weeks of age. The baby that is smaller at birth obviously will require a somewhat longer time to reach a weight that will enable him to go through the night without the usual two o'clock feeding.

FAMILY PARTICIPATION

Although the remarks in this chapter are directed primarily to the mother-infant feeding situation, it is often desirable for other family members to have the opportunity to feed the baby. Some fathers enjoy the sociability that comes when they assist with a feeding. Usually older children are delighted by an occasional chance to feed a baby. Of course, the degree of responsibility delegated to siblings should be consistent with their capability and maturity. Even a very young child, however, can help under close adult supervision.

It is a wise mother who encourages other family members to play a role in feeding the baby if they wish. The closeness of meal time shared with the newest family member seems to quickly draw the newly expanded family together, and may help to relieve feelings of apprehension or jealousy.

VITAMIN NEEDS

Supplements

During early infancy, milk is the sole source of nutrients, but milk alone does not actually provide all of the vitamins and minerals needed by the infant for optimum nutrition. Therefore, it is frequently the practice to supplement the milk diet with a liquid vitamin mixture tailored to the needs of young children. This vitamin supplement is particularly appropriate during the period when the young baby is consuming quite a small volume of milk each day. The vitamins that need to be supplemented during this period of time before the infant is consuming a quart of milk a day include vitamin A, thiamin, riboflavin, niacin, ascorbic acid, and vitamin D. In addition, the premature infant should have a supplement of 0.5 mg of vitamin E per kilogram of body weight to offset the low vitamin E level that accompanies prematurity. He should also have a folate supplement. When the child begins to drink a total of a quart of milk a day the vitamin supplement becomes less necessary because the increased quantity of milk, coupled with the gradual addition of solid foods, supplies an adequate amount of many of the vitamins and minerals needed by the child.

Regulation of Intake of Vitamins A and D

It is important to realize that two vitamins, namely vitamins A and D, are harmful when supplemented in the diet in large amounts. They are harmful to older children and adults when they are included in excessive quantities, but the problem is exaggerated in the infant and young child because of the significantly smaller body size. Excess vitamin A continued over a period of time has caused cases of mental retardation. Massive doses of vitamin D cause excessive deposition of calcium and phosphorus and eventually may be fatal. It is extremely important to the health of the infant that large doses of these two vitamins not be given in the vitamin supplement. It should be emphasized that these harmful effects of vitamins A and D only occur when large supplemental doses of these two substances are being consumed; the levels of vitamins A and D naturally occurring in foods are not toxic.

The apparent need for vitamin A has been established at 1400 International Units (I.U.) for the newborn to 6 months of age, at which time the recommendation is increased to 2000 I.U. (Table 6.1). This amount should not be greatly exceeded for optimum health. Since 1400 I.U. of vitamin A are provided by one quart of whole cow's milk, this vitamin can be supplied almost entirely by milk once the infant consumes a quart of milk each day.

Table 6.1   Recommended daily dietary allowances for infants [a]

Nutrient	Recommended allowances for:	
	Infant[b]	Baby[c]
Energy (kcal)	kg x 117	kg x 108
Protein (g)	kg x 2.2	kg x 2.0
Vitamin A activity (I.U.)	1400	2000
(retinol equivalents)	420[d]	400
Vitamin D (I.U.)	400	400
Vitamin E activity (I.U.)	4	5
Ascorbic acid (mg)	35	35
Folacin (ug)	50	50
Niacin (mg)	5	8
Riboflavin (mg)	0.4	0.6
Thiamin (mg)	0.3	0.5
Vitamin B_6 (mg)	0.3	0.4
Vitamin B_{12} (mg)	0.3	0.3
Calcium (mg)	360	540
Phosphorus (mg)	240	400
Iodine (ug)	35	45
Iron (mg)	10	15
Magnesium (mg)	10	15
Zinc	3	5

[a]From the 1974 revision of the daily dietary allowances as recommended by the Food and Nutrition Board of the National Research Council, National Academy of Sciences.

[b]Age 0 to 6 months, weight is 6 kg or 14 pounds, and height is 60 cm or 24 inches.

[c]Age 6–12 months, weight is 9 kg or 20 pounds, and height is 71 cm or 28 inches.

[d]Assumed to be all as retinol in milk during the first 6 months of life.

The recommended allowance for vitamin D is 400 I.U. and the intake of this vitamin also should be maintained at levels of approximately this value. The need for this vitamin is effectively met once the infant begins to consume a quart of irradiated milk per day because a quart of cow's milk, when irradiated, contains 400 I.U. of vitamin D. Breast-fed infants, however, will need a vitamin D supplement.

Ascorbic Acid

Milk frequently has been described as nature's most perfect food, but it should be emphasized that it is not a perfect food and ascorbic acid (vitamin C) is one nutrient that is definitely inadequate in quantity in cow's milk. The amount of ascorbic acid in human milk is related to the nutritional adequacy of the mother's diet, but it may be necessary to supplement the intake of this vitamin.

Any normal infant's need for ascorbic acid can be met simply by including one-fourth cup (two ounces) of orange juice in the diet each day. This juice frequently is included regularly in the diet as early as one to two weeks of age. If orange juice is not well tolerated by the infant, strained apple juice, fortified with ascorbic acid, may be a satisfactory substitute. Another alternative is to give ascorbic acid in a vitamin supplement. The important thing is that some means of providing ascorbic acid should be included in the diet plan for the young infant.

To summarize, the young infant will need a vitamin supplement until one quart of milk a day is being consumed. Ascorbic acid will need to be provided by juice or a vitamin supplement regardless of the amount of milk being consumed since this vitamin is very low in quantity in cow's or human milk. A vitamin D supplement of 400 I.U. is necessary daily for the breast-fed infant; such supplementation is unwise for infants consuming one quart of irradiated or vitamin-D enriched milk each day.

MINERAL NEEDS

Milk is a valuable source of minerals needed by the infant for optimal growth. The two minerals that will be in inadequate amounts in the diet without supplementation are iron and fluoride. A full term infant delivered by a well nourished mother with an adequate intake of iron during the pregnancy will be born with a reserve of iron sufficient to last for approximately 3 months. Therefore, iron supplementation in the infant's diet is needed prior to depletion of this reserve. Such supplementation often is provided through use of an iron-enriched formula or iron-fortified instant cereals.

The fluoride can be provided through the use of fluoridated water. If the mother is drinking fluoridated water, a limited amount of the fluoride will be excreted via her milk to her infant. This mineral should be administered daily to infants if it is not being provided in the diet. Liquid supplements are available, to be given via dropper. Fluoride during the preschool period, including infancy, is of value in developing teeth with a minimum of dental caries.

SOLID FOODS

Cereal

Although milk alone is adequate for the very young infant, it will fairly soon become apparent to the mother that it is desirable to add other foods that will help to prolong the feeling of satisfaction. This need is particularly noticeable at the night-time feeding. Mothers who have been getting up to give late-night feedings for several days or weeks begin to develop a strong desire for an uninterrupted night's sleep. In many instances this can occur more quickly if an infant is given some cereal at the last feeding before the mother wishes to go to bed.

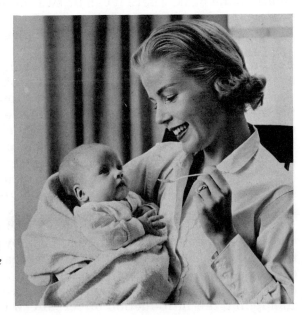

Cereal, when diluted with milk, can be fed to the infant with the aid of a small spoon which fits the baby's little mouth.

The addition of cereal should be done at first in very small amounts, beginning with one-fourth to one-half teaspoon and then gradually increasing to approximately a tablespoon. With the pregelatinized, enriched cereals that are now available for babies, one can easily prepare as little as a teaspoon of this cereal by diluting the dehydrated cereal product either with milk or with some of the baby's formula.

Adults ordinarily expect hot cereals to be quite thick, but this consistency is difficult for a young baby to manipulate in his mouth and swallow. It seems easiest to first introduce the baby to this food by mixing sufficient milk to make a very, very thin cereal that is not a great deal different in consistency from the milk to which the infant is accustomed. By using a small (demitasse) spoon that fits the baby's mouth, it is quite easy to feed this very fluid food to the baby. The technique is to simply allow the cereal to flow off the spoon into the baby's mouth. The slightly thicker product plus the new experience of the spoon may be quite a surprise to the baby! Even though some of the cereal may run out of his mouth, this does not mean that the baby does not like the cereal. It simply shows that he needs a little bit of practice in eating. The ability to move food from the front of the mouth to the back, where it can be swallowed, will gradually be developed.

Usually when solid foods are first placed in the baby's mouth, much of the food comes right back out on the baby's lips because he is not accustomed to moving food to the back of the mouth and swallowing it. This problem can be partially solved by trying to place the food toward the back of the tongue. Even then, some food will move forward and out on the lips and face. Then simply use the spoon to gather together the food around the baby's mouth and once again place it in on the back of the tongue. If this is done several times, he will soon begin to get the idea of how to manipulate solid food and swallow it. The problem is greatly simplified, however, if the initial solid foods are fairly fluid.

The addition of cereal to the baby's diet occurs at different times, depending on the individual baby, the mother, and the doctor. Some infants will receive cereal as early as ten days to two weeks of age; other babies may not be fed cereals until they are about two months old. From a nutritional standpoint, the introduction of cereal can be delayed satisfactorily until at least 6 weeks of age; milk and the supplements previously suggested will provide the nutrients needed for this period of time. This is later than many persons apparently add cereal to the diet. A reasonable guideline to use in determining when cereal should be added is to begin to add cereal when the infant is no longer satisfied with a quart of milk or formula in a 24-hour period. This suggestion needs to be based on actual infant demand and not upon the overfeeding that some adults encourage.

Today's enriched cereals for babies are important dietary sources of thiamin, riboflavin, niacin, and iron. The iron enrichment is particularly significant because of the low iron level in milk. In addition, cereals are valuable for the textural difference they provide, a difference that helps to expand a baby's range of experience. Any of the cereals specially marketed for babies will be a suitable and convenient choice to introduce solid foods. The dehydrated, pregelatinized cereal products presently available on the market include single-grain cereals (rice, barley, oatmeal), mixed cereals, and high protein cereal. Single-grain cereals generally are recommended for the first cereal to be introduced. Rice cereal is preferred by many because its protein generally is tolerated well by most infants. By introducing single cereal grains, it is possible to identify the specific type of grain causing the difficulty should an allergic response be triggered by the cereal. Yet another type of cereal product now is on the market. This is the pregelatinized cereal plus freeze-dried fruit. The addition of this type of fruit to cereal is quite expensive and certainly is not necessary from the nutritional standpoint.

The patterns of adulthood frequently may be transferred to the feeding of infants and children. A case in point is the preparation of cereals for feeding infants. As mentioned previously, a much thinner product than that preferred by adults is the best way to introduce this new food experience. Secondly, infants do not need to have sugar added to the cereal. They will learn to enjoy cereals for their own distinctive flavors without developing a need for the sweetness added by sugar.

The addition of cereal to the diet provides an important source of iron, a source that will continue to be needed. Purvis (1973) found that cereals were contributing very substantially to the iron intake of infants in the United

States by the age of 1 month. He found that the intake of cereals began to decline at approximately 6 months of age, a change that caused the iron intake to fall well below the recommended allowance throughout the remainder of the year. On the basis of his study, emphasis should be given to insuring that iron needs are being met, either by cereals or in some other manner.

Fruits and Vegetables

Usually the next foods added after the introduction of cereal will be fruits or vegetables. Many people prefer to use fruits as the next food group to augment the cereal and milk diet, but others feel that vegetables are more readily accepted if the baby has not yet become acquainted with the sweet flavors of fruits. This decision usually is made by the mother and the doctor together. Fruits and/or vegetables are most commonly introduced between the ages of one and four months; occasionally these foods are added even before a baby is a month old. Opinion regarding the best time for the

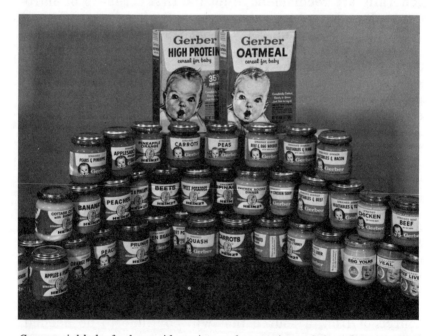

Commercial baby foods provide variety and convenience. Salt and monosodium glutamate levels have been reduced to improve nutrition of infants.

addition of fruits and vegetables is somewhat divided. Although it has been shown that month-old babies can safely consume fruits and vegetables, some physicians still prefer to wait until the age of three or four months before including these foods in the diet.

Despite the fact that pureed fruits are very well received by most infants, the addition of new fruits should be done very gradually. Usually one-half teaspoonful will be an appropriate amount to serve the child the first day that a new fruit is served. The next day the portion may be increased slightly. The amount of fruit, however, is never large for the young infant; approximately a tablespoon of fruit at a feeding is the maximum reasonable amount.

It is apparent from the preceding paragraph that, when new foods are introduced to the young infant, it will be impossible to finish the jar or can while the food is still fresh. Therefore it is important that mothers develop the attitude of expecting to throw away some of the baby food rather than keeping it around until it is of questionable quality. As the baby grows, his larger appetite and increasing familiarity with foods will make it possible for him to consume the contents of a container within a couple of days and waste food no longer will be a problem.

In order to preserve the wholesomeness of canned baby foods, the amount of food to be used at one feeding should be removed and the remainder of the contents should be covered tightly and immediately refrigerated in the original commercial container. There is less likelihood of contamination when the food is stored in its commercial package than there is if it is transferred to a home storage container. Prompt refrigeration of the leftovers retards bacterial growth.

From the baby's standpoint, it is wise to introduce a variety of fruits rather than to concentrate on the feeding of only one or two. The early period of life is a highly experimental time for the infant, and the variety of experiences that can be provided through food should not be ignored. Many fruits and combinations of fruits are available for mothers at this time, and it is wise to help develop the baby's range of taste experiences by providing many of these different fruits. It is to be expected that the baby will show preference for certain fruits over others, but the general pattern for fruits will probably be one of excellent acceptance.

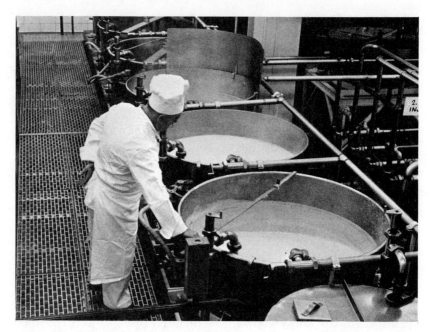

Baby food being processed by direct injection of steam to quickly and uniformly heat the product, a technique designed to retain the nutritive value of the food.

If fruits have been added to the baby's diet before vegetables, fruits should be served about 2 weeks before vegetables are introduced. Fruits should be continued along with the new vegetables in the day's menu. Although the pureed vegetables for babies are generally tasty, some babies will accept fruits more readily than vegetables. Most babies, however, will eat vegetables when they are presented in a pleasant manner that indicates that the baby will enjoy the food.

Baby foods will taste rather bland to the adult palate. Consequently, baby food manufacturers had begun to add flavoring components, notably salt and monosodium glutamate. As a result of inquiries into the desirability of this practice, the use of monosodium glutamate has been dropped and salt levels have been reduced. These changes are of significance for the infants because of the increased renal solute load. The intake of salt appears to have primarily a negative nutritional value. Sufficient sodium and chloride are available without added salt.

Some fruits and vegetables may be prepared easily at home with the use of a blender. These pureed foods are useful for feeding infants and may provide substantial savings in some instances. Cooked vegetables and fruits are prepared simply by removing any peelings, seeds, or highly fibrous material and then pureeing them in the blender. In many cases, it will be necessary to add some water to reach the necessary fluidity required by young babies. The water can be the cooking water used in preparing the fruit or vegetable for blending. With this approach, it would not be necessary to buy commercial pureed baby foods. However, many people may not be willing to take the time to prepare the foods at home as needed. In most situations, it probably would be wise to keep some commercial foods on hand so that by the time the baby is about three months old his total food needs will be met on a regular daily basis.

The range of pureed vegetables like the range of fruits is wide, and again it is advisable to offer the baby many of these vegetables during the early period of babyhood rather than specializing in just peas and beans. Not only does a variety of fruits and vegetables expand the baby's range of experiences, but it also aids in meeting the infant's need for a variety of vitamins and minerals. Although no one vegetable or fruit satisfactorily meets the body's need for minerals and vitamins, a variety of these foods will provide significant amounts of most of these nutrients.

Manufacturers of baby foods now produce combinations of vegetables and meats which are marketed as "dinners." Such products are basically a vegetable flavored with a bit of meat, and therefore are not to be considered as an adequate protein source. In assessing daily food intake, these "dinners" should be classed as a vegetable.

Protein Foods

Although there is a trend toward early supplementation with meat (sometimes even before cereals), it is still common practice to withhold meat and egg yolks until fruits and vegetables are well established in the diet. Certainly by the time the baby is three months old these foods need to be added to the diet, for meat and egg yolks are valuable sources of iron, the mineral that becomes increasingly important for the infant after the age of three months. The early addition of meats and egg yolks is of value in helping to check the drop in hemoglobin value which occurs as the fetal store of iron becomes inadequate for the infant's needs.

Again, as with other types of baby foods, a wide variety of pureed meats is available. Adults may find that they feel a distinct bias against the meats prepared for babies because the strained product is so different, both in texture and in flavor, from the meats to which they are accustomed. This rejection on the part of the adult may be communicated to the baby unless the mother realizes that the baby has no previous experience with meat to provide a comparison. In this case the baby's lack of experience is a definite asset in promoting acceptance, and mothers need not be apprehensive about offering the pureed meats.

The availability of strained meats is a real boon to mothers and babies alike. Conscientious mothers used to cook and scrape meat to make it suitable for infants; many mothers did not go to this trouble and infants were frequently in need of the B vitamins, iron, and copper which the meat could have provided.

Canned egg yolks for babies are useful not only because of their iron content, but also because of their reduced allergenicity. During the sterilization process, the intense heat and increased pressure cause denaturation of the proteins. This change in the proteins effectively reduces the likelihood that the infant will have an allergic response to the egg proteins. Another side benefit of commercially canned egg yolks is that there is no longer a need to find ingenious ways to use excess egg whites. The addition of whites is recommended later in the first year; whites in early infancy are more likely to produce an allergic reaction than are the yolks.

High meat dinners and cottage cheese are also available as strained baby foods and may be served occasionally as the main course. These foods may be used to add greater variety to the diet of a hungry baby; babies with a small capacity usually should have the regular strained meats, which are a more concentrated source of protein. In a 4½ – ounce volume the average protein content of these products is 8.5 grams of protein, whereas the plain baby meats contain approximately 19.1 grams of protein in 4½ ounces of strained meat.

Breads and Pastas

The use of bread, crackers, and cookies as baby foods warrants discussion from two angles. First, such foods contribute useful amounts of the B vitamins when they are made with enriched flour. Also in their favor are the facts that (1) the hardness of breads like zwieback may provide a brief comfort to teething babies, and (2) these foods are easy for the infant to manage when he begins to wish to feed himself. On the negative side, it must be admitted that some mothers use these foods as pacifiers to the point where the infant's appetite is so poor at meals that he fails to eat the foods he needs. In answer to the need to improve the nutritive value of such snacks, a baby cookie is now being marketed that is suitable for teething problems and that contains additional B vitamins and twice the usual amount of protein found in teething biscuits. Even with these nutritional enhancements, however, it is still wise to limit the consumption of these cookies to a maximum of four, and preferably fewer, each day.

Since potatoes and pastas such as macaroni are quite filling foods, it is customary to wait to introduce these foods until the baby becomes approximately six months old or perhaps at even a later date. From that time on, small servings of these foods are perfectly appropriate as part of the diet, as long as other foods are being included at normal levels.

Desserts

During the first year of life the baby's nutritional needs are proportionately great in comparison to his relatively small capacity. Therefore, it is necessary to be sure that the foods being fed to an infant are foods that offer excellent nutritional advantages. The most appropriate desserts for a baby will be fruits, custards, or other nourishing foods that are not too sweet. There is no requirement that babies need a dessert. In fact, this is a pattern that well could be avoided.

Daily Scheduling of Solid Foods

The times at which solid foods will be offered during the day depend somewhat on a family's schedule and routine.

If a mother is involved in getting her husband and other children off to job and school early in the morning, it is difficult for her to attempt to do a reasonable job of feeding the infant in the midst of the confusion. She may wish to give the baby only milk during this rush period and then offer the other foods later in the day when there is less confusion in the household.

Although it is not necessary to plan a perfectly rigid schedule for a baby's meals, both mother and baby will find mealtime goes more smoothly if a workable plan is generally followed. A regular meal pattern helps to ensure a hearty appetite. At each meal a planned part of the day's solid foods may be served. The use of a preplanned meal pattern aids in determining that all the necessary foods have been included daily.

PREVENTION OF OBESITY

Overfeeding of infants and the development of overweight to obese babies has been receiving increasing attention in the United States recently. Research on obesity has highlighted the developmental pattern of obesity. Adipose or fat cells are developed in number during childhood. The concern of overfeeding in early childhood is based on the fact that the obese child will have a greater number of fat cells than will the child of normal weight. These fat cells then will increase in size (but not in number) during adulthood. If an individual has developed an excessive number of fat cells during childhood, he thus has the potential for increasing the size of these extra fat cells during adulthood, and obesity becomes a lifelong problem for him. The recommendation at this point is to avoid developing these extra fat cells in babyhood and early childhood.

There is a very human tendency to compare the development of one baby against another, and proud parents may feel that their baby's rapid weight gain is a reflection of their excellence as parents. This is but one of the psychological factors that may encourage parents to overfeed their babies. The incidence of bottle feeding is considered to be one of the factors in overfeeding because the amount of milk consumed is measured so readily. Also, there is the tendency to encourage a baby to finish all of the formula in the bottle. Many parents have themselves been raised

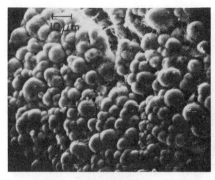 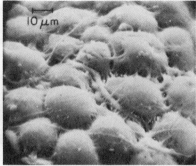

Scanning electron micrograph of adipose tissue from male Sprague-Dawley rats: left, 2 days old; right, 8 weeks old.

with the theorem that food should not be allowed to go to waste, a theorem which they quickly transfer to their offspring.

Another factor is often cited as a contributing force in overfeeding of infants. This is the early introduction of baby foods and over-generous servings of them in the daily diet. Although there are reasons for including some of the baby foods in the diet, as discussed above, the urge to finish the serving of these solid foods should be controlled. With today's sanitary conditions and preventive medicine, there is little reason to follow the dictum that a fat baby is a happy, healthy baby. This picture is to be avoided by nourishing infants at proper dietary levels. Control of caloric intake is best managed by using relatively small servings of the solid foods and including regular strength formula or whole milk up to a maximum of a quart daily. The preferred solid foods will include iron-fortified baby cereals, pureed fruits and vegetables (without additives such as cereals), strained meats, and egg yolks. The high meat dinners, desserts, and wet pack cereals are not needed in the diets of infants.

Another facet of weight control in infancy is that of exercise. If babies have an opportunity to roam rather freely within a home, they will get considerably more exercise than they will when they are confined for long periods of time in a playpen. This greater freedom to explore may be less convenient for parents, but it does aid in developing the baby. The added benefit of this approach is that a parent

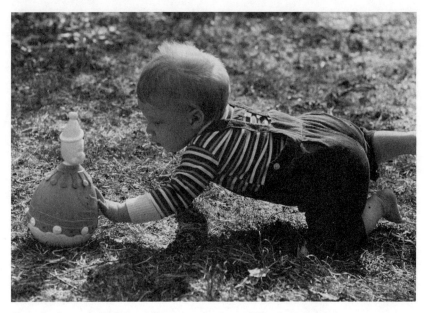

Exercise is an important adjunct to good nutrition for babies as well as adults.

also gets more exercise while supervising the activities of a crawling or walking baby.

Of course, weight gains will vary from one baby to another, but an average rate of weight gain during the first six months is about six ounces weekly. Many babies double their birth weight at about four months and triple their birth weight by one year. The rate of gain during the last half of the first year is slower than the first half. Tables of gain in both height and weight are in the Appendix, Tables 1 and 4. These can be of some assistance in monitoring the rate of gain in an individual child.

Planning the Day's Menus

With the recommendations on avoiding excessive weight gain to prevent the formation of large numbers of fat cells and the importance of providing opportunity for exercise in mind, plans need to be developed that will provide a well balanced diet for the baby. These plans need to aid in developing acceptance of a range of foods without encouraging overeating. By the age of three or four months, most infants will be consuming the wide range of foods commonly consumed by adults. Although babies will be consuming their food in a somewhat different form, these foods may be viewed as being equivalent to the adult foods. The spectrum of the diet for infants by the age of four months can be evaluated by using the Basic Four as a check list.

The overall diet for the day should be examined to be certain that all necessary nutrients are being included. This is the responsibility of parents, physicians, and dietitians. Babies cannot be counted upon to indicate the foods that they need. The suggestion that they can is encountered frequently, but babies apparently are no more gifted in sensing what they need than are adults in consuming diets based on impulse rather than calculated need. The research by Davis in the 1930's which suggested that infants might be able to select a diet that was nutritionally sound was structured in a way that virtually insured that the diet would be adequate. This is not sufficient proof to support such an approach to planning the diets of infants and young children.

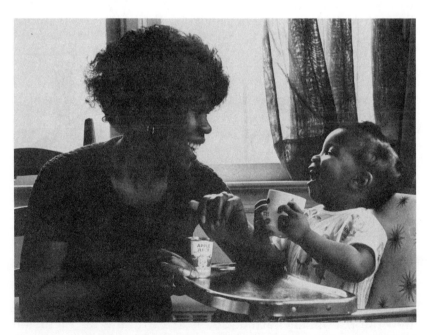

To avoid overfeeding, small servings can be given at first; a small additional serving can be given when the appetite is hearty.

The size of servings to use for babies will vary somewhat depending upon the size and age of the infant as well as upon the total variety and quantity of food planned for the day. The size of baby food containers may suggest that these foods are packaged in serving size. Actually, a considerably smaller serving often will be more appropriate for the baby. Again, the amount of food to serve needs to be gauged according to the infant's appetite and his rate of gain. As he grows, it is natural for a baby gradually to desire larger servings of all of the foods and his intake should be increased accordingly. One limitation does need to be imposed on his diet; the intake of milk should be limited to a quart (32 ounces) daily in order to leave room for the other foods needed for growth. His appetite can be sated by increasing the amounts of fruits, vegetables, and protein foods until he is satisfied.

JUNIOR FOODS AND TABLE FOOD

The form in which foods are served to a baby late in the first year varies from family to family. Most babies by about the age of ten months are ready for the commercial junior baby foods or for some foods from the family table. Chopped junior foods and soft table foods provide a new and important experience for babies as they approach this age. The textural changes provided by these foods present a gradual transition to the variety of textures present in the preschool child's diet.

With a bit of planning and care it is possible to change to table foods without the intermediate step of the junior foods. In many families this early introduction to table foods is a convenience because there is then only one menu to prepare for the entire family. If the baby is not yet eating according to the family meal schedule, it may be simpler for the mother to elect to use junior foods for three or four months.

Some adults may begin to feed babies soups late in the first year. These soups are not suitable replacements for servings of vegetables and meats, yet they often seem to be used in this manner. The practice may also be carried into the preschool period. Soups are suitable for inclusion when a child has a capacity that will enable him to eat meats, fruits, and vegetables, along with a small serving of soup.

Yet another use of commercial soup concentrates has been noted with concern. This is the feeding of the undiluted soup concentrate as a replacement for junior foods. Soup concentrates are quite high in salt and should not be used in undiluted form to provide a serving of food in the diet of young children.

A suggested pattern for feeding the infant approximately a year of age is as follows:

BREAKFAST	egg
	toast sticks
	milk
	cereal (if desired)
SNACK	orange juice
LUNCH	chopped liver
	green beans
	mashed potato
	milk
SNACK	small glass of milk
	enriched animal cookie
DINNER	cottage cheese
	carrots
	bread (if desired)
	banana
	milk

THE MEAL SETTING

Some of the problems that parents express regarding the feeding of the preschool child really stem from problems that begin to develop during the feeding of the child under a year of age. The mealtime environment for the baby needs to be considered carefully. Ideally, feeding time is a pleasant, sociable time for the infant, a time at which he gets to know his family better while enjoying the satisfaction of eating. The feeding situation should be as pleasant as possible and should seem neither hurried nor harried. If a baby is helped to adjust to a feeding schedule that fits in with the other demands of the family, mealtime usually will be a calm and pleasant time without hurry and confusion.

The feeding will proceed more smoothly if the room is reasonably quiet and if both participants are comfortable. Although they cannot understand what is said, babies respond to a warm voice and seem to enjoy some pleasant conversation; often they enjoy songs or some soft music in the background, just as adults like a quiet, pleasant atmosphere for eating.

The feeding of solid foods will be simpler and more comfortable for the child if suitable silver is used. A demitasse spoon works well for the first eight to ten months because it is sufficiently small to be comfortable in a young baby's mouth. Such a small spoon is not satisfactory, however, when the baby begins to feed himself. At that time a spoon with a slightly larger handle will be easier for the baby to manage.

The wise parent will be certain that these preceding conditions have been met and that the food is attractive in color and flavor combinations. Then people who may be with the baby at a meal will avoid urging him to keep eating when his interest begins to lag. This general urging of food is frequently the prelude to a regular pattern of conflict at meals; soon the baby begins to feel that he is eating for others rather than for himself, and eventually refusal to

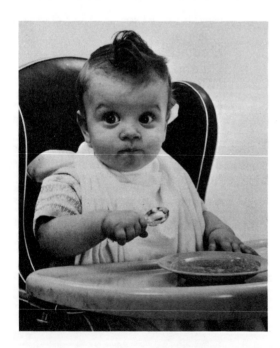

*Feeding oneself is
exciting when the spoon
and plate are designed
for small hands.*

eat may be used as a device to get his own way. The pattern can be prevented if a parent can feel relaxed about the quantity of food that is eaten at each meal and suppress any tendency to urge a child to eat when he has had all he wants. Healthy children, when they are allowed to select their own foods, will consume the necessary amount of food without being urged. Their appetites will show considerable variation from day to day, but this is normal and should not be of concern.

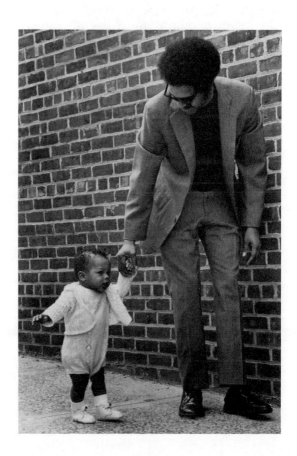

A well nourished baby will grow normally and develop the coordination and vigorous spirit needed to begin to explore the world.

SUMMARY

During the first year, infants will meet much of their nutritional need through breast feeding or a suitable formula. However, this is also the period when new experiences in texture and flavor may be introduced. The usual pattern is to add cereal to the diet by at least two months of age. The next additions will be pureed fruits and vegetables, followed by egg yolks and strained meats.

Attitudes toward food are being formed during this first year. This period has been identified as an important one to introduce variety in the diet without encouraging overeating. Attention should be given to avoiding development of overweight because this is the time when new fat cells are being formed. An excessive number of fat cells will make weight control more difficult throughout the remainder of life. Effort should be directed toward meeting nutritional needs and establishing a comfortable attitude toward food, an attitude that promotes enjoyment of food without placing undue emphasis on its role in life.

BIBLIOGRAPHY

Anderson, T.A. and S.J. Fomon, 1971. Commercially prepared infant cereals: nutritional considerations. *J. Pediat.* 78: 788.

Anderson, T.A. and S.J. Fomon, 1971. Commercially prepared strained and junior foods for infants. *J. Amer. Dietet. Assoc.* 58: 520.

Anonymous, 1970. Nutrition and cell growth. *Dairy Council Digest* 41, No. 6: 1.

Bakwin, H., 1961. The overuse of vitamins in children. *J. Pediat.* 59: 154.

Beal, V.A., 1961. Dietary intake of individuals followed through infancy and childhood. *Amer. J. Pub. Health* 51: 1107.

Caddell, J.L., 1965. Magnesium in the therapy of protein-calorie malnutrition of childhood. *J. Pediat.* 66: 392.

Committee on Nutrition, American Academy of Pediatrics, 1965. Vitamin D intake and the hypercalcemic syndrome. *Pediat.* 35: 1022.

Darby, W.J., 1964. The rational use of vitamins in medical practice. *Med. Clin. N. Amer.* 48: 1203.

Davis, C.M., 1964. Self selection of diets by newly weaned infants. *Amer. J. Dis. Children* 46: 743.

Fomon, S.J., 1971. Pediatrician looks at early nutrition. *Bull. N.Y. Acad. Med.* 47: 569.

Fomon, S.J., 1974. *Infant Nutrition*, 2nd ed. Saunders. Philadelphia.

Fomon, S.J. and T.A. Anderson, 1972. *Practices of Low-Income Families in Feeding Infants and Small Children with Particular Attention to Cultural Subgroups.* U.S. Dept. of Health, Education, and Welfare. Health Services and Medical Health Administration. Maternal and Child Health Service. Rockville, Md.

Fomon, S.J., et al., 1970. Acceptance of unsalted strained foods by normal infants. *J. Pediat.* 76: 242.

Greenwaldt, E., et al., 1960. The onset of sleeping through the night in infancy: relation to introduction of solid food in the diet, birth weight and position in the family. *Pediat.* 26: 667.

Hirsch, J., et al., 1960. Studies of adipose tissue in man. *Amer. J. Clin. Nutr.* 8: 499.

Hulme, J.M., 1966. Some observations on infant feeding. *Nutr.* 20 (Summer): 50.

Jelliffe, D.B., 1962. Culture, social changes and infant feeding: Current trends in tropical regions. *Amer. J. Clin. Nutr.* 10: 19.

Knittle, J.L., 1972. Obesity in childhood: Problems in adipose tissue cellular development. *J. Pediat.* 81: 1048.

Knittle, J.L. and J. Hirsch, 1968. Effect of early nutrition on development of rat epididymal fat pad: Cellularity and metabolism. *J. Clin. Invest.* 47: 2091.

Mayer, J., 1969. Physical activity and food intake in infants, children, and adolescents. In *Nutrition in Preschool and School Age.* Ed., G. Blix. p. 92. Swedish Nutrition Foundation. Uppsala.

Meyer, H.F., 1960. *Infant Foods and Feeding Practice.* Thomas. Springfield, Ill.

Nutrition Foundation, 1967. Solid foods in the nutrition of young infants. *Nutr. Reviews* 25: 233.

Nutrition Foundation, 1973. Overfeeding in the first year of life. *Nutr. Reviews* 31: 116.

Purvis, G.A., 1973. What nutrients do our infants really get? *Nutr. Today* 8, No. 5: 28.

Puyau, F.A. and L.P. Hampton, 1966. Infant feeding practices, 1966: Salt content of modern diets. *Amer. J. Dis. Child* 111: 370.

Roe, D.A., 1966. Nutrient toxicity with excessive intake. I: Vitamins. *N.Y. State J. Med.* 66: 869.

Shank, R.E., 1965. Is there a need to fortify infant foods? Amer. J. Pub. Health 55: 1188.

Smith, C.A., 1960. Overuse of milk in the diets of infants and children. *J. Amer. Med. Assoc.* 172: 567.

Smith, N.J., 1972. *Challenge of Obesity*. Ross Laboratories. Columbus, Ohio.

Stern, J.S. and M.R.C. Greenwood, 1974. Review of development of adipose cellularity in man and animals. *Fed. Proc.* 33: 1952.

Whitten, C.F., 1972. TLC and hungry child. *Nutr. Today* 7, No. 1: 10.

Winick, M., 1974. Childhood obesity. *Nutr. Today* 9, No. 3: 6.

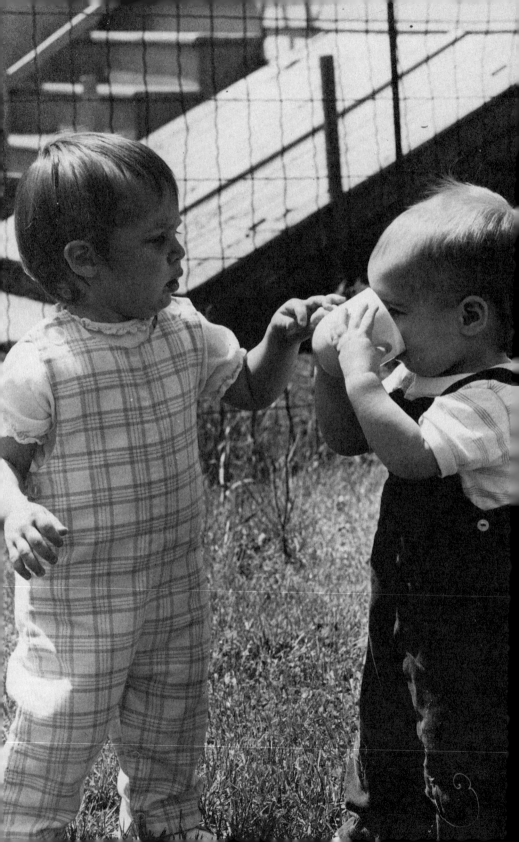

Chapter 7
Preschool Children

From the age of a year until school age is a formative period in the development of a person's food habits. Some distinct changes begin to take place at approximately the age of a year or a little later, for this is the time when babies graduate from baby foods to table foods; formulas and bottles are discarded in favor of milk from a cup; and self-feeding becomes the youngster's delight (and sometimes the mother's despair). Many children become regulars at the family's meals soon after the age of a year. This period of transition can proceed very smoothly if one understands and adjusts to the changing dietary needs.

CHANGING PATTERNS

Probably the greatest concern of most mothers is the reduced food intake of the typical one-year-old. The child who may have been ravenous during his first year may develop a diminutive appetite soon after his first birthday. These changes assume monumental significance to some mothers and become the cause of feeding conflicts.

One of the chief reasons for this change in food patterns is that, although growth continues, the rate of growth becomes somewhat slower; consequently, nutritional demands do not increase at as fast a rate as they did during the first year. Therefore it really is not surprising that a child who has previously had a very large appetite will rather suddenly begin to eat less food. When one observes this natural change taking place, there is no reason to be alarmed, but there is reason to be particularly careful about the foods being eaten so the total nutrient intake will be adequate.

NUTRITIONAL NEEDS OF THE PRESCHOOLER

Even when the growth rate decelerates in the second year, there is a continuing need for a well-balanced diet that supplies the nutrients required for growth and maintenance (Table 7.1). Notice that the recommended allowances for calories, protein, vitamin A, the B vitamins (folacin, niacin, riboflavin, thiamin, vitamin B_6, and vitamin B_{12}), and ascorbic acid gradually increase throughout the preschool period. These increases reflect the gradual growth in body size during this period. Diet at this time is important not only to achieve optimum growth and development, but also to instill basically sound dietary habits for life.

The wise parent will continue to use the Basic Four Food Plan (milk and dairy products, meat and fish, fruits and vegetables, and breads and cereals) as the basis for planning the child's meals during the preschool period. This plan, although basically the same as that outlined in Chapter 4, should be considered with the development of the young preschooler in mind.

Milk continues to be an important source of calcium and phosphorus for bones and teeth formation. The need for these minerals continues despite the normal slowing of growth rate during the preschool period. Since considerable emphasis has been given to the importance of milk during the first year of life and, indeed throughout childhood, most parents in the United States are aware of the importance of milk in the diets of their children, but they may be uncertain about the amount needed. It is generally recommended that the preschool child between the ages of one and five should consume a minimum of two cups of milk per day, and preferably the intake should be approximately three cups. The value of milk, however, should not be magnified out of proportion; it does not mean that milk should occupy the major part of the diet at the expense of other foods.

The second group, the meat group, is of particular importance to the preschool child; special consideration in this group needs to be given to the problems of the one- to two-year-old child because of his difficulty in chewing the meats that might be regular family fare. Usually by the age of two, or certainly by the age of three, the average child will be able to chew most meats that are served at the table, but it

Table 7.1 Recommended daily dietary allowances for preschool children[a]

Nutrient	Recommended Allowance for Child:	
	Age 1–3	Age 4–6
Weight, kg. (lb.)	13 (28)	20 (44)
Height, cm. (in.)	86 (34)	110 (44)
Energy, kcal.	1300	1800
Protein, g.	23	30
Vitamin A, I.U.	2000	2500
Vitamin D, I.U.	400	400
Vitamin E activity, I.U.	7	9
Ascorbic acid, mg.	40	40
Folacin, μg.	100	200
Niacin, mg.	9	12
Riboflavin, mg.	0.8	1.1
Thiamin, mg.	0.7	0.9
Vitamin B_6, mg.	0.6	0.9
Vitamin B_{12}, μg.	1.0	1.5
Calcium, mg.	800	800
Phosphorus, mg.	800	800
Iodine, μg.	60	80
Iron, mg.	15	10
Magnesium, mg.	150	200
Zinc, mg.	10	10

[a]From the 1974 revision of the daily dietary allowances as recommended by the Food and Nutrition Board of the National Research Council, National Academy of Sciences.

is the younger child who sometimes will receive an inadequate amount of meat when he is fed at the family table.

The amount of meat has been recommended as two servings for the food plan, but actually, how large is a serving of meat for the preschool child? Although the specific amount that is needed will vary from one child to the other, a serving size equal to one tablespoon of the food for each year of life is a workable guideline. Thus an appropriate serving of meat for the average two-year-old child will be two tablespoons of meat, while four tablespoons is average for the four-year-old. This, as indicated, is intended to serve only as a guideline. Larger servings may be provided for children who are growing rapidly or are very active. Servings of meat that are particularly desirable for the preschool child include such items as sauteed strips of liver, hamburgers, meat loaf, lightly seasoned luncheon meats, tender steaks, well-done pot roast, or any other type of meat that is chewed easily. Fish is excellent for young children if care has been taken to remove all bones. The main thing to consider when planning meats for this age child is that the meat be tender enough so that the child with few teeth can chew the meat and enjoy having meat in his meal. Eggs and cheese are other rich protein sources that are particularly useful during this period.

The third food group, the fruit and vegetable group, should number four or more servings per day including the specified serving of a fruit high in ascorbic acid and a vegetable high in vitamin A on alternate days. Again, the suggested size of these servings can follow the rule of thumb previously stated, namely that a serving consists of a tablespoon of the food for each year of age. The four-year-old child thus would consider one-fourth cup of carrots (four tablespoons) as a serving of vegetable.

Fruits and vegetables need to be prepared by methods which make them easy for a child to chew. For example, carrot sticks and crisp, unpeeled apples are difficult for the one-year-old child to chew easily and there is some danger of choking; cooked carrots or apple sauce are easily managed, however. Uncooked fruits such as bananas or peeled ripe peaches and cooked vegetables of most any type are all appropriate for even the rather young child in this group. The more chewy fruits and vegetables should be added as more teeth erupt; most children can manage any fruit or vegetable by the age of four. It is easy to drift into the habit of serving only soft fruits and vegetables and to perpetuate such practices as peeling apples, but it is wise to gradually increase the chewy foods as the chewing ability increases. Otherwise some children become so accustomed to a soft diet that they may develop a block against eating crisp or chewy foods.

A definite effort should be made to expand the young child's familiarity with a wide selection of fruits and vegetables during the preschool period in order to capitalize on the interest that young children feel in the world about them. If a breadth of tastes, textures, and color experiences with fruits and vegetables is introduced during the formative years, most children will develop a wide range of food preferences that will provide pleasure to them as they grow older. With a reasonable expenditure of effort, fruits and vegetables can be prepared in a variety of ways to add considerable interest to the menu of the preschool child. Imagination in the preparation of these foods is well rewarded.

The bread and cereal group requirement is four or more servings per day, as it is for all other age groups. It is not difficult usually to meet this recommendation for the preschool child because most of the foods in this group are easily chewed, well accepted by the child, and easily prepared. Perhaps the acceptance and utilization of this particular food group is greater than any of the other food groups for the preschool child. In fact, it may be necessary to curtail the intake of these foods because some children will eat bread and related products to the exclusion of other foods needed in the diet.

Now let's look at the actual nutritional needs of the child and see how these are met by the Basic Four Food Plan

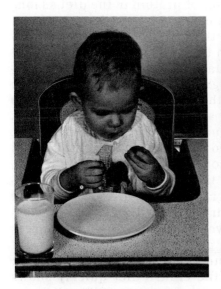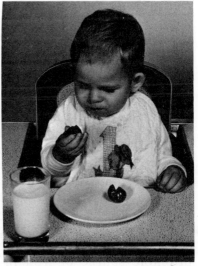

Armed with one cherry tomato in each hand, this one-year old boy carefully examines the strange food. The new food tastes different from anything he knows, but he did try a bite of each tomato. Next time he may eat a whole one.

(Table 7.1). One of the nutrients of greatest concern during this period is protein. The preschool child is building muscle tissue, and optimum development of muscle tissue can occur only with an adequate supply of protein. The amount of protein that is recommended for the preschool child is divided into the age group from one to three and the group from four to six. The recommended allowance for the average child in the former group is 23 grams and for the latter group, the four to six-year-olds, is approximately 30 grams.

These figures become more meaningful when they are interpreted in terms of the recommended food intake in the Basic Four Food Plan. Since an 8-ounce serving of milk provides approximately 8 grams of protein per glass, the child who is drinking two glasses (16 ounces) receives 16 grams of protein from the dairy group. If he eats an egg as one of his servings in the meat group, another 6 grams of protein are provided by the egg. A serving of meat usually will provide at least 10 grams of protein. These figures total 32 grams of protein for two glasses of milk per day, and the child drinking three glasses of milk per day receives about 40 grams of protein. Clearly, it is not difficult to include an adequate amount of protein in the diet as long as the Basic Four Food Plan is being followed.

Studies also have shown that one pint of milk per day produces adequate growth in the normal, healthy preschool child who is eating a well-balanced diet. It should be understood here that a child who is growing at a faster than average rate might need more than the minimum suggestion of two glasses of milk per day, but apparently three cups of milk per day are certainly adequate for children of this age.

The amount of iron needed by the preschool child is still a matter of discussion among nutritionists. The recommended allowance of iron in this age group is 10 to 15 milligrams per day. Fifteen milligrams of iron are recommended for the child from one to three; 10 milligrams are recommended for the four to six-year-old child. Dietary sources of iron are necessary for the growing child despite the fact that the body conserves and reuses iron. A look at the probable source of iron in the child's diet quickly shows that the recommended amounts of iron are difficult to include in the menu. For instance, a serving of meat usually contains a maximum of 3 milligrams of iron, and an egg, the yolk of which is a good source of iron, provides less than 2 milligrams.

When the preceding values are compared with the recommended servings of these "iron-rich" foods in the Basic Four Food Plan, it becomes apparent that most children are not receiving the recommended amount of iron, and yet these children frequently do not show iron-deficiency symptoms. There are two plausible explanations for the failure to develop an iron deficiency on a seemingly inadequate diet. One is that the child who has little iron in the diet, but who has need for iron in his body, will tend to utilize the iron in the food that is offered more efficiently than he will if he has a large amount of iron available in the diet. Second, it appears that the child, as he approaches the age of a year, actually has adequate storage deposits of iron in his body as a result of eating the various iron-fortified baby foods during his first year of life. Therefore it would be possible for him to continue to draw on these stores of body iron until they are depleted, and he would not immediately show the iron-deficiency condition that slowly may be building up in his body.

The potential problem of iron deficiency can also be countered by continuing the daily use of breakfast cereals fortified with iron. An iron supplement is another alternative if other measures are not adequate.

Fluoride is a very important mineral in the diet because of its protective role in reducing the incidence of dental caries. Well controlled studies, including the classic study conducted in Newburgh and Kingston, New York, have demonstrated that fluoridation of city water supplies is an effective measure in helping to protect against caries if the fluoride is available during the early period of life. In the case of the deciduous teeth, fluoride should be available from birth throughout the early years. To gain maximum protection for the permanent teeth, fluoride needs to be present in the diet by at least the age of two.

The most practical way to provide fluoride is to fluoridate the city water supply (or use fluoridated bottled water) so that any water children consume will contain this important mineral. The level of fluoride recommended for fluoridation of water is 1 ppm, i.e., 1 part fluoride per million parts of water. This level has been shown to be sufficient to provide

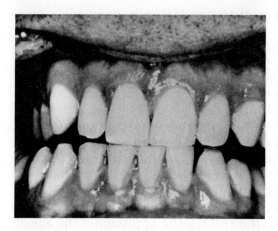

Fluoridated water during the early years is an aid in reducing the incidence of dental carries. This 44-year-old man drank water with a fluoride content of 1 ppm in childhood. He has no decayed, missing, or filled teeth.

the desired protection and is well below the level that can cause mottling of teeth. Before any mottling will occur, the level would have to be at least 2 ppm. Actually, mottling will only occur if high levels of fluoride are available regularly at the time that the tooth is forming and before it erupts. Once a tooth has erupted, fluoride will continue to be deposited in the enamel matrix as fluorapatite. The incorporation of fluoride in enamel crystals results in somewhat larger, well shaped crystals that are quite resistant to acid.

Some communities have not elected to fluoridate their water supplies. Children in these communities should be given fluoride by some alternative means. This can be done by topical applications of fluoride by dentists, using fluoride-containing toothpastes, or fluoride drops or lozenges. For children younger than three, 0.5 milligrams of fluoride ion per day will provide a suitable protective effect. After age three, the level should be increased to 1.0 milligrams per day. When a child is old enough to suck on a lozenge, this is the preferred way of administering the fluoride because the lozenge bathes the teeth in the fluoride as well as permitting some of the fluoride to be absorbed in the system.

IMPROVING FOOD INTAKE

Food Preparation

We have taken some time to look at the particular foods that are recommended for the young child, but recommendations and actual intake all too often may be two different

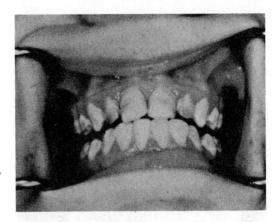

The mottling of these teeth was the result of prolonged consumption of water containing fluoride at 5.5 ppm, a level five times greater than the amount recommended.

sets of figures. It is not enough simply to know what a child should eat. It is also necessary to examine the factors that may influence achievement of optimum nutrition. It may seem hard to realize this, but the young child often is a reasonably good judge of the quality of foods served to him. Therefore, even though he is eating a meal separately prepared for him rather than eating at the family table, it still is important that the food be prepared carefully. The food that is served should have an attractive appearance, a mild aroma, and taste appeal for the child.

Most children are highly experimental at this age; they will be very much interested in trying new food flavors and enjoying the flavors and textures of different foods. Parents can capitalize on this interest by expanding the child's experience while his mind is wide open and receptive to the new foods being offered. The preparation of food should be geared toward maintaining or achieving maximum color and beauty. It is certainly more inviting to serve a highly colorful food than one that has no particular color appeal.

Vegetables. This matter of color coupled with texture is one reason that vegetables may sometimes become a bit of a problem during this preschool period. Vegetables, as they naturally occur, are perhaps one of the most colorful food groups that we have. They are certainly more attractive in color than meats, and yet there is much less talk about problems with meat acceptance than there is about acceptance of vegetables. To resolve this, it may be necessary to look a little more carefully at vegetables as they actually are served to the child, for vegetables rapidly lose their

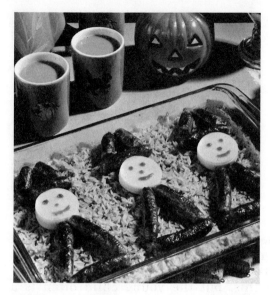

This Halloween main dish of rice, sausage links, and cheese rounds creates a festive atmosphere. Even if a child is not acquainted with these foods, he probably will want to sample this.

color appeal through poor cooking practices. The tendency to overcook vegetables seems to be a general habit. Probably the green vegetables suffer the most in the kitchen; when they are overcooked, the attractive, natural green color gradually changes to a drab, yellow-green that is much less inviting to the child (and also to adults).

Not only does prolonged cooking change the color of a green vegetable, but it also has a harmful effect on the texture of any vegetable. The soft, mushy vegetable that results from overcooking has little feel in the mouth other than a very smooth mass. Remember that the baby has been eating very soft foods since early infancy. There is considerably more interest in eating a vegetable that has texture characteristics different from the smoothness of the baby foods. Vegetables cooked just until they lose crispness and begin to soften provide a distinctly more interesting texture than a very mushy vegetable.

Proper cooking of vegetables not only ensures color appeal and a more interesting texture, but also it improves the aroma and flavor. When vegetables are overcooked, both flavor and aroma are adversely affected. Vegetables with cabbage-like flavors (cabbage, Brussels sprouts, cauliflower, and broccoli) gradually will develop stronger and stronger flavors and odors with extended cooking. Although these vegetables are often well accepted by the preschool group when properly cooked, it is not unusual to find less enthusiastic acceptance when they are overcooked. The strong flavors and aromas of the overcooked vegetables frequently repel rather than attract. In contrast, some of the mild-flavored vegetables such as carrots will be poorly accepted when overcooked because their flavor becomes too weak. Mild flavor and aroma are gradually lost with extended cooking time. Vegetables will be tempting when cooked just until they can be cut easily.

A few suggestions on cooking will make it easier to prepare vegetables that are enjoyed by the young child as well as by the older members of the family. Green vegetables retain their color best if they are cooked in an uncovered pan. This helps to retain the bright green color that is so appealing in these vegetables. Strong-flavored vegetables have a milder, more pleasing flavor if they are cooked without a cover, for some of the strong flavoring substances will escape from the uncovered pan while the vegetables are boiling.

In order to retain the maximum amount of the water-soluble vitamins in boiled vegetables, it is usually wise to use a relatively small amount of water so that the vitamin loss in the cooking water will be minimized. Ordinarily, vegetables should be boiled in just enough water to bubble up over the vegetable. In the strong-flavored vegetables, such as those in the cabbage family, however, the flavor is improved when it is weakened by boiling the vegetables in enough water to extend about one-half inch above the vegetable.

The preceding recommendations for vegetable cookery are designed to gain wide acceptance of vegetables. They are based on the premise that food left on the plate provides no nourishment for the child even though it may contain many needed vitamins and minerals. In vegetable cookery it is prudent occasionally to sacrifice a bit of the vitamin content in order to achieve greater palatability and acceptance.

Fruits. Fruits require less comment and preparation, partially because children often consume raw fruits. Fresh fruits generally are a little softer than vegetables and are more easily chewed by the young child. A possible exception to this is skin on an apple, which might present a chewing problem to the young preschooler. Occasionally adults get in the habit of peeling apples for young children and forget to break the habit as the child grows older. It certainly is true that an apple is less nourishing when it is peeled, because the peeling is an excellent source of the vitamins in the fruit. Therefore, as soon as the child has adequate teeth to chew the skin of the apple, it is no longer necessary or appropriate to continue peeling the fruit.

Meat. Preparation of meat for the young child is quite simple, but the chewing difficulties of the younger child (one to three) in the preschool age group should be considered when planning menus. Pot roast or flank steak, which may sound like rather chewy pieces of meat, actually can be prepared so that they are perfectly suitable for the very young child. It is important, however, that the cooking time for all less tender cuts be sufficient to adequately tenderize the meat. Otherwise, if chewing problems are too great, the child gets tired of chewing and loses interest in his meal before he has had an opportunity to consume the amounts that he needs.

Meats have the most pleasing flavor and the greatest tenderness if they are cooked carefully at reasonably low temperatures. The less tender cuts of meats require long periods of slow cooking in a covered pan with moisture added. The trapped steam slowly converts some of the tough connective tissue into gelatin, which obviously makes the meat easier to chew. It should be pointed out that the liquid for cooking these meats does not always need to be water. Pleasing tastes and color changes can be accomplished by using other liquids such as fruit juices, tomato juice, or occasionally sour cream to provide variety in the meat course of a meal.

Milk. In most instances milk is consumed as the liquid beverage. Various food products made with milk, however, can be useful in increasing the milk consumption of children who tend to drink inadequate amounts of milk. Cream soups, usually popular with children, may be varied by using different vegetables. One of the favorite foods of many children is pudding. Puddings contain a large amount of milk and therefore are an excellent dessert choice. If egg yolk is added to the pudding, the dessert is called a cream pudding and is still more nourishing than the plain cornstarch pudding. Ice cream and custards are two other possible foods that are high in milk and are well accepted by the preschool child.

Meals for the Day

A particularly effective means of increasing or satisfactorily meeting the nutritional needs of the child each day is the maintenance of a reasonable schedule of meals. This schedule need not be completely inflexible, but it should be sufficiently rigid to provide security to the child and aid him in establishing practical dietary habits. Appetites at meals usually are best when a fairly regular interval is maintained between meals.

Most families find that it is sensible to have a good breakfast in the morning. The preschool child usually has had a long night's sleep and is quite hungry within half an hour after he wakens. At this time a well-planned and carefully prepared breakfast should be prepared for the child. A suitable breakfast might include: a glass of orange juice, a bowl of cereal, one soft-cooked egg, and a glass of milk.

If breakfast has been eaten at 7:00 or 8:00 in the morning, the preschool child frequently will feel hungry and perhaps a bit tired and irritable between 9:30 and 10:30. A snack is appropriate when these signs appear. This snack in the middle of the morning need not, in fact should not, be large. A small glass of fruit juice or milk is suitable; other good possibilities are fresh fruit or a slice of cheese. This mid-morning snack should be nourishing, but should be small enough so that the child is hungry for lunch, which should be a well-balanced meal. If a child's appetite is poor at meals, snacks should be reduced or even eliminated to improve consumption at meals.

Usually by noon the preschool child is hungry for a good lunch, such as a grilled cheese sandwich, broccoli, apple wedges, and a glass of milk. If he is still hungry, a piece of sponge cake may be added for dessert. A satisfying lunch sets the stage for a nap or rest time.

One of the happy traditions in many homes is a light snack after the afternoon nap. This is a particularly nice time to have a little party with the preschooler. For most children the afternoon snack should provide the lift needed to maintain a comfortable feeling till dinner, but should not inter-

fere with the appetite for dinner. A suitable afternoon
snack might be a small serving of gelatin with fruit in it.

Dinner in the evening may or may not be with the family,
depending on the scheduling problems of the various family
members. The preschool child is usually ready for supper by
5:30 or 6:00. This should be a complete meal and might
include: meat loaf, baked potato, buttered carrots, sliced
tomato, and a glass of milk. Dessert may be served if a child
is still hungry when he has finished the main course.
Desserts, however, are not always necessary or desirable.

The foregoing suggestions for a typical day's meals and
snacks are summarized below:

BREAKFAST	orange juice
	cereal
	soft-cooked egg
	milk
SNACK	milk
LUNCH	grilled cheese sandwich
	broccoli
	apple wedges
	sponge cake (optional)
SNACK	gelatin with fruit
DINNER	meat loaf
	baked potato
	buttered carrots
	slice of tomato
	milk

Meals for the preschool child should be scheduled at
times when he is hungry, but should not be delayed until
he becomes so tired and hungry that he loses his appetite.
It is far better for the preschool child to have an early supper at 5:00 or 5:30 when he is hungry than it is to stall him
with crackers and have him eat with the family at 8:00 at
night. Sometimes it is practical to feed the preschooler an
early dinner and then serve him a light snack with the rest
of the family.

Families who get up either earlier or later than the average family can easily shift the times suggested for this meal pattern. The time spacing that has been suggested, however, is typical for the preschool child and could be followed with reasonable variations to fit the individual family.

Physical Arrangements

The physical arrangements for feeding the preschool child need to be considered rather carefully if one is to establish good eating habits at this age. Usually the preschooler will be eating at least one meal with the family. The sociability of family meals can be of great value to the developing child. To the rest of the family, however, the presence of the youngster may be less than enjoyable unless the physical setup is designed to enable the young child to fit into the group easily.

There is nothing much more annoying and chaotic than to have milk spilled regularly at each meal. It is apparent that glass design is one of the obvious features to consider in planning for the child at the table. Since the young child's hand is rather small, it is sensible to give him a small glass that fits comfortably into his hand rather than expecting him to manage the large glasses used by the adult members of the family. Fewer spills usually occur if a glass has a weighted bottom so that the full glass tips less readily. It will be easier for a child to handle a glass that is filled only half way rather than giving him a full glass each time. This practice also helps to avoid the spills that happen when he tips up the glass for a drink before the glass reaches his lips. A small pitcher of milk at the table is convenient for refills.

The table arrangements for young children should be relatively simple, yet attractive, and the chairs should be designed for comfort at the table. If adults had to eat a meal with their feet hanging in mid-air, they would soon realize the discomfort a child feels when he is on a chair that is too high for him. The preschooler's ideal chair should meet two criteria: (1) it is the proper height for him to comfortably reach the table, and (2) it has a foot rest in a convenient position so that his feet will not dangle in space. Well-designed junior chairs meet these requirements.

Silverware should be designed and sized with the young child in mind. Since a salad fork is smaller than a dinner fork, salad forks often are provided for the preschooler's convenience. Junior silverware sets are usually a very comfortable size for the preschool child to use.

Generally it is easier when the young child is at the table if the plates are served in the kitchen or if the table is arranged so that it is not necessary to pass foods across and in front of the youngster. This distraction often will provide too much confusion at the table for the young child and interest will be shifted from his own plate to the general group at the table.

Manners

When a child is comfortable at the table and is served a well-planned meal that is tastefully prepared, it would seem that he would be well nourished. Unfortunately this is not always true because of interactions within the family. The social environment at the table should be one of pleasure and pleasant conversation rather than a time for family arguments and tirades.

When the young child begins to eat with the family, his manners certainly will not be perfect, but it is important that he be accepted as a family member and not be singled out for constant criticism over his table manners. This does not mean that a child should be totally ignored in his eating habits, but these habits can be trained slowly. The important thing when a child first joins the family at meals is that he learn to eat the food that is served at the table and to enjoy the family fellowship. Refinements of manners can come as the family meal routine becomes a little less stimulating than it is when the child first begins to join the family at the table.

PITFALLS IN FEEDING THE PRESCHOOLER

Variable Appetite

The typical preschool child will have days when he eats quite a large amount of food and on other days his food intake will be surprisingly small in comparison with the average intake. An examination of the food eaten by Charlie during two consecutive days (Table 7.2) illustrates this point.

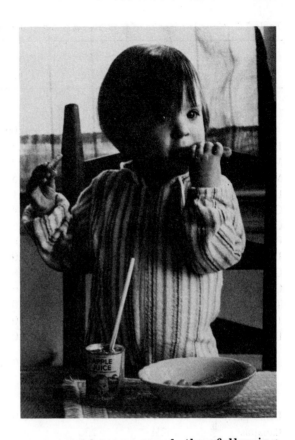

Pleasure in eating a good breakfast is of primary importance; table manners are developed gradually.

Charlie, a typical one-year-old, consumed the following foods on the first day:

BREAKFAST	9:00	2 tbsp. applesauce
		1½ bananas
		½ slice toast with jam
		8 oz. milk
SNACK	10:15	1 marshmallow
SNACK	11:30	8 oz. milk
SNACK	12:30	1 doughnut
LUNCH	1:30	1 slice bread
		1 slice corned beef
		1 egg omelet
		¼ cucumber

Table 7.2   Charlie's intake of food over a two-day period

Food	Measure	Calories	Protein g.	Calcium, mg.	Iron, mg.
		First Day			
Apple sauce	2 tbsp.	23	0.06	1.0	0.1
Bananas	5½	484	6.6	44.0	0.33
Marshmallow	1	22	0.2	0.0	0.0
Milk	40 oz.	830	42.5	1440.0	1.0
Doughnut	1	136	2.1	23.0	0.2
Corned beef	1 slice	37	3.4	8.0	0.4
Cucumber	¼	12	0.8	10.0	0.4
Potato salad	¼ cup	25	0.6	3.5	0.2
Lamb roast	1 slice	115	10.0	0.5	1.3
Omelet	1 egg	106	6.8	50.0	1.3
Cupcake	1	161	2.6	58.0	0.2
Toast	½ slice	31	1.0	9.0	0.2
Jam	1 tsp.	18	0.03	0.6	0.03
Bread	1 slice	63	2.0	18.0	0.4
Totals		*2063*	*79.69*	*1665.6*	*6.06*
		Second Day			
Lamb patty	½ med.	178	10.0	5.0	1.15
Bananas	2½	220	3.0	10.0	2.2
Milk	10 oz.	208	10.5	360.0	0.3
Apple juice	4 oz.	62	0.1	8.0	0.6
Marshmallows	3	65	0.06	0.0	0.0
Chicken sticks	4	95	12.5	7.0	0.8
Pudding, banana	½ cup	141	6.1	141.0	0.6
Noodle casserole	½ cup	53	1.9	3.0	0.4
Toast	½ slice	31	1.0	9.0	0.2
Totals		*1053*	*32.16*	*543.0*	*6.25*

Table 7.2 (Continued)

Vitamin A, I.U.	Thiamin, mg.	Riboflavin, mg.	Niacin, mg.	Ascorbic Acid, mg.
		First Day		
10	0.006	0.004	0.01	0.4
2365	0.22	0.25	0.385	55.0
0	0.0	0.0	0.0	0.0
1950	0.45	2.1	1.5	15.0
40	0.05	0.04	0.4	0.0
Tr.	0.007	0.045	0.7	0.0
0	0.04	0.04	0.2	8.0
5	0.03	0.01	0.3	4.0
0	0.06	0.11	2.2	0.0
640	0.05	0.17	Tr.	0.0
50	0.01	0.04	0.1	0.0
0	0.02	0.02	0.25	0.0
Tr.	Tr.	Tr.	Tr.	0.3
0	0.06	0.04	0.5	0.0
5055	*1.003*	*2.869*	*6.045*	*82.7*
		Second Day (continued)		
0	0.07	0.08	2.3	0
0	0.07	0.17	4.0	0
488	0.10	0.52	0.4	4
45	0.025	0.035	Tr.	1
0	0.0	0.0	0.0	0
0	0.02	0.08	2.4	0
420	0.06	0.25	0.1	0.5
30	0.11	0.05	0.8	0
0	0.02	0.02	0.25	0
983	*0.475*	*1.205*	*10.25*	*5.5*

SNACK	3:30	8 oz. milk
SNACK	6:00	8 oz. milk 1 banana
DINNER	6:30	1 slice lamb roast ¼ cup potato salad 2 bananas
SNACK	8:30	8 oz. milk 1 banana 1 cupcake

The following day Charlie's appetite was considerably smaller and his menu included:

BREAKFAST	9:30	½ lamb patty 1½ bananas ½ slice white enriched toast 6 oz. milk
LUNCH	12:30	1 banana 4 baby chicken sticks 4 oz. apple juice
SNACK	5:00	3 marshmallows
DINNER	6:30	½ cup beef and egg noodle casserole ½ cup banana pudding 4 oz. milk

Of particular interest is a comparison of the caloric intake for the two days (Table 7.3) for it dramatically reflects the variability in a child's appetite at this age. The average caloric intake for the two days is higher than the recommendation. The fact that Charlie is a little too heavy for his height (34 pounds and 33 inches) indicates that this average caloric excess is probably typical of his eating pattern. Charlie's nutritional status could be improved by giving more careful attention to menu planning and by feeding him his dinner earlier. The use of cupcakes, marsh-

Table 7.3 Comparison of Charlie's intake with the allowances recommended
for the one-year-old child

Intake	First Day	Second Day	Recommended Allowances[a]
Calories	2063	1053	1300
Protein, g.	79.69	32.16	23
Calcium, mg.	1665.6	543	800
Iron, mg.	6.06	6.25	15
Vitamin A, I.U.	5055	983	2000
Thiamin, mg.	1.003	0.475	0.7
Riboflavin, mg.	2.869	1.205	0.8
Niacin, mg.	6.045	10.25	9
Ascorbic acid, mg.	82.7	5.5	40

[a]From the 1974 revision of the daily dietary allowances as recommended by the Food and Nutrition Board of the National Research Council, National Academy of Sciences.

mallows, and doughnuts should be curbed and a wider variety of fruits and vegetables introduced. It is not necessary, however, to try to get Charlie to eat the same amount of food each day for this would focus too much attention on food and might cause Charlie to become a "problem eater."

A quick look at Charlie's menu also shows that children sometimes do go on food jags; bananas seem to play a significant role in Charlie's list of food likes at this time. Such food jags usually are short-lived and fade as quickly as they appear. To a point, it is all right to indulge these whims, but it is still important that a child eat a variety of foods each day in order to be well nourished.

His low intake of iron should be corrected, preferably by adding an iron-fortified cereal. Also, ascorbic acid needs to be available daily since it is not stored well in the body.

Indulgence in Snacks

Examination of a couple of day's menus in the life of Karen, a two-year-old child, quickly reveals some of the problems that are common at this age when snacks are large and mealtimes erratic. In this particular example the problem was compounded because Karen was visiting relatives on one of the days, but the pattern tended to persist at home also. Karen's menu the first day was as follows:

SNACK	8:30	6 potato chips 2 candy cigarettes (given to her by her aunt)

BREAKFAST	9:30	1 egg and cheese omelet
		1 piece cheese
		¼ piece toast (white enriched
		  bread) with jam and pea-
		  nut butter
		4 oz. milk

SNACK	12:00	5 marshmallows
LUNCH	1:30	2 all-beef frankfurters 2 baby all-meat franks (taken from her brother) ½ dill pickle
SNACK	4:00	4 marshmallows 4 oz. apple juice
DINNER	6:30	½ lamb taco ½ cheese enchilada 2 tbsp. green salad 2 scoops vanilla ice cream
SNACK	8:45	3 marshmallows 2 oz. milk

The menu for the second day, which was spent at home, again indicates Karen's tendency to consume excessively large quantities of food low in nutrients and high in calories. The day's menu included:

BREAKFAST	9:00	¼ sliced banana ½ slice toast with jam 1 bowl cold cereal with milk 4 oz. milk
SNACK	10:15	4 marshmallows

SNACK	12:30	1 doughnut
LUNCH	1:30	1 slice corned beef
		½ slice white enriched bread
		1 egg omelet
		1 dill pickle
		¼ cucumber
		4 oz. milk
		2 pieces candy
SNACK	3:30	1 small piece celery
SNACK	4:00	2 pieces candy
DINNER	5:30	¼ cup potato salad
		2 small slices lamb roast
		½ tomato
		2 oz. milk
		1 scoop vanilla ice cream
SNACK	8:30	2 cupcakes

Tables 7.4 and 7.5 summarize the nutrients included in Karen's two-day diet. Karen is consuming more calories than she actually needs, yet she is not consistently meeting the recommended allowances for her age group. To overcome possible shortages of nutrients, she should eat more fruits and vegetables. Attention should be given to including a food high in ascorbic acid each day and an adequate source of iron. To promote good dental health and to avoid excessive weight gain, it would be wise to reduce markedly the amounts of candy in Karen's diet and increase the consumption of milk, fruits, and vegetables. The dietary patterns Karen is establishing as a preschooler are likely to persist unless she is helped to change them during this formative period.

Another area of concern when dietary patterns, such as the one revealed by Karen, develop is that there is an increased likelihood of developing dental caries. Carbohydrates, particularly sucrose, promote the formation of dental plaque by serving as food for *Streptococcus mitis*. These microorganisms convert dietary carbohydrates into glycogen-like polysaccharides which constitute a part of

Table 7.4   *Karen's food intake for two days*

Food	Measure	Calories	Protein, g.	Calcium, mg.	Iron, mg.
		First Day			
Potato chips	6 large	100	1.0	5.0	0.3
Candy cigarettes	2	31	0.4	13	0.25
Toast	¼ piece	16	0.5	5.0	0.1
Jam	1 tsp.	18	0.0	0.6	0.03
Peanut butter	1 tsp.	30	1.4	4.0	0.1
Omelet, cheese	1 egg	106	6.8	50.0	1.3
Milk	6 oz.	126	7.5	216.0	0.2
Cheese	1-in. cube	105	6.6	191.0	0.3
Apple juice	4 oz.	62	0.1	8.0	0.6
Marshmallows	12	264	2.0	0.0	0.0
Frankfurters	2	248	14.0	6.0	0.12
Tomato	¼	8	0.4	4.0	0.2
Baby all-meat franks	2	62	5.5	2.0	0.3
Pickle	½ large	8	0.5	17.0	0.8
Enchilada, cheese	½	267	16.5	236.0	1.7
Taco, lamb	½	30	1.0	10.0	0.3
Lettuce salad	2 tbsp.	2	0.1	1.3	0.025
Ice cream	2 scoops	129	2.5	76.0	0.1
Totals		*1612*	*64.9*	*844.9*	*6.725*
		Second Day			
Banana	¼ piece	22	0.3	2.0	0.15
Jam	1 tsp.	18	0.03	0.6	0.03
Toast	½ slice	31	1.0	9.0	0.2
Ice cream	1 scoop	64	1.25	38.0	0.05
Milk	10 oz.	208	10.5	360.0	0.3
Lamb roast	2 slices	130	20.0	0.9	2.6
Doughnut	1 plain	136	2.1	23.0	0.2
Tomato	½ med.	16	0.7	8.0	0.5
Pickle	1 large	15	0.9	34.0	1.6
Egg omelet	1 egg	106	6.8	50.0	1.3
Bread	½ slice	31	1.0	9.0	0.2
Corned beef	1 slice	37	3.4	8.0	0.4
Cucumber	¼	12	0.8	10.0	0.4
Cupcakes	2 iced	262	5.2	124.0	0.4
Chocolate creams	4 pieces	220	2.2	–	–
Marshmallows	4	88	0.8	0.0	0
Celery	1 sm. piece	3	0.2	8.0	0.06
Potato salad	¼ cup	25	0.6	3.5	0.2
Totals		*1424*	*57.78*	*688.0*	*8.59*

Table 7.4 (Conti...

Vitamin A, I.U.	mg.		Niacin, mg.	Ascorbic Acid, mg.
		First Day		
9	0.03	0.02		2
9	0.0075	0.025		0
0	0.01	0.01	0.1	0
Tr.	Tr.	Tr.	Tr.	0
0	0.007	0.007	0.9	0
640	0.05	0.17	Tr.	0
276	0.07	0.30	0.2	2
370	Tr.	0.12	Tr.	0
45	0.025	0.035	Tr.	1
0	0	0.0	0.0	0
0	0.16	0.18	2.6	0
416	0.02	0.015	0.2	8
0	0.04	0.045	0.6	0
210	Tr.	0.045	0.05	4
7	0.085	0.25	2.7	6
Tr.	0.3	0.025	3.0	Tr.
34	0.0025	0.005	0.05	0.5
320	0.03	0.12	0.1	1
2336	0.7970	1.372	11.05	24.5
		Second Day (continued)		
107	0.01	0.01	0.2	3
Tr.	Tr.	Tr.	Tr.	0.3
0	0.02	0.02	0.25	0
160	0.015	0.06	0.05	0.5
488	0.10	0.52	0.4	4
0	0.12	0.4	4.4	0
40	0.05	0.04	0.4	0
820	0.04	0.025	0.4	17
420	Tr.	0.09	0.1	8
640	0.05	0.17	Tr.	0
0	0.02	0.02	0.25	0
Tr.	0.007	0.045	0.7	0
0	0.04	0.04	0.2	8
100	0.02	0.06	0.2	0
0	0	0	0	0
0	0.01	0.006	0.06	1
5	0.03	0.01	0.3	4
2780	0.532	1.516	7.91	45.8

Table 7.5 Comparison of Karen's intake for two days with the recommended allowances [a]

Intake	Saturday	Sunday	Recommended Allowances[a]
Calories	1612	1424	1300
Protein, g.	64.9	57.8	23
Calcium, mg.	844.9	688	800
Iron, mg.	6.7	8.6	15
Vitamin A, I.U.	2336	2780	2000
Thiamin, mg.	0.797	0.532	0.7
Riboflavin, mg.	1.372	1.516	0.8
Niacin, mg.	11.05	7.91	9
Ascorbic acid, mg.	24.5	45.8	40

[a]1974 recommendations of the Food and Nutrition Board of the National Research Council, National Academy of Sciences.

the plaque forming in the crevices along the gum line. Carbohydrate-containing foods that tend to stick to the teeth for a period of time present the greatest problem because of the length of time that they are present in the mouth. Caramels and other sticky candies are particularly noteworthy for their ability to adhere to the teeth.

The carious lesion in a tooth begins with decalcification of a small area of the enamel. This break permits the invasion of the tooth by *S. mitis.* Cavitation continues by this microorganism. The original decalcification is promoted by the presence of organic acids that are produced from sugars by bacteria. Dietary sugars are able to penetrate into the plaque formed on the teeth so that the acids can be formed and then come in contact with the actual enamel of the tooth.

The protection of deciduous teeth against dental caries is important so that these teeth will remain in position and allow for the normal development of the permanent teeth. Young children are notably inept in doing a thorough job of brushing their teeth. Consequently, even this hygienic measure is not very effective in helping to remove food residues that would tend to contribute to formation of plaque and dental caries. An important and effective means of helping to control dental caries in young children is through good dietary management. This means that fluoridated water should be used if at all possible, but it also means avoiding the use of sugar-containing snacks. In fact, the intake of sucrose and other sugars should be infrequent and low. This includes honey, raw sugar, sugar-coated cereals, and sugar-containing beverages such as soda pops and ades. Starch has been shown to be less caries-inducing in its action than sugars, but brushing of teeth after eating is still an important protective measure. A classic study of the caries-inducing effect of various dietary regimens is one done in Sweden (the Vipeholm study, 1954).

Too Much Milk

Suzie's eating habits are generally poor, but the most outstanding problem is that of unusually high milk consumption. Her meals are irregular in quantity and timing. Also she frequently receives a bottle rather than a solid meal although she is 15 months old. Some of the causes for her poor eating habits are:

1. Since she is the youngest of six children, her mother is busy and it is quick and easy to give her a bottle.
2. Suzie is slow at teething and at present has only four teeth.
3. Suzie is at the point where she wants to try to feed herself. Her mother feels this is too time-consuming and messy. The result is a scanty meal on a bottle.
4. Suzie's father is always concerned that she will choke on solid food. This is a major reason why she did not begin solid foods at an earlier age to replace the bottle.

The examination of the menus for Suzie will quickly show the problems involved with excessive milk consumption. Her menu for the first day included:

6:00 A.M.   2 oz. milk in bottle

7:30 A.M.   1 tsp. tuna

8:00 A.M.   1 soft-cooked egg
             ½ slice bread

10:30 A.M.	4 oz. milk in bottle
1:00 P.M.	8 oz. milk in bottle 2 large jellybeans
4:30 P.M.	2 tbsp. chopped liver 5 oz. milk 3 tbsp. peas 1 diced apple 1 scoop ice cream
6:00 P.M.	6 oz. milk in bottle
7:30 P.M.	8 oz. milk in bottle
2:00 A.M.	8 oz. milk in bottle

The menu for the following day was:

6:00 A.M.	3 oz. milk in bottle
8:00 A.M.	1 scrambled egg 6 tbsp. farina 2 oz. milk
9:30 A.M.	4 oz. milk in bottle
11:30 A.M.	½ peanut butter, jelly sandwich 2 oz. milk
12:00 P.M.	8 oz. milk in bottle
4:30 P.M.	1 small bowl tomato soup ½ peanut butter, jelly sandwich 4 oz. milk
7:00 P.M.	1 scoop ice cream 8 oz. milk in bottle
12:00 A.M.	8 oz. milk in bottle

The accompanying tables (Tables 7.6 and 7.7) illustrate the problems present when milk occupies such a prominent place in the diet. Notice the low values for ascorbic acid and niacin intake. Notice also that, without the farina in the diet, the iron intake would be extremely inadequate. The niacin intake could be enhanced significantly, along with the iron, by increasing the use of meats and fortified cereals and decreasing the quantity of milk.

It is apparent that Suzie's diet is decidedly inadequate, but these simple suggestions for dietary modifications will not be sufficient to correct the problem. Before she can be helped, it is necessary to interpret Suzie's nutritional needs to both her father and her mother in a clear and meaningful way. Her father will need to understand the importance of more solid foods to provide necessary iron and vitamins. It also will be necessary to allay his fear of Suzie choking because his anxiety will communicate itself to Suzie and make it difficult for her to adjust to a variety of solid foods. This adjustment in attitude may require some time and considerable patience.

Suzie's mother apparently does not realize that her child is not receiving an adequate diet. The importance of meat, fruits, vegetables, and cereals in the preschooler's diet should be emphasized to her. It also may be necessary to help her work out a schedule that encourages Suzie toward three meals and two snacks a day. Certainly it should be possible to eliminate the night feeding by changing the evening meal to 5:30 and offering a greater quantity of solid foods at that time. Suzie is old enough to be drinking from a cup. This transition should be accomplished as soon as possible. It is likely that the bottle is still being used simply because Suzie's mother has not taken the time to wean Suzie to the cup. If Suzie seems to gain comfort from the bottle, some warm attention from her mother should facilitate the weaning.

Problems of Interaction Between Mother and Child

The case of Gary is not a normal situation, but it does serve to point out how complications may arise as a result of antagonism between mother and child. Gary is a four-year-old boy whose parents expect a great deal of him. Throughout his lifetime there has been considerable emphasis on forced feeding at mealtime. Thus the feelings at mealtime have grown progressively stronger and more antagonistic between

Table 7.6 Suzie's food intake for two days

Food	Measure	Calories	Protein, g.	Calcium, mg.	Iron, mg.
		First Day			
Milk	41 oz.	841	43.6	1476	0.5
Tuna	1 tsp.	19	2.9	1	0.14
Egg (soft cooked)	1	77	6.1	26	1.3
Bread (enriched)	½ slice	31	1.0	9	0.2
Liver, chopped	2 tbsp.	17	1.7	1	0.6
Peas	3 tbsp.	28	2.0	9	0.8
Apple, diced	1 tbsp.	7	–	–	0.04
Ice cream	1 scoop	207	4.0	123	0.1
Jelly beans	2 lg.	36	2.0	–	–
Totals		*1263*	*63.3*	*1645*	*3.68*
		Second Day			
Milk	50 oz.	1000	56.0	1700	0.6
Egg, scrambled	1	110	7.0	51	1.1
Farina	6 tbsp.	50	1.7	71	6.0
Peanut butter & jelly sandwich	1	243	8.2	49	1.1
Tomato soup	½ cup	45	1.1	12	0.5
Ice cream	1 scoop	207	4.0	123	0.1
Totals		*1655*	*78.0*	*2006*	*9.4*

mother and son. The problem has deepened until, at the age of four, the boy is suffering from milk anemia and general lack of calories. Obviously something needs to be done to correct this situation immediately. The food ingested during the past week is as follows:

Monday	BREAKFAST	1 scrambled egg
		1 8-oz. cup milk
	LUNCH	1 cup chicken noodle soup
		4 crackers
	DINNER	4 crackers
		1 tbsp. pork
		2 tbsp. broccoli
		1 cup milk

Table 7.6 (Continued)

Vitamin A, I.U.	Thiamin, mg.	Riboflavin, mg.	Niacin, mg.	Ascorbic Acid, mg.
		First Day (continued)		
1850	0.42	2.15	0.5	10.5
8	–	0.01	1.28	–
550	0.05	0.14	Tr.	–
–	0.03	0.02	0.02	–
3731	0.02	0.26	1.0	2.0
267	0.1	0.05	1.0	6.0
11	Tr.	Tr.	0.02	0.6
520	0.04	0.19	0.1	1.0
–	–	–	–	–
6937	*0.66*	*2.82*	*3.92*	*20.1*
		Second Day (continued)		
2290	0.50	2.57	0.6	12.5
690	0.05	0.18	Tr.	–
–	0.07	0.01	0.2	–
Tr.	0.14	0.10	3.6	–
615	0.01	0.50	0.3	5.0
520	0.04	0.19	0.1	1.0
4115	*0.81*	*3.55*	*4.8*	*18.5*

Tuesday	BREAKFAST	1 scrambled egg
		1 cup milk
	LUNCH	1 cup chicken gumbo soup
		4 crackers
	DINNER	2 crackers
		1 tbsp. fried pork
		2 tbsp. broccoli
		1 cup milk
Wednesday	BREAKFAST	1 scrambled egg
		1 cup milk
	LUNCH	1 cup chicken gumbo soup
		4 crackers

Table 7.7 *Comparison of Suzie's intake for two days with the recommended allowances* [a]

Intake	Monday	Tuesday	Recommended Allowances[a]
Calories	1263	1655	1300
Protein, g.	63.3	78.0	23
Calcium, mg.	1645	2006	800
Iron, mg.	3.68	9.4	15
Vitamin A, I.U.	6937	4115	2000
Thiamin, mg.	0.66	0.81	0.7
Riboflavin, mg.	2.82	3.55	0.8
Niacin, mg.	3.92	4.8	9
Ascorbic acid, mg.	20.1	18.5	40

[a]1974 recommendations of the Food and Nutrition Board of the National Research Council, National Academy of Sciences.

	DINNER	2 crackers
		1 tbsp. beef
		2 tbsp. cauliflower
		1 cup milk
Thursday	BREAKFAST	1 scrambled egg
		1 cup milk
	LUNCH	1 cup chicken gumbo soup
		4 crackers
	DINNER	2 crackers
		1 tbsp. beef
		2 tbsp. broccoli
		1 cup milk
Friday	BREAKFAST	1 scrambled egg
		1 cup milk
	LUNCH	1 cup chicken gumbo soup
		4 crackers
	DINNER	2 crackers
		1 tbsp. chicken
		2 tbsp. broccoli
		1 cup milk

Saturday	BREAKFAST	1 scrambled egg
		1 cup milk
	LUNCH	1 cup chicken gumbo soup
		4 crackers
	DINNER	2 crackers
		1 tbsp. beef
		2 tbsp. spinach
		1 cup milk
Sunday	BREAKFAST	1 scrambled egg
		1 cup milk
	LUNCH	1 sliced chicken sandwich
		2 tbsp. potato salad
		1 orange
		½ cup ice cream
	DINNER	2 tbsp. rice
		3 tbsp. turkey
		2 tbsp. green peas
		1 piece apple pie
		1 cup milk

Two things are readily apparent when the menus and information in Table 7.8 are examined. First, the menus throughout the week, with the exception of the last day, are extremely repetitious and monotonous for the child. This may be interpreted as a lack of interest on the part of his mother. The next point of interest is the food consumed at lunch and dinner on Sunday. Why is the food intake suddenly so much greater and more varied on that day? The answer to this proved to be that Gary had gone to a friend's house after breakfast and had spent the rest of the day there.

The correction of the problems that exist in this family is not an easy matter. The attitude and habits of mother and son have been built up over a period of time and therefore probably will require a rather long time for correction. Since the boy did eat a reasonable amount of food when he was visiting others, it appears that the food intake is a problem between his mother and himself, and is not an actual physical problem.

The most obvious changes to be made are an increase in the size of servings and greater variety in the menu. He needs to have many different foods included in his diet at this age.

Table 7.8 *Comparison of Gary's intake for seven days with the recommended allowances*

Intake	Mon.	Tues.	Wed.	Thurs.	Fri.	Sat.	Sun.	Recommended Allowances[a]
Calories	615	593	592	721	607	595	1322	1800
Protein, g.	37.3	38.3	36.5	38.5	36.4	37.3	69.5	30
Calcium, mg.	979	901	1139	952	999	1229	2526	800
Iron, mg.	4.9	4.57	5.67	6.27	4.94	6.26	7.36	10
Vitamin A, I.U.	3052	2283	2271	3115	2483	4055	2367	2500
Thiamin, mg.	0.59	0.30	0.35	0.36	0.56	0.40	0.66	0.9
Riboflavin, mg.	1.73	1.11	1.19	1.25	1.61	1.26	2.38	1.1
Niacin, mg.	4.97	4.74	4.67	4.55	5.14	4.46	8.67	12
Ascorbic acid, mg.	42	31	18	42	28	16	107	40
Vitamin D, I.U.	200	200	200	200	200	200	200	400

[a]1974 recommendations of the Food and Nutrition Board of the National Research Council, National Academy of Sciences.

He particularly needs to be consuming a broader range of meats and other foods; his menu should be expanded to include a wider variety of fruits and vegetables. Fruits have been totally lacking in his diet at home. He also should be receiving various enriched cereal products rather than limiting his experience to crackers.

Such a problem is most readily remedied when an outsider helps to correct the situation. At the age of four, it might be possible for Gary to attend a nursery school where he would gradually learn to enjoy food by watching the example of the other children. The greater variety of food served at the school would also help to broaden his range of food preferences.

Nursery school personnel would help Gary's mother, too. She would be able to discuss her problem with the nursery school teacher and gain her counsel in coping with the problem. The nursery school provides a valuable change in environment and routine from the situation that enabled this problem to develop in the first place.

If it is not possible to enroll Gary in a nursery school, perhaps Gary's mother could consult a doctor or county nutritionist. In order to solve Gary's nutritional difficulties, it is necessary to help his mother understand the nutritional needs of her four-year-old and to interpret these needs in practical terms. She may desire and need help on such facets of the total problem as: planning nutritious meals with child appeal; preparation techniques to make food more tempting; and understanding the abilities and emotional needs of her child. Gary's situation can be corrected, but it will require considerable patience and time because the underlying attitudes have been developing over a period of many months.

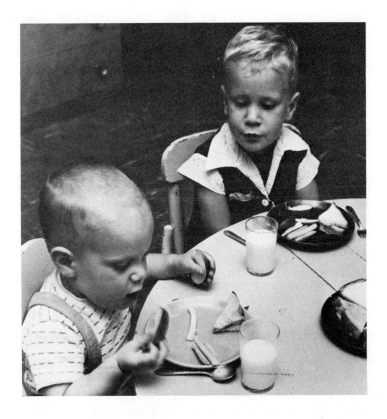

Small servings encourage young children to eat a good meal.

SUMMARY

The preschool child will undergo periods of varying appetite; these changes in appetite should not cause concern because they are usually short-lived. The important thing to remember when feeding the preschool child is that this is a period when dietary habits are being firmly established. Efforts should be made to offer the preschooler a wide range of foods to broaden his experiences. The mealtime setting should be geared toward the comfort of the child.

Wise parents will take time periodically to analyze what their children are eating so that they can correct nutritional deficiencies that may be occurring. Such a check can be made by comparing the diet plan for the preschooler with the Basic Four Food Plan. If shortages appear to exist, an immediate effort should be made to correct the situation.

Frequently the parents themselves will be able to correct feeding problems that may exist for their children. Sometimes, however, outside help may prove to be the most suitable method for correcting existing conditions within the family.

BIBLIOGRAPHY

Ast, D.B., et al., 1956. Newburgh-Kingston caries – fluorine study. XIV: Combined clinical and roentgenographic dental findings after ten years of fluoride experiments. *J. Amer. Dent. Assoc.* 52: 314.

Beal, V.A., 1961. Dietary intake of individuals followed through infancy and childhood. *Amer. J. Pub. Health* 51, No. 8: 1107.

Blayney, J.R., 1960. Report of thirteen years of water fluoridation in Evanston, Illinois. *J. Amer. Dent. Assoc.* 61: 76.

Council on Foods and Nutrition, 1960. *Symposium 8: Nutrition in Tooth Formation and Dental Caries.* American Medical Assoc. Chicago.

Eppright, E.S., et al., 1969. Eating behavior of preschool children. *J. Nutr. Ed.* (Summer): 16.

Food and Nutrition Board, 1964. *Pre-School Child Malnutrition.* National Research Council of the National Academy of Sciences. Washington, D.C.

Fox, H.M., et al., 1970. North Central Regional Study of Diets of Preschool Children. 1. Family Environment. *J) Home Ec.* 62: 441.

Fox, H.M., et al., 1970. North Central Regional Study of diets of preschool children. 2. Nutrition knowledge and attitudes of mothers. *J. Home Ec.* 62: 327.

Glass, R.L., 1974. Diet and dental caries: dental caries incidence and consumption of ready-to-eat cereals. *J. Amer. Dent. Assoc.* 88: 80.

Gustafsson, B., et al., 1954. The Vipeholm dental caries study: effect of different levels of carbohydrates intake on caries activity in 436 individuals observed for five years. *Acta Odont. Scand.* 11: 232.

Lindquist, B., 1969. Nutritional needs in preschool and school age. In *Nutrition in Preschool and School Age.* Ed., G. Blix. p. 50. Swedish Nutrition Foundation. Uppsala.

Lowenberg, M.E., 1948. Food preferences of young children. *J. Amer. Dietet. Assoc.* 24: 430.

McWilliams, M., 1974. *Food Fundamentals.* 2nd ed. Wiley. New York.

Madson, K.O., 1966. Oral food residues and tooth decay. *Food Nutr. News* 37, No. 5: 1.

Meyer, H.F., 1960. *Infant Foods and Feeding Practice.* Thomas. Springfield, Ill.

National Research Council, 1966. *Pre-School Child Malnutrition: Primary Deterrent to Human Progress.* Publ. 1282. National Academy of Sciences. Washington, D.C.

Nizel, A.E., 1972. *Nutrition in Preventive Dentistry: Science and Practice.* Saunders. Philadelphia.

Nutrition Foundation, 1966. Subsequent growth of children treated for malnutrition. *Nutr. Rev.* 24: 267.

Scrimshaw, N.S., 1963. Malnutrition and health of children. *J. Amer. Dietet. Assoc.* 43: 203.

Smith, C.A., 1960. Overuse of milk in the diets of infants and children. *J. Amer. Med. Assoc.* 172: 567.

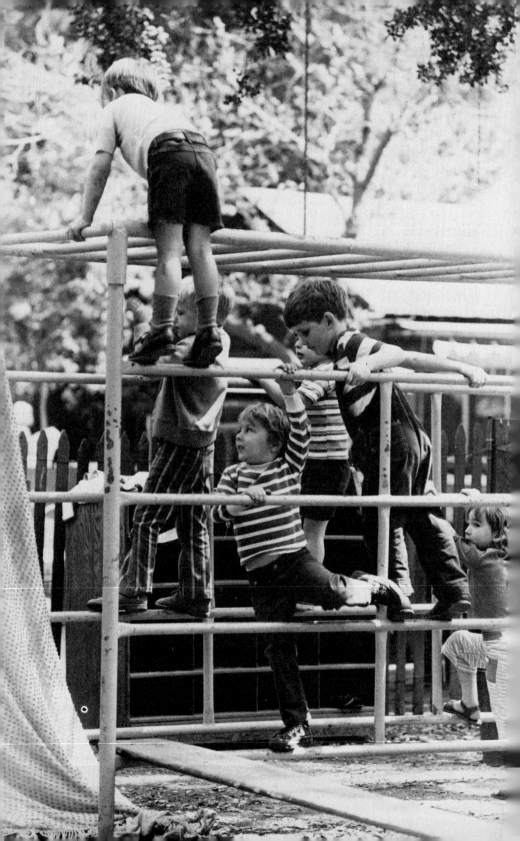

Chapter 8
Nursery School Children

Nursery schools and children's centers offer unique situations for developing excellent nutrition habits. Three basic attitudes underlying the philosophy of a nursery school provide the key to building these habits:

1. The attitude of continuous curiosity and exploration encourages the children to learn by feeling and tasting a wide variety of foods.
2. The attitude that a child's way of doing things is acceptable makes it easy for a child to thoroughly examine and then to enjoy his food.
3. The attitude of expectancy in the school motivates a child to develop confidence that he can do many things, including eating his lunch and trying new foods.

When these attitudes are fostered and developed to their fullest, a nursery school can provide a sound basis for a lifetime of good nutrition. The extent to which this potential is utilized, however, varies from one school to another.

Often it is easier to introduce new foods successfully and to expand appreciation of familiar foods in a nursery school situation than it is in the child's home, for at school he not only sees adults other than his parents who enjoy and appreciate the food, but also he has the example of his nursery school peers to set the stage for acceptance of foods. The combination of the example set by others and the child's own natural curiosity about new foods often make it very simple to gain approval of the new food.

The keys to a successful nursery school feeding program are good original planning of the menus, tasteful and careful preparation of the food, attractive service, and a comfortable environment within the dining situation itself.

MENU PLANNING

Careful menu planning for the nursery school nutrition program ensures that a wide spectrum of foods will be introduced into the preschool child's diet, and such a variety can serve well as a basis for a diet of wide diversity throughout life.

Plans for the nursery school menu should be considered from the standpoint of differences in texture, color, combination of flavors, interesting shapes, and familiarity with the food. The first four factors, considered earlier as they influenced the planning of family meals, may be applied directly to menu planning in the nursery school. The familiarity of the foods is also an important consideration when working with young children.

Ideally the menu should include a wide variety of foods that are familiar to the children in the group to promote a feeling of security and comfort at the meal. This means that some staple foods in the diet will vary somewhat from one section of the country to another. Hominy and grits may play an important part in the nursery school menu in the southern United States, but these foods are not commonly consumed by families in many other areas of the country. Other examples of food common in specific areas or population groups include tortillas in the Southwest and rice among Oriental groups. Such familiar foods, when included in the nursery school menus, provide the springboard for a child to seek new experiences with food. The wise nutritionist will use the nursery school as an opportunity to expand a child's acquaintanceship with various foods.

New foods can be included in all nursery school menus. Preschoolers are ready to become acquainted with meats such as turkey or liver loaf that may be new to them. In the dairy products category children often will enjoy trying some new kinds of cheese. The holes in Swiss cheese are a fascinating curiosity which encourage a close examination with the hands and eyes, to be followed by an experimental taste. Parmesan cheese in a shaker can is fun for children to sprinkle on spaghetti or lasagne, and it also adds to the nutritional value of the meal. Variety is easy to achieve when serving breads and cereals; corn bread, bread sticks, hot baking powder biscuits, spoon bread, or hot yeast rolls would tempt any child to try them.

It is particularly interesting to emphasize the variety available in fruits and vegetables. With a bit of imagination, these foods can be served in many intriguing ways to invite exploration. For example, raw turnip slices become an item of interest when cut into different shapes; the ceremony of pulling off the leaf of an artichoke and dipping it in a little butter or salad dressing provides another entree into the vegetable world. Radish roses, cross-sectional slices of mushrooms, and small flowers of cauliflower are tempting when served raw as finger foods.

One of the problems encountered in the use of fresh produce is the cost. By watching the seasonal variation in price, however, it is possible to include a reasonable variety of fruits and vegetables without exceeding the budget for the nursery school lunch programs. Refrigerator space, work space in the kitchen, and the labor required to prepare fresh produce also need to be considered when the menus are being planned.

The menus served in children's centers and nursery school settings vary from only a small snack in the middle of the morning or afternoon to the types of menus suitable for providing much of the day's nutrition for the child. Many all-day centers provide a mid-morning snack, lunch, and a mid-afternoon snack; some also serve breakfast. Dinner, however, is not ordinarily included in the typical preschool program.

Breakfast

Nursery schools and children's centers whose student populations consist primarily of children whose mothers work full time may need to plan to serve breakfast to the children soon after they arrive. When breakfast is served, it regularly should consist of at least citrus fruit, milk, and cereal or toast, and preferably should also include either meat or an egg.

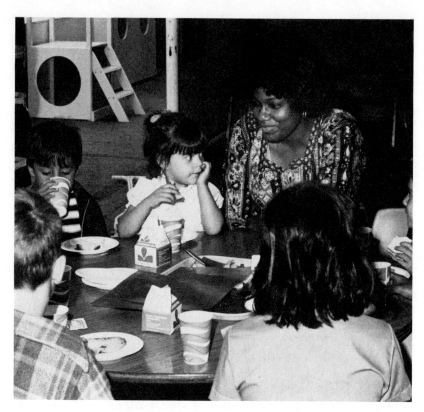

Children at this center are ready for a large snack soon after they arrive because they often do not have time for breakfast at home.

Snacks

The mid-morning snack is intended to provide the energy necessary to avoid the late-morning slump. When children become overtired or overhungry, their appetites are often poor at a meal. This problem can usually be avoided by serving an informal snack about ten o'clock. The type and quantity of food served should be geared to the specific nursery school situation.

To avoid the possibility of an inadequate intake of ascorbic acid, a snack of tomato juice, citrus juice, or other fruit juices that contain adequate amounts of this vitamin either naturally or synthetically should be served frequently. Of course, orange and grapefruit juices do naturally provide the quantities of ascorbic acid needed by the young child, but it is also possible to use some other fruit drinks that will meet this need by commercial addition of the synthetic vitamin. Several canned fruit juices are now being marketed to which ascorbic acid has been added in significant, practical amounts. The use of Kool-aid and other similar products is inappropriate because of the high sugar content and low nutritive value of such beverages.

In some situations, a larger mid-morning snack is appropriate. When the children are very active throughout the morning or when there is a long interval between breakfast and lunch, it is often wise to serve something in addition to the fruit juice. The larger snack in such cases actually improves lunchtime appetites because the children are less likely to be too fatigued or hungry to eat. Snack foods that often are enjoyed by children include raw vegetables such as carrot sticks, turnip slices, celery curls, green pepper strips, or radishes. Toast sticks made from enriched bread also would be suitable to serve with the fruit juice.

Lunch

The lunch meal should be planned carefully to provide a serving of meat or a casserole containing a high proportion of meat, at least two fruits or vegetables (dark green, leafy or yellow vegetable every other day), and bread, rice, noodles, or similar foods. Milk should be the beverage served at the meal. If desired, a simple dessert such as fruit, custard, or sponge cake may be included.

At least one-third of the day's nutritional requirements should be furnished by the lunch. Attention in planning the menus should be directed toward providing good sources of protein in adequate amounts for the children. The tendency to serve large amounts of breads and pastas and small quantities of meats should be avoided despite the obvious economic temptation.

The menus for lunch ideally will include favorites of the children as well as new foods. When planning nursery school menus, it is necessary not only to keep in mind the food preferences of the children, but also to consider various physical limitations such as preparation time, work space, oven space, refrigeration facilities, and availability and cost of foods. Obviously this is a large order. Unfortunately, even when these criteria are met and the meals are also esthetically and gustatorily satisfying, there will be some persons who will not like everything that is served.

It is important for the person in charge of the nursery school nutrition program to eat lunch with the children. Through conversation with the children and observation of the plates at the end of the meal, she can quickly glean information that will help in future planning; by actually eating with the children, she can more readily and accurately evaluate the menu planning and the preparation of the foods. In addition, she is in a position to help the children develop good attitudes toward food.

It is usually practical to very carefully plan a complete set of nursery school lunch menus for a time interval of at least four weeks and then to use these tested menus as the basis of a repeating pattern. Each meal in the series should be carefully and critically evaluated, with changes being made when necessary. Substitutions for fresh produce, of course, will need to be made according to seasonal availability.

Table 8.1 contains menus suitable for preparation in a nursery school with limited facilities. Table 8.2 presents a month's menus as served in one nursery school program with a good physical arrangement. If kitchen facilities are limited, it may be necessary to decrease the variety slightly, but at least the basic pattern of meat or meat substitutes, vegetables or fruits, a bread or bread substitute, and milk should always be included.

Afternoon Snack

In many situations the children may go home shortly after lunch, but if full daytime care is provided, a snack should be served after the nap. The types of foods mentioned in the preceding discussion on morning snacks are also suitable for afternoon. Thirst quenchers such as milk or juice are particularly popular at this time.

CARE IN THE KITCHEN

Sanitation

Food preparation for the nursery school should be carefully controlled to ensure not only that the food is palatable

Table 8.1 *Menus for a nursery school with limited kitchen facilities*

Day	Menu
Monday	Meat Loaf Buttered Peas, Baked Squash Whole-Wheat Bread, Butter Fruit Cup Milk
Tuesday	Hurry-up Hot Dogs Baked Beans, Carrot Sticks Enriched White Bread, Butter Seedless Grapes Milk
Wednesday	Fish Sticks French-Cut Green Beans Waldorf Salad, Toast Triangles Angel Cake Milk
Thursday	Sausage Links Spoon Bread, Broccoli Cherry Tomatoes Apple Sauce, Crunchy Oatmeal Cooky Milk
Friday	Tune & Noodle Casserole Buttered Carrots, Apple Wedges Toast Sticks Chocolate Cream Pudding Milk

and attractive, but also that it is safe for consumption. Every nursery school should have a supervisor who is qualified to oversee the entire spectrum of events dealing with food from the planning and purchasing through the preparation, service, and cleanup. It is essential that she insist on strict sanitation in the kitchen.

The cook should have an adequate physical checkup to ensure that she is in good health and is not transmitting any communicable disease to the children via the food that

Table 8.2   Sample lunch menus for a nursery school

Day	Week 1	Week 2
Monday	Cheese & Rice Casserole Green Beans Celery Stuffed with Peanut Butter Enriched Toast, Butter Apple Crisp Milk	Hamburger Stew (with Potato) Celery Sticks, Carrot Sticks Green Beans Whole-Wheat Toast Oatmeal Cookies Milk
Tuesday	Porcupine Meat Balls Corn Fresh Fruit Enriched Toast, Butter Chocolate Pudding Milk	Spanish Rice with Bacon Chips Broccoli Cottage Cheese Whole-Wheat Toast Angel Food Cake Milk
Wednesday	Spaghetti & Meat Sauce Buttered Broccoli Carrot Sticks Enriched Toast, Butter Pears Milk	Liver Strips Saute Parsley Potatoes Buttered Carrots Fresh Fruit Rolled Wheat Cookies Milk
Thursday	Baked Heart Mashed Potato Cauliflower in Cheese Sauce Fresh Fruit Salad Oatmeal Cookies Milk	Ham Rice Pilaf Buttered Peas, Tomato Wedges Whole-Wheat Toast Fruit Jello Milk
Friday	Scrambled Eggs Oven-Browned Potatoes Buttered Beets, Dried Apricots Whole-Wheat Toast Gingerbread Milk	Salmon Loaf Buttered Rice, Spinach Tomato Wedges Whole-Wheat Toast Ice Cream, Ginger Cookies Milk

she prepares. It also is extremely important that the cook be aware of the necessity of maintaining a sanitary kitchen: work surfaces should be clean; the floor should be scrubbed regularly; and the kitchen must be free of bugs and rodents.

The cook and any assistants should be thoroughly schooled regarding the importance of careful handwashing because unclean hands can spread food-borne illnesses. Cooks should form the habit of placing a taste spoon in the dishwashing area as soon as it has been used. Under no

Table 8.2 (Continued)

Week 3	Week 4
Cheese & Ground Beef Pizza Buttered Corn Fresh Fruit Salad Ice Cream Milk	Frankfurters Stuffed with Cheese Buttered Rice Spinach Ice Cream & Bananas Milk
Swedish Meat Balls Mashed Potato, Milk Gravy Broccoli Cornmeal Bread with Honey Fresh Green Grapes Milk	Liver Loaf Vegetable Relish Plate, Lima Beans Cottage Cheese & Pineapple Salad Rolled Wheat Muffins Butterscotch Pudding & Banana Milk
Oven-Fried Chicken Creamed Rice, Green Beans Raw Cabbage Wedges Cornmeal Bread Melon Milk	Roast Turkey Southern Spoon Bread Bunny Salad, Brussels Sprouts Whole-Wheat Toast Sticks Watermelon Milk
Split Pea Soup with Ham Fresh Fruit Salad Rolled Wheat Muffins Baked Custard Brownies Milk	Beef Loaf Mashed Potato with Milk Gravy Buttered Peas Stuffed Celery Fresh Green Grapes Milk
Fish Sticks Broccoli Jellied Carrot & Pineapple Salad Cottage Cheese, Toast Triangles Rolled Wheat Spice Bars Milk	Baked Halibut Noodles au Gratin, Green Beans Carrot & Raisin Salad Whole-Wheat Toast Sticks Fresh Fruit Milk

circumstance should the food be tasted either with a spoon that has been used previously or with fingers. Often this is a precaution that requires considerable monitoring until the cook is thoroughly trained in the problems of sanitation in the nursery school. Other personal habits of the cook, such as rubbing her mouth and nose with her hand or coughing and sneezing without covering her nose and mouth, will need to be corrected when they exist.

It is important that the cook be fully aware of the need

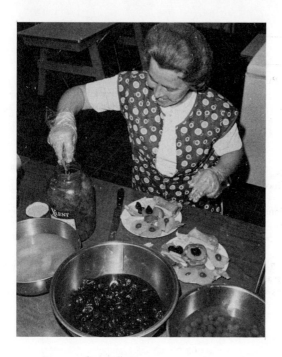

*A hair net and plastic
gloves help to insure
sanitary preparation of
food.*

for extremely careful washing of all fruits and vegetables
that will be consumed raw. Of course, it is also necessary
to wash fresh produce that will be cooked, but the hazards
are greater in the food to be consumed raw.

Storage

Food should be stored carefully at all times to avoid
growth of harmful microorganisms. These microorganisms,
capable of causing food-borne illnesses, flourish in readily
perishable foods in the temperature range between 40°F
(4°C) and 140°F (60°C), with the greatest growth occurring
between 60°F and 120°F. Hazard is greatly reduced by either
refrigerating perishable foods or holding them in a warming
oven at 140°F or higher. Room temperature storage is dangerous! Foods that are particularly dangerous include
meats, fish, poultry, egg products, foods containing mayon-
naise, and creamed dishes or other foods containing milk.

Dishwashing

Good dishwashing practices are essential. They can be maintained if the following requirements are met.

1. Adequate space for the dishwashing operation, including space for prerinsing, draining, and drying.
2. Food preparation area separate from the dishwashing operation.
3. Adequate equipment and supplies.
4. Covered storage space for clean dishes away from the dishwashing space.
5. Good physical working conditions (clean, adequately lighted, comfortable temperature, and well ventilated).

Many nursery schools have facilities only for hand washing of the dishes. When dishes are washed by hand, detergent should be added until the water feels slippery. The wash water should be changed often and kept at 110° to 120°F. Rinsing is best accomplished by immersing racks of the washed dishes several times in clean water at 120°to 140°F. The rinsed dishes can be satisfactorily sanitized in hand-washing operations by submerging the rack of dishes in hot water (at least 180°F) for a minimum time of one-half minute. This temperature should be checked with a thermometer. Chlorine, iodine, and quaternary ammonium compounds, when used according to directions, are suitable sanitizing agents. Any dish drying towels should be freshly laundered for each use.

Machine dishwashing also should be carefully checked. The machine should maintain a 0.25 per cent detergent concentration — that is, one ounce of detergent for each three gallons of water, during the washing cycle. The water for all operations in the machine should be held between 160°F and 165°F. Since the design of the many machines available today is highly variable, it is best to observe the specifications for installation and maintenance as set forth by the manufacturer.

More extensive information on either hand or machine dishwashing may be obtained from most city and county health departments.

SETTING THE STAGE

Schedule

For optimum food acceptance, the physical facilities and routine should be appropriate for the children. One important consideration is the time schedule for meals and snacks. The timing of the first snack depends heavily on the morning routine at home. Children who eat a good breakfast before coming to nursery school will be ready for a small snack at approximately 10 A.M., whereas a child who has had no breakfast will welcome a large snack as soon as he arrives. The morning program at the school will function more effectively if the snack is appropriate to the needs of the children, both in quantity and in time of service.

After the snack, a play period followed by a quiet activity will help to ensure a good appetite for lunch. A quiet activity before lunch provides a smooth transition between active play and the meal situation. Usually a planned story time at which the children sit and listen is an effective bridge between morning play and lunch.

An appropriate time for lunch is approximately 11:45, although certain nursery school schedules may require an adjustment in the time. Children's appetites are generally better when lunch is served at the same time each day.

Ideally the time for the afternoon snack will be flexible to coordinate with the nap period. Many children are thirsty when they waken from a nap so it is often practical to let the individual children have a snack as they get up from their naps.

Physical Arrangements

The habit of washing hands carefully before eating needs to be emphasized with nursery school children. If the teachers carefully set the example and assist the children in developing this habit, there will be much less likelihood of spreading colds and other communicable diseases in the school. The regular school routine should include adequate time for all children and teachers to wash just before the meal. Adequate facilities should be provided for hand-washing so that this operation can be done effectively. Any preschool center should have warm (but not hot) water and

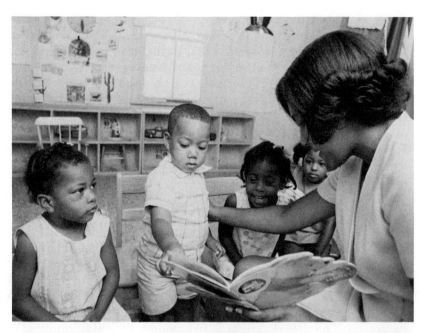

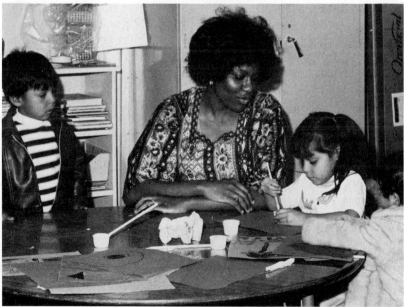

Story time (above) or a quiet activity (below) are effective transitions from active play to eating.

soap available in the quantities necessary to ensure that all children are able to wash before the meal. Soap should always be available, not simply left to the whims of the janitor.

It is ideal to have the furniture in the dining area proportioned to fit the preschooler. The tables should be low so the children can reach their food easily, and the chairs should permit the children to rest their feet comfortably on the floor. When possible, it is desirable to have only a small group of children and an adult at each table. A table that seats from four to six children and an adult is practical for food service and conversation.

Seating arrangements may be informal, with children sitting in any empty chair, or they may be assigned. This decision should be worked out by the teachers. Some children may enjoy the mealtime more if they have a particular place to sit each day. This may help them to feel that they are a definite part of the group, thus promoting the feeling of security necessary for a happy mealtime. Such seating arrangements could be done orally or each child might have his own place card. Since many preschool children cannot read their names, these place cards might actually be pictures or colors rather than names.

The seating arrangement can be varied from time to time, but it is helpful if one adult can be at the same table with a child long enough to establish some continuity in the mealtime pattern. As the teacher becomes aware of the individual child's attitudes and eating patterns, she can more effectively assist each child in achieving good nutrition habits. In seating arrangements an effort should be made to plan compatible groupings. Often it is possible to seat a child who is enthusiastic about food next to a child who may be less interested in eating. The good example beside him may help the reluctant child to begin to eat better.

In most situations the tables may be set with the serving dishes of food, a milk pitcher, and the empty plates placed at each teacher's cover; a glass, silverware, and a napkin can be arranged at each child's place before the children come to the dining area.

AT THE TABLE

While the children are seating themselves at the table, the adult can quickly serve the individual plates that have

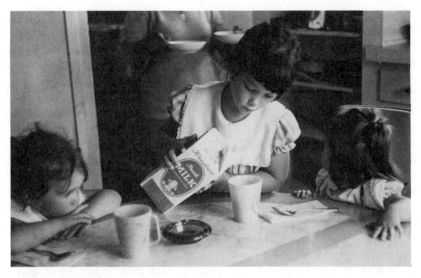

Children enjoy helping by pouring milk while the food for lunch is being served.

been stacked at her place. The children can pour their milk from a small pitcher while the plates are being served.

Sometimes it is wise for the adult to ask a child how large a serving he wishes. At other times it may be preferable to offer small servings originally and provide second helpings if they are desired. Small servings appear to be the best way to encourage many young children's appetites. A small serving may be interpreted as approximately a one-ounce meat patty, a floweret of cauliflower, or one carrot stick. Servings this size encourage the child with a small appetite to at least try the food, whereas large servings may overwhelm him and discourage him from even attempting to find a place to begin.

As the adult at the table becomes better acquainted with the appetites of the various children, she can tailor the size of the servings to the individual children. Children with big appetites may prefer to be served a larger quantity initially. A rule of thumb for amounts of food is approximately three tablespoons for the three-year-old with a good appetite and four tablespoons per serving for the hungry four-year-old.

Additional servings are appropriate when they are desired, but adults may wish to encourage children to eat some of each food served at the meal before seconds are provided. This does not mean that there should be a fixed rule that plates must be cleaned before second servings may be obtained, but it does help children realize that many different foods are important for their bodies.

Children who have a very narrow range of food likes are less likely to be well nourished than are those who eat a wide variety; therefore they should be encouraged to learn to like more foods. The nursery school teacher can help to expand a child's food preferences both by her example and by subtle suggestion. If she enjoys and eats her portions of all of the food served at the meal, the children are likely to follow her example. The nursery school teacher who has narrow food preferences will find her role difficult at mealtime. With a concerted effort, however, she should be able to overcome this attitude and set a positive example for the children.

When a teacher notices that a child is ignoring a particular food, she may pleasantly and subtly suggest that he try the new food. For example, this might be done simply by saying, "Johnny, do you know what crisp means? Try this green pepper and see." A remark such as this, when said in a relaxed manner, is usually sufficient to create enough interest to taste the food. Certainly it is unwise for the teacher to make an issue of a particular food at the table, for this may create resistance within the child and reduce acceptance of the food by other children at the table.

The nursery school teacher will be most successful in the mealtime situation if she is able to:

1. Objectively examine her own food preferences and attitudes and then reduce her food prejudices as much as she can.
2. Adopt the philosophy that it is desirable for children to like a wide variety of foods, but that there will be some foods that an individual may find simply tolerable rather than truly enjoyable.
3. Maintain a relaxed and comfortable atmosphere at the table.
4. Quietly encourage children to try new foods.
5. Feel a genuine interest in the nutrition habits of the individual children.

The foregoing list may give the impression that the teacher has to be extremely concerned about the food habits at the table. She should take considerable interest in the nutrition of each child in her care, but this concern should be maintained in its proper perspective. A worrisome adult only communicates tension and apprehension to the children. The constructive teacher will make herself aware of the habits of the individual children and then, in an objective manner, evaluate the individual's pattern of food intake. From this objective basis it is possible for the teacher to unemotionally aid and encourage each child to build good nutrition habits. Nursery school teachers can be much more effective in this role when they have had a good basic nutrition course and a course in child nutrition at the college level.

Good nutrition habits usually are achieved only with patience and persistence over a period of time. Even in preschoolers whose habits are being established, existing dietary attitudes are relatively resistant to change. Therefore, wise adults will expect the changes to be slow and will patiently and without pressure continue to work toward good nutriton habits.

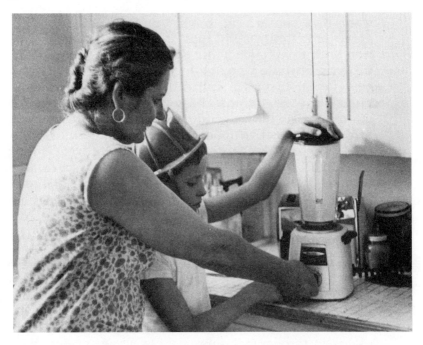

When a child helps to prepare a new food, he will be interested in testing it.

All adults in the dining room need to be in agreement on policy regarding matters at the table. Usually it is a good idea for all adults who are involved to discuss problems together and to arrive at a mutually satisfactory way of approaching them. When possible, such a discussion should be led by a qualified nutritionist. Then the teachers have the charge of applying the suggestions in the classroom. Policies and guidelines can be developed together to aid the teacher in effectively promoting good nutrition. Some of the types of questions that may require discussion among the group are reviewed below:

1. The desirable scheduling of snacks and meals may require input from the entire group of adults. Similarly, there may be a wide variety of opinions on the manner of serving the children and the seating arrangements.
2. One problem that will probably require clarification is that of the introduction of new foods. In most instances it is desirable to encourage children to try at least one bite, but there may be isolated instances when it is impractical to insist on this. If the teachers agree on a philosophy that encourages experimentation with new foods while still permitting some flexibility in attitude when children seem fearful of trying new foods, they will individually feel competent in a variety of situations and will find it fairly easy to maintain a relaxed attitude while they are still striving to develop positive food attitudes in the children. A new food may be more tempting to children if they have had an opportunity to see it growing or to help prepare it. Several suitable suggestions are included in the next section. With this type of introduction, many children will be eager to try the new food.
3. Usually lunch proceeds more smoothly for the children if traffic around the room is somewhat controlled. One child from each table may be appointed to pass the bread basket so that the children have an opportunity for social learning, too. The other children may reasonably be expected to sit at the table during the first course. The routine of taking their lunch plates to the central supply table when through with the first course and returning to their places with

dessert affords children the opportunity to stretch, thus helping to divide the sitting time at the meal.

4. Lunch is more relaxed and pleasant if children eat at their own rate and are free to proceed to dessert when through with the main course. If each child is excused from the table when he is through eating, the slow eater will not be distracted by children who are unoccupied and fidgeting at the table. When the children are excused from the table, they may wash and then proceed to a quiet, supervised play area away from the dining room.

5. Many preschool children are fascinated by pouring liquids. By permitting children to pour their own milk from an easy-to-manage pitcher, this interest may be utilized to increase milk intake.

NUTRITION EDUCATION IN THE NURSERY SCHOOL

There are various ways in which nutrition education may be coupled with other facets of the nursery school program; for example, colors may be taught using foods as illustrations. When a particular color is being emphasized, a food of the appropriate color may be prepared by the children for a snack, and the lunch menu can spotlight additional kinds of food of the same color. The pleasing bright colors of fruits and vegetables serve both as an effective introduction to the observation of different colors and as an attractive invitation to taste the illustrative material. An imaginative teacher will be able to think of many ways in which nutrition education may be used effectively to enrich the nursery school program as well as to improve the students' nutrition habits.

The coordination of color study with nutrition education can be worked out in various ways[1]. For example, the color "green" may be taught by setting up a tray at snack time so that the children can sample green foods with a variety of flavors. Such a tray would present considerable taste as

---

[1] Some of the suggestions on color in this section are adapted from material developed by Margaret Irene Coleman, kindergarten teacher for El Rancho Unified School District, and Miriam P. Bates, director of La Mirada Baptist Nursery School, P.O. Box 546, La Mirada, Calif.

well as color interest if it contained an assortment of green foods. Green grapes, romaine, parsley, butter lettuce, sweet and dill pickles, green pepper, and avocado slices are but a few of the foods that might be used. Obviously there are many other green foods that would lend themselves equally well to a sampling party. To prevent consumption of too large a snack between meals, it may be possible to arrange to have a different green snack tray each day for several days and serve two or three foods each day.

Interest in the color "green" also can be expanded to include the idea of the importance of seeds in the production of food. When fresh peas in the pod are available, children would be fascinated to shell the peas and then have them boiled and buttered as a part of lunch. This is one time when a vegetable will really vanish quickly at the table. Some nursery school children would be interested to have the "pea lesson" continued by seeing samples of canned and frozen peas. In the spring, the children could help with the planting and growing of a packet of seeds.

Blue can be taught to the children by using blueberries to illustrate the color. Children will particularly enjoy preparing blueberry muffins to be served for lunch. Another good illustration for this color is blueberry pancakes, which the children could help prepare in a portable electric skillet.

Grape juice at snack time can be a good introduction to purple. Another purple food, which probably is unfamiliar to many of the children, is eggplant. After being used as the centerpiece on the service table one day, it could be fried or stuffed and served as the lunch vegetable on the following day. Fresh plums are a popular, although seasonal, food to illustrate purple in food.

The bright, sunny effect of yellow makes this a particularly delightful color to present to the children. Foods that are appropriate for this color include Golden Delicious apples, lemons, grapefruit, sweet corn, crook-neck squash, butter, margarine, pineapple, and cornmeal. With this wide variety of foods, taste trays again may be used effectively as snacks.

Projects also can be used well with some of the yellow foods. Children are amazed to watch cream turn from its characteristic color into the yellow lumps of butter when they churn it in a small churn. If the school has no churn,

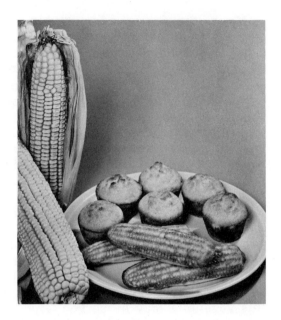

Nursery school children can learn about yellow colors by seeing an ear of corn and then making cornmeal muffins themselves. Corn sticks also provide an interesting shape that will attract the children.

butter can be made by the children individually by vigorously shaking a little cream in a jar, or the teacher can quickly beat the cream with an electric mixer until the butter appears. After the butter is removed from the liquid and squeezed to force out additional whey, a little salt is added and the children are then ready for a snack of crackers spread with homemade butter. Lemons could be squeezed to make lemonade, or cornmeal muffins might be made by the children. The lemonade is an excellent afternoon drink for a snack and the cornmeal muffins add pleasing color and texture to a lunch.

One of the colors that lends itself particularly well to coordinated projects is orange. Oranges obviously are excellent to illustrate the color, and these can be prepared in several ways to delight the children. The fresh fruit could be featured in a centerpiece and the sectioned or sliced oranges can be used as a snack food or as a salad at lunch. Orange juice or orange rolls are very popular with both children and adults. Today's nursery school children may never have seen orange juice being squeezed from the pulp, and this makes an interesting project for them. The seeds from the oranges may be planted and carefully tended for the children to observe.

Many other fruits and vegetables also are various shades of orange and thus present other possibilities in the presentation of this color. Acorn squash, yams, apricots, and carrots may interest children when they learn that these foods contain provitamin A, a substance that helps them to see better at night. A sweet potato may be grown in water with spectacular results.

Carrots are inexpensive and afford many teaching opportunities in the nursery school. Krauss' book *The Carrot Seed* can be read or the record of the book can be played to introduce the idea of fun with carrots. Then the teacher can make thin slices of the carrot which the children can make into carrot curls to be served at snack time. Another project that is fun for the children (using supplies previously sliced by an adult) is to insert thin pickle slices into a ring hollowed out from a slice of a big carrot. Carrots could also be included in the lunch menu in a different form for a few days to help the children see the variety of ways in which this vegetable may be served. The first day a crisp grated carrot and raisin salad could be served, followed on succeeding days by buttered carrots, a whole carrot baked in a meat loaf, parsley carrots, and carrots with lemon butter. The children also might cut off the top portion of the carrot and sprout it in a bit of water.

The foods selected to teach the color red will be influenced both by the season of the year and by the population group. Red chilies are a familiar food to Mexican American children in the Southwest. Other foods, however, may be more easily obtained in many regions. Fresh sour cherries or strawberries in season are a beautiful red and may be eaten raw or made into pie or jam for the children. Uncooked jam[1] made from frozen strawberries can be prepared in the classroom and served on biscuits that the children have helped cut out. This type of jam is a particularly luminous red which illustrates well the color being taught.

Red apples are available most of the year and may be coordinated with a story session in the school. The teacher may tell the story of the little boy who was asked to find the little house with no doors and no windows and a star inside.

---

[1] "Uncooked jams from frozen fruits," mimeo, Purdue University School of Home Economics, Lafayette, Ind. 1953.

He went all around town looking and looking, but he could not find the house. The teacher then can ask the children to help the little boy. When there are no more suggestions from the children, the teacher can help the children find the answer by cutting a red apple horizontally to reveal the star in the bright red house with no doors and no windows (the apple).

These are some ideas for the ways in which food can be used to illustrate and broaden concepts the teacher may wish to develop in the nursery school. Certainly many other opportunities will present themselves to the creative teacher when she attempts to integrate nutrition into the nursery school program.

WORKING WITH PARENTS

Informal Conferences and Meetings

Frequently parents will comment to nursery school teachers that Johnnie won't eat liver or some other food, and yet the teacher may have observed him eating the supposedly disliked food with great enthusiasm at nursery school. When the parents learn about the difference between food acceptance in the nursery school and at home, they are often very much interested in learning how the nursery school

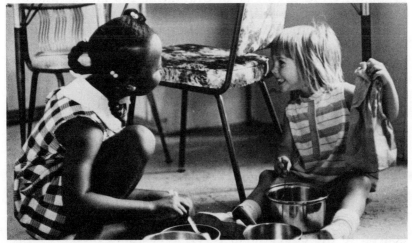

The strong interest children have in food is reflected in their play. This interest provides a good foundation for teaching nutrition.

teacher accomplishes this difference in attitude. Such queries offer excellent opportunities to begin to help parents to better understand their children at the family meal table. Informal teacher-parent conferences are often helpful to parents because it is easier for the teacher to objectively view a child's mealtime attitudes and habits than it is for the parent who has been in a close relationship with the child for a long time. The teacher, who is in a position to be a qualified observer, can often provide constructive suggestions based on unemotional observations.

Parent-teacher conferences, either formal or informal, are one means of assisting the parent who wishes to learn more about child nutrition. If parents are naturally interested in their children and relate readily to the teacher, such person-to-person talks may be very meaningful and helpful. In some situations, however, group meetings of parents with a qualified nutritionist or a teacher who has had some formal nutrition training may provide the best approach and meet with the desired acceptance. Formal meetings dealing with nutrition and other topics of interest in child development are often a regular part of nursery school programs.

Many parents find nutrition more interesting, understandable, and practical if the Basic Four Food Plan is used as the basis of the initial presentation. This plan was developed to simplify the problems of evaluating the menus planned for an entire day. Familiarity with this plan will help parents in their planning. With this plan in mind, it is valuable to outline the nutrition program conducted in the nursery school and then show how this may be continued in the home. Emphasis should be placed on the environmental factors that influence the nutrition of a child.

Ample opportunity should be provided for questions. Usually the points particularly significant in the feeding of preschoolers will be brought out in questions asked by the parents themselves. When these are answered adequately, parents will have a sound, practical basis for improving the nutrition program in their own home. Question-and-answer sessions are definitely more meaningful when the lecturer knows the background of the group so that answers can be geared to the educational level, needs, and interest of the parents. The nursery school can provide a valuable service by sending home weekly menus and recipes to be served

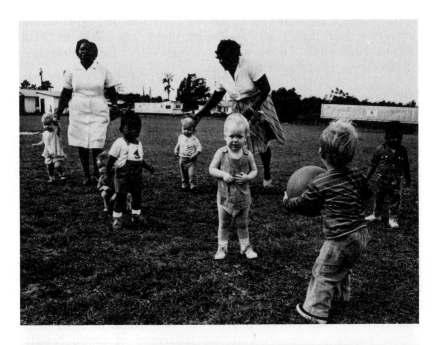

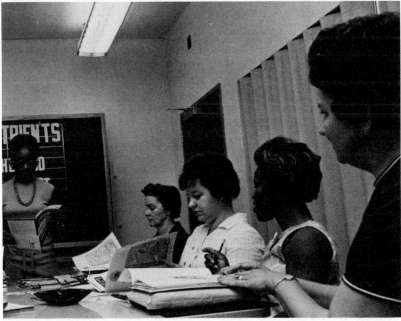

While their children are engaged in active, supervised play (top) mothers can direct their attention to a nutrition education program designed to answer their questions (below).

at the school. A mother can do a better job of planning the family's other meals if she knows what her child is being served at school. These menus also should be posted in a conspicuous place at the school.

Nutrition Surveys

Dietary records completed by parents can be a valuable aid for the person in charge of the nutrition program in the nursery school. When these records for the entire group have been gathered and analyzed, they provide a practical basis for planning school menus that effectively complement the existing nutrition patterns of the children. These surveys can serve as an important guide for helping a parent work with the individual child. Such records are more accurate and also more acceptable to the cooperating parents if the survey is planned to be as brief and as easy to complete as is practicable. Table 8.3 illustrates one such form.

After the survey is completed, each record should be analyzed to determine individual shortages of nutrients. Those parents who wish to be informed of these results can then have a conference with the nutritionist, at which time any problems in the diet can be identified and practical suggestions for overcoming deficiencies can be given.

School Visits

Parents can learn a great deal about child nutrition by visiting the nursery school at lunchtime. Such visits should be encouraged by the nursery school personnel. When parents sit on low chairs at tables designed for children, they begin to see meals from a child's perspective, a vantage point quite different from their adult view. The opportunity to observe the interaction of teacher and students at the table and to experience a meal setting specifically designed to meet the needs of the preschooler often will generate ideas for parents to try in their own homes.

SPECIAL PROGRAMS

Nutrition programs for preschoolers are operated under many different circumstances and for children from different cultural and socioeconomic backgrounds. To plan a

Table 8.3 Dietary record form suitable for recording food eaten by nursery school children at home

Name of child_____ Age_____

Usual time for: Breakfast_____ Snack_____

                Dinner   _____

Breakfast eaten: Alone_____ with family_____ with siblings only_____

Dinner eaten: Alone_____ with family_____ with siblings only_____

Day	Breakfast	Dinner	Snacks
Monday			
Tuesday			
Wednesday			
Thursday			
Friday			

suitable and effective nutrition program for a specific setting, the background of the student's families needs to be
considered. Cultural and economic factors will be particularly important considerations if the nutrition program
is to meet the children's needs. Project Head Start programs
provide valuable illustrations of nutrition planning and
education tailored to meet the needs of specific families.

Plans for nutrition programs in Project Head Start should
be considered with three thoughts firmly in mind. The
first is that good nutrition can be achieved through diets
that are not based on the classical ideas of the good, all-
American diet. Second, good nutrition is more difficult to
achieve when money for food is very limited, and thus suggestions for modification of diets need to be based on the
practical consideration of cost of the food as well as the
nutrients provided in a food. Third, and perhaps most important, is the recognition that familial and cultural habits
are strong and resistant to change; little dietary improvement can be expected on a daily basis unless suggested
changes in food habits are consonant with their existing
traditions.

Situations are certainly as varied in low-income groups
as they are in families with higher incomes. Some observations based on the Los Angeles area, however, may find
application in many other parts of the country and suggest
opportunities for working with related dietary concerns.

Realistically, meals in the homes of some families are not
necessarily the family gathering envisioned by the typical
middle-class nursery school teacher, but rather they may be
a "catch-as-catch-can" arrangement with the family members
helping themselves to a pot of beans that is constantly
available. There may be several reasons for this situation.
Often the family will not have enough chairs for everyone to
sit down to a meal together. There may not be enough dishes
and silverware to serve everyone at once. The family may
have only one pan for cooking, a fact that automatically
greatly limits the food that can be prepared and served. If
the mother is working away from home, she cannot afford to
hire an adult to help, and the children are left to fend for
themselves. All of these are actual reasons why some Project
Head Start children are inadequately fed at home.

Nutrition for Project Head Start children is best
approached in relatively simple ways as a part of the regular
program. Breakfast, as well as lunch, is an important part of

some Head Start programs because many of the children may arrive without having eaten anything. Breakfast helps to make the day go more smoothly, and it also helps children learn more about food. The discomfort from hunger during the morning certainly would not facilitate learning from the experiences provided at school.

Since the diets of these children are more likely to be less adequate in fruits and vegetables and milk than in the other food groups, breakfast and lunch menus can profitably concentrate on wide and imaginative use of these foods. Although one of the purposes of Head Start is to broaden the experiences of the children, it also seems wise to give particular attention to the introduction of relatively inexpensive but carefully prepared foods that would help to supplement their usual diets. For instance, carrots are an outstanding source of the precursor of vitamin A, a nutrient that may well be inadequate in the average diet of Mexican-American children participating in Project Head Start. This vegetable could become an important addition to their diets because of its year-round availability and its low cost.

It is important for the teacher to show acceptance of the foods normally served in the children's homes. Usually it is possible to instill ideas for small changes in habits; far better results are obtained when minor improvements or changes are made in the diet than when the usual dietary patterns are ignored and a totally foreign diet encouraged. The Mexican-American diet typically relies heavily on tortillas and beans. If these foods are retained as a basis of the diet and some cheese is melted on the refried beans, the children's nutrition will be improved. Two other ideas that may need to be fostered to help to receive maximum nutrition from this typical diet are:

1. It is wise to encourage the use of the corn rather than wheat tortillas because the liming process in the production of corn tortillas adds valuable calcium to the diet.
2. If less lard is added when beans are refried, the family will likely have less trouble with unwanted weight gains.

These subtle suggestions indicate that the teacher appreciates the dietary pattern of her group and that she is genuinely interested in maintaining the cultural heritage while helping to promote the welfare of the children. Her suggestions thus are less likely to be received with suspicion by the mothers. These ideas are simply illustrations of ways to modify food patterns without creating obstacles to acceptance. All dietary patterns can be studied in this manner.

Obviously the parroting of middle-class ideas on good nutrition will be of little value in this totally different situation. Practical suggestions on food shopping on a limited income can help considerably. Guidance on obtaining Food Stamps also may be appropriate. These suggestions usually need to be coupled with some information regarding the nutritive value of different foods. For instance, sometimes it is possible to persuade people that dried skim milk powder is not only much less expensive than fluid whole milk, but it is also much more valuable for the bones and teeth of their children than are the artificial fruit drink powders that are purchased so frequently. Rapid acceptance rarely occurs, and it is important to repeat the ideas many times if they are to be gradually accepted. Sometimes it is possible to help these families change their purchasing patterns slightly so that money used for candy is diverted to buy more nutritious foods. A 1966 survey emphasizes this problem. It reported that families with very limited income spent more money for candy than any other population group except newlyweds. These are just two illustrations of the need for better understanding of nutrition so that money can be utilized to the best advantage at the market. Others will become readily apparent as the nutritionist or teacher works with Project Head Start families.

Programs for improving the nutritional status of preschoolers and their families need to be based on an accurate assessment of the actual nutritional practices of the participating families if such programs are to be effective. Larson, et al., 1974, reported a study of Mexican-American migrants' dietary patterns in the Lower Rio Grande Valley of Texas. In this study, data regarding living conditions and various demographic items were gathered to help provide the context in which the dietary patterns were set. The survey of nutritional status for different age groups and frequency of eating various types of foods also were studied. This is the type of information which allows nutrition programs to be planned that will benefit the participants in preschool settings.

An important aspect of nutrition programs for preschoolers that merits considerable attention is ways of working with mothers of the children to help improve the nutritional habits at home as well as at school. An effective illustration of this type of approach is provided in Missoula, Montana by Zimmerman and Munro, 1972. These workers used group discussions to identify the overall dietary patterns that seemed to be common among the mothers of Head Start children in the Missoula Head Start Program. Based on this background, the group learned how a favorite food could be improved nutritionally by adding powdered milk in one instance and soy flour in another example. This initial success in modifying a familiar food in a way that was accepted by their families developed the confidence level of the mothers to the point where they were ready to learn about positive reinforcement methods that they could use to help their children build better food habits. Through the participation of the mothers and their input in developing the nutrition education program, an effective program was developed that benefited the children and their families. This is but one example of the importance of tailoring programs to meet the interests and needs of a specific group.

Although more research is needed in identifying dietary habits and assessing nutritional status of preschool children from many cultural and socioeconomic backgrounds, interest in this field has been expanding with gratifying increases in the amount of information that is being published to help workers in the field of nutrition education. There is a need to not over-generalize the findings from one group into related, yet different settings. For example, the very useful and informative study of food patterns of Indians in an Indian reservation in the Dakotas (Bass and Wakefield, 1974) can serve as a useful guide to the types of information that should be studied. However, the patterns these workers found in this specific Indian group cannot be transposed directly to Indian groups in Arizona or New Mexico.

SUMMARY

Nutrition is an important part of preschool programs in public and private settings. These programs should be planned to provide good nutrition at snacks and mealtimes while the children are at the centers. Ways of promoting acceptance of nourishing foods have been presented. The practical aspects of feeding children in group settings have been considered. These programs will be most effective when nutrition education is a part of the curriculum, parents are included in the program, and when the cultural and socioeconomic factors of food patterns are understood and incorporated in programs.

BIBLIOGRAPHY

Bass, M.A. and L.M. Wakefield, 1974. Nutritient intake and food patterns of Indians on Standing Rock Reservation. *J. Amer. Dietet. Assoc.* 64: 29.

California State Dept. of Public Health. *Dishwashing in Commercial Establishments.* Sacramento, Calif., undated.

Fomon, S.J. and T.A. Anderson, 1972. *Practices of Low-Income Families in Feeding Infants and Small Children.* U.S. Dept. of Health, Education, and Welfare, Maternal and Child Health Services. Rockville, Md.

Frankle, R.T., et al., 1967. Project Head Start – a challenge in creativity in community nutrition. *J. Home Econ.* 59, No. 1: 24.

Hille, H.M., 1960. *Food for Groups of Young Children Cared for during the Day.* Publ. No. 386. U.S. Dept. of Health, Education and Welfare, Children's Bureau. Washington, D.C.

Larson, L.B., et al., 1974. Nutritional status of children of Mexican-American migrant families. *J. Amer. Dietet. Assoc.* 64: 29.

Los Angeles County Health Department, 1963. *You Can Prevent Foodborne Illness.* Div. of Public Health Education. Los Angeles.

Nutrition, Better Eating for a Head Start, 1965. Office of Economic Opportunity. Washington, D.C.

Nutrition Guidelines for the Project Head Start Centers Feeding Program, 1965. Office of Economic Opportunity. Washington, D.C.

Sadow, S., 1965. *Food Buying Guide and Recipes for the Project Head Start Centers Feeding Program.* Office of Economic Opportunity. Washington, D.C.

Schulz, L., 1965. *Study of Food Preferences of Children in Nursery School.* Unpublished report. California State University, Los Angeles.

Sims, L.S. and P.M. Morris, 1974. Nutritional status of pre-schoolers. *J. Amer. Dietet. Assoc.* 64: 592.

Sweeny, M.E. and M.F. Breckenridge, 1951. *How to Feed Children in Nursery Schools.* Merrill-Palmer School. Detroit, Mich.

Zimmerman, R.R. and N. Munro, 1972. Changing Head Start mothers' food attitudes and practices. *J. Nutr. Ed.* 4: 66.

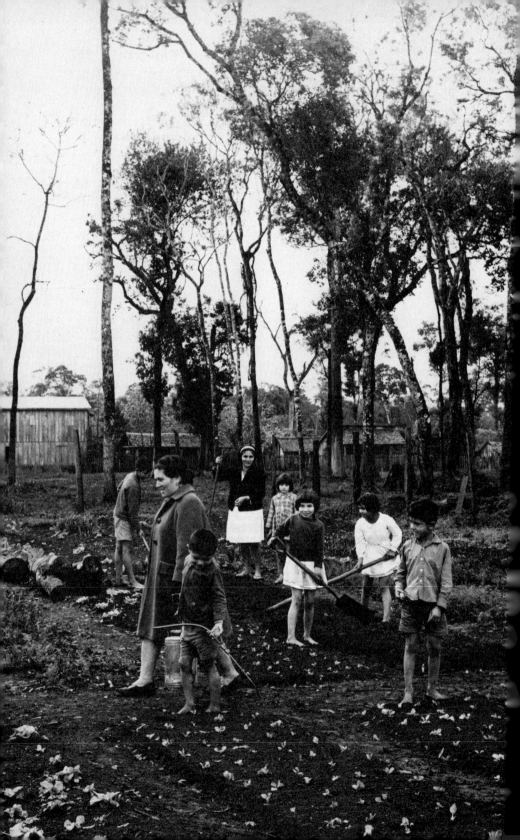

Chapter 9
Preadolescents

The elementary school years are significant nutritionally because they provide a time to build up body stores of nutrients in preparation for the rapid growth of adolescence. This is also a period when it is appropriate to give continuing emphasis to nutrition education and to direct attention toward developing good nutrition habits that are self-motivated.

CHANGING NUTRITIONAL NEEDS

Gradual Changes

The elementary school child is growing, but the growth rate is distinctly less than that of infancy and certainly does not approach the spectacular change in height and weight that normally occurs in adolescence. If observable growth rates are used as the only criterion on which to base nutritional needs, one may erroneously conclude that nutrition does not play a very significant role in the development of the child during this period of time. Actually this is far from true. The elementary school child has a continuing need for an adequate diet to:

1. Provide building materials for growth.
2. Furnish the energy needed for the vigorous physical activities of this age group.
3. Help to maintain resistance to infections.
4. Ensure that adequate body stores of nutrients are available for the growth demands of the teens.

Attention should be given during these years to developing the habit of eating a good diet. By the time a child reaches adolescence, he should be accustomed to regularly eating a good diet and should have a good understanding of the reasons why he needs to be well nourished. Good habits, coupled with knowledge, will help greatly in maintaining good nutritional status during adolescence.

During ages 7 through 10 of the elementary school years, nutritional needs are increased somewhat from the needs of the preschool child. An examination of the complete table of recommended daily dietary allowances (Table 4.4) will reveal that there is a gradual increase in the need for calories from birth through the elementary school period, to be followed by an increasing need during the adolescent period. As one would expect, there is also an increased need for protein, iodine, magnesium, vitamin A, the B vitamins and vitamin E. The recommended allowances for calcium, phosphorus, iron, zinc, ascorbic acid, and vitamin D remain the same for the elementary school child as they were for the preschooler. It is apparent from this summary (see Table 9.1) that the elementary school child has need for somewhat more food that the preschooler, but the changes are not startling. The normal, healthy child will naturally increase his intake during this period if good nutrition habits are encouraged quietly and well-planned, tasty meals are served. Perhaps it is necessary to mention the importance of exercise in maintaining good appetites. Active physical play develops healthy appetites, but too much television viewing or other sedentary activity fosters poor nutrition. Frequently children who watch television a great deal nibble while watching and completely spoil appetites for meals.

Sex Differences

As shown in Table 9.1, no sexual distinction is made between the nutritional needs of boys and girls until the age of 11. Boys between the ages of 11 and 14, however, have a greater need for calories, vitamin A, thiamin, riboflavin, niacin, iodine and magnesium than do girls of the same age. These differences reflect the greater muscle development and physical activity of boys in contrast to the slightly greater fatty deposits and lesser physical activity of girls. The greater

Table 9.1 Recommended daily dietary allowances for children of elementary school age[a]

	Age 4–6	Age 7–10	Age 11–14 Male	Female
Weight, kg. (lb.)	20 (40)	30 (66)	44 (97)	44 (97)
Height, cm. (in.)	110 (44)	135 (54)	158 (63)	155 (62)
Energy, kcal.	1800	2400	2800	2400
Protein, g.	30	36	44	44
Vitamin A, I.U.	2500	3300	5000	4000
Vitamin D, I.U.	400	400	400	400
Vitamin E activity, I.U.	9	10	12	12
Ascorbic acid, mg.	40	40	45	45
Folacin, μg.	200	300	400	400
Niacin, mg.	12	16	18	16
Riboflavin, mg.	1.1	1.2	1.5	1.3
Thiamin, mg.	0.9	1.2	1.4	1.2
Vitamin B_6, mg.	0.9	1.2	1.6	1.6
Vitamin B_{12}, μg.	1.5	2.0	3.0	3.0
Calcium, mg.	800	800	1200	1200
Phosphorus, mg.	800	800	1200	1200
Iodine, μg.	80	110	130	115
Iron, mg.	10	10	18	18
Magnesium, mg.	200	250	350	300
Zinc, mg.	10	10	15	15

[a]From 1974 revision of the table of daily dietary allowances as recommended by the Food and Nutrition Board of the National Research Council, National Academy of Sciences.

need for some of the B vitamins is related to the greater quantity of food that will be ingested by boys than will be ingested by girls of the same age.

Nutrients of Special Concern

Nutrition surveys have been conducted on a national basis at intervals during this century. The most recent of these was the 10-State Nutrition Survey, a survey conducted in 1969 in the states of California, Kentucky, Louisiana, Massachusetts, Michigan, New York (including a special survey in New York City), South Carolina, Texas, Washington, and West Virginia. This study, which was directed toward districts within these states where many families were living on low incomes (the majority with incomes of less than $3000 per year), revealed a number of nutritionally-based problems for individuals of all ages. Dental problems, retarded growth, and evidence of low serum levels of ascorbic acid, protein, riboflavin, thiamin, calories, iron, vitamin A, and also vitamin C were found in numerous individuals. Tangible evidence of improved nutritional status (increased stature, body weight, advanced skeletal and dental development, and earlier maturation) was correlated positively with increasing per capita income.

This survey, although directed toward a somewhat selected sample, supports the broader findings of the national survey of food intake and nutritive value of diets conducted in 1965. These data were evaluated in relation to the recommended dietary allowances, 1968 revision. The results of the survey indicated that elementary-age school children up until the age of 9 were receiving adequate amounts of protein, calcium, iron, vitamin A, thiamin, riboflavin, and ascorbic acid. Between the ages of 9 and 11, boys were found to be better nourished than girls; boys were low in their intake of calcium, but girls were considerably lower than boys in their intake of calcium and, in addition, were also very low in their consumption of iron and slightly low in ingestion of thiamin.

THE MOTHER'S ROLE

Meal Preparation

The nutritional needs of large numbers of elementary school children will be met only partially at home because most rural and city schools commonly have a lunch program. It is apparent that the mother still maintains an important role, because she usually is responsible for two meals and an after-school snack each day. It is also essential, however, that the school recognize its responsibility for the lunch meal.

If a child is to be well nourished during the elementary school period, it is essential that the mother continue to maintain a very conscientious effort in planning and serving meals. She can meet this responsibility by preparing appetizing, nourishing meals on a schedule convenient for her family. In today's urban societies, there appears to be a growing tendency for family meals to be less and less a family affair. With fathers gone from the home many hours a day and school children involved in various activities, mothers may feel less responsibility toward meal preparation and the feeding of their children. It still is necessary, despite all the convenience foods, to spend some time planning an adequate menu and then preparing it. The temptations are great for the modern mother to let children help themselves to ready-to-eat convenience foods that they can fix whenever they are hungry. Unfortunately, this type of helter-skelter approach does not lead to a well-nourished child.

Few elementary school children are capable of planning a well-balanced diet each day without some adult assistance, nor are they usually able to prepare complete meals that will meet their needs. The mother still needs to retain the final responsibility for the family's meals. If the mother is working outside the home, it may be appropriate to have school age children or a domestic helper do some meal preparation, but the mother still should be certain that the meals are nutritionally adequate and appetizing.

It is as important for children to have a nourishing breakfast and lunch as it is for them to have a good dinner. In the modern family, the greatest tendency toward skimping on nutrition probably occurs at breakfast and lunch. Since the father is at home for dinner, it is usually far more adequate than the other meals of the day. Good breakfast habits are likely to be maintained in families who have a formal breakfast together. Unfortunately, the staggered scheduling in some families may make this arrangement impractical. The mother, however, can still encourage her children to eat a good breakfast if she gets up early enough to fix an appetizing meal and eats with the children, both on school mornings and during vacations.

Supervisory Capacity

The role of the mother now begins to assume a slightly different character from that which she performed when her child was younger. The supervisory role begins to gain in importance as children go through elementary school. Mothers need to check periodically to be sure that their children are eating the types of foods in the quantities necessary to maintain their growing bodies during this period. It is not enough simply to feed a child sufficient calories to prevent hunger; it is also necessary to be sure that the diet includes adequate amounts of milk, breads and cereals, meats, fruits, and vegetables to provide the necessary protein, vitamins, and minerals. During the elementary school period there is an increasing tendency to consume more foods that are low in nutritive value and high in calories. Children of this age begin to be increasingly independent, particularly in regard to snacks. The small amount of financial independence resulting from allowances, odd jobs, and paper routes enables boys and girls to buy candy or pop, both of which fill little nutritional need and are superfluous in the elementary school child's diet.

It is the conscientious mother's responsibility to be certain that her school-age child has an adequate diet. It will be necessary for her to make a deliberate effort to be aware of the foods her child actually consumes during the entire day, including school lunches and snack foods. Many schools make it a practice to have their school lunch menus published weekly in the local newspaper, a practice

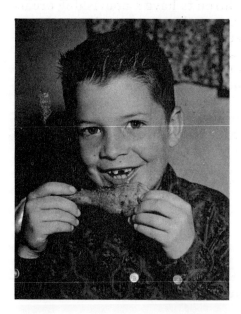

A piece of fried chicken, cold from the refrigerator, makes an appetizing snack that is high in protein. If one piece is eaten right after school, dinner appetite will still be good.

that makes it easier to correlate family meals with those eaten at school.

Children are usually very hungry after school and do need a snack. The snack, however, should be eaten as early as possible and should be sufficient to ease the immediate hunger without squelching the appetite for dinner. When necessary, mothers should help children plan more nourishing food for snacks, and they may also need to make suggestions regarding the quantity of the snack eaten after school. The amount of the after-school snack is impossible to suggest here because of the individual variation in children's appetites and the differences among families in their traditional time for the evening meal. It is important, however, that snacks not interfere with dinner appetites, because a well-planned dinner will provide many necessary nutrients that may be lacking in a snack.

THE FATHER'S ROLE

Although the father in a family traditionally does not have the primary responsibility for his family's nutritional status, he can make important contributions in this matter. As head of the family, the example he sets will influence his children at the table. If he likes the foods served at a meal and eats them with enthusiasm, his children usually will emulate him and contentedly eat their food. He can also help by complimenting his wife when food is well prepared. Such praise encourages excellence in meal preparation because the effort required is appreciated. The net result is a well-nourished family. Fathers also can encourage children to be active and participate in sports. A conscious effort is needed to increase the level of physical activity by both children and adults.

PRACTICAL APPLICATIONS

Breakfast

The dietary pattern for the elementary school child should include a broad variety of foods selected to meet the child's needs for growth, maintenance, and activity. Attention certainly should be given in the home to consumption of an adequate breakfast. Children will perform better in school when they have an adequate breakfast before starting the day's school work. Such a breakfast should include a citrus fruit or other good source of ascorbic acid, with a good source of protein such as bacon or an egg, cereal or toast, and a glass of milk. This breakfast is adequate for the young elementary school child, but the quantities will need to be increased considerably to satisfy a boy's appetite by the time he reaches the sixth grade. A typical sixth-grade boy's breakfast might include a four-ounce glass of juice, an eight-ounce glass of milk, a large bowl of cereal and milk, two pieces of toast, and bacon, weiner, or egg.

Lunch

Whether lunch is eaten at home or at school, it is again important that a good source of protein be available in adequate quantities. The protein at lunch could be from either animal or vegetable sources; cheese, eggs, meat of any type, poultry, fish, kidney beans, lima beans or other legumes are all appropriate. It is important to realize that soups containing a small amount of meat are definitely inadequate as the sole source of protein at a meal. Soups have their place in a meal, but they should be supplemented by another food high in protein in order to meet the need for protein at the lunch meal. Soup, combined with a meat sandwich, would adequately meet the body's need for protein at lunch. The lunch menu should also include two or more vegetables and/or fruit, a serving of bread or bread substitute, and a glass of milk. Many elementary school children, particularly the older boys, may need more food than this and they may desire additional servings or a greater variety of food at lunch.

If a child carries his lunch to school, it is still important that the lunch be well prepared and appetizing. Simply taking a jelly sandwich and calling it lunch is not adequate for any elementary school child. Again, protein should be included in the sack lunch every day. The protein food can be varied from day to day by including such foods as cold fried chicken, a slice of cold meat loaf, slices of cold cuts, a hard-cooked egg, cheese, or other meats. Sack lunches often contain a high proportion of bread and baked products and inadequate amounts of protein foods, fruits, and vegetables. Fruits and raw vegetables are quite adaptable to use in a sack lunch. Milk usually can be purchased at the school, but it could be taken in a thermos bottle when necessary.

Dinner

Dinner in most families is probably reasonably adequate. Attention at this meal should be centered on pleasant service of an attractive, well-balanced meal. Dinner usually provides the best opportunity for mothers to be creative in the kitchen and to consciously attempt to expand a child's experiences with new foods, including a variety of seasonings and spices. Children of elementary school age are able to experiment with a wide range of seasonings because the gastrointestinal tract is less easily irritated, and they are able to digest more highly seasoned foods than the pre-schooler can manage.

This is a good time to expand the family menus to include many things that may not have been prepared previously for the children. She may wish to establish the tradition of having a meal typical of a different foreign country one night each week. The children could learn a little about the various countries in this way and the entire family could enjoy such a project. Appropriate table decorations can be made by the children. Menus and recipes from foreign countries are readily available, and most of the ingredients needed can be found in supermarkets or specialty shops.

THE SCHOOL LUNCH

Although the school lunch is a government-subsidized program operated in the public schools, it still seems wise for parents and teachers to have an opportunity to learn something about the purpose of the program and its operation. An interested involvement on the part of parents in the community is vital to a vigorous, effective school lunch program. The ensuing discussion pinpointing some of the key factors involved in successful operation of school lunch programs is intended to develop a greater understanding of some of the problems schools face in this area.

Legislation

The National School Lunch Program developed from a federal program that was launched in 1935 to distribute some surplus foods to schools to be used in free lunch programs. Eight years later, in 1943, schools received payments through the Unites States Department of Agriculture to help meet part of the costs of foods that were purchased locally for school lunches. Formal support of the concept of school lunch program was provided in 1946 when the National School Lunch Act was passed. Its purpose was defined: "to safeguard the health and well-being of the Nation's children and to encourage the domestic consumption of nutritious agricultural commodities and other food, by assisting the States, through grants-in-aid and other means, in providing an adequate supply of foods and other facilities for the establishment, maintenance, operation, and expansion of nonprofit school lunch programs". Subsequent legislation has added to the program to improve the nutrition of the nation's children. An amendment in 1970 stipulated that every American school child who was needy (according to specified guidelines) should be served meals free or at reduced cost. States were charged with the responsibility of bringing this program to every school.

The Child Nutrition Act of 1966 was significant because it authorized a 2-year pilot program for a School Breakfast Program. Extensions of this effort were provided in 1968 and 1971. In 1973 the breakfast program became available to all schools wishing to apply. The reimbursement rate for the program in late 1973 provided a payment of 29.5 cents of federal funds for each free breakfast served, 24.25 cents for each reduced-price breakfast, and 8.5 cents for each paid breakfast. Participation in this aspect of school feeding programs has increased from 330,000 students in 1969 to a projected 1.8 million in 1974.

The National School Lunch Program is now operated under the original act with a number of amendments extending and modifying the original legislation. The 1973 amendment authorized federal reimbursement to the states at the rate of 10 cents per lunch, with an additional 45 cents average for free lunches served. With an eye toward the inflationary trend in food prices that was evident in 1973, the legislation provided for semi-annual review of costs and

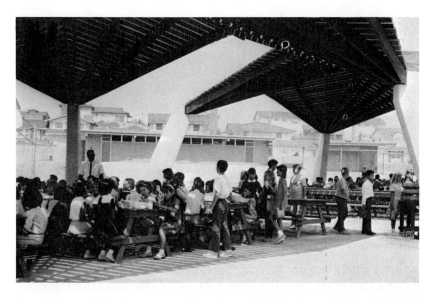

The National School Lunch Program is operated in many different physical settings ranging from this outdoor, shaded area in California to school gymnasiums in colder climates.

adjustments to be made as necessary. This escalation clause was already utilized when support in the last half of 1974 was increased to 10.5 cents for lunches and 47.25 cents for free lunches. The school lunch, as supported by federal funds, reaches increasing numbers of children. In 1972 more than 25 million school children participated in the program. Free or reduced-price lunches were served to 8.7 million needy children in 1972, and almost 9 million were reached, according to estimates, in 1973. As a consequence of increasing costs, many schools have raised the price of the lunches. The United States Department of Agriculture reported that a 1 cent increase in the cost of the lunch resulted in a 1 percent decrease in participation.

Another aspect of federal support for nutrition is found in the 1968 amendment to the National School Lunch Act, the amendment which established a 3-year pilot Special Food Service Program for Children. Under this amendment, coverage was extended to cover day care centers, settlement houses, and recreation programs operated as public and non-profit institutions. Summer recreation programs for

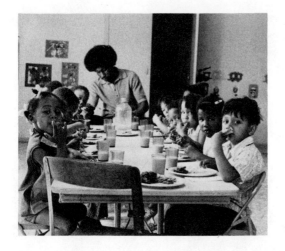

Under the Special Food Service Program for Children amendment to the National School Lunch Act, day care centers are entitled to federal assistance in providing good nutrition for preschoolers.

school children in low income areas were included. Year-round programs for the children of needy working mothers, preschool as well as older children, are included for support. Coverage may include support for breakfast and/or lunch and/or dinner and/or between-meal supplements. Up to 100 percent of the daily dietary allowances may be provided under this program. This program has been extended beyond the original 3-year period and is estimated to have reached approximately a million children in the 1973 summer program and more than 220,000 in the year-round phase.

Milk programs to provide milk to school children trace their history to the early 1940's. Support for the Special Milk Program, which was provided in the 1966 Child Nutrition Act, has been quite controversial. The growth of other aspects of the National School Lunch Program has caused some opponents to recommend cutting back the Special Milk Program to aid only schools where no other type of food service was available. This argument has been defeated, at least for the present, and the Special Milk Program has support at least through 1974.

Planning the Menus

Planning a school lunch is a real challenge for any nutritionist despite the fact that the school lunch supervisor is assisted in her planning by the requirements set forth under the National School Lunch Program. The Type A lunch must meet these requirements and provide approximately one-third of the RDA.

1. Eight ounces (one-half pint) of fluid types of unflavored milk or low-fat or skim milk or cultured buttermilk meeting State and local standards for such milks and flavored milks made from milks meeting such standards.
2. A protein-rich food: two ounces of cooked or canned lean meat, fish, or poultry; or two ounces of cheese, or one egg; or one-half cup cooked dried beans or peas; or four tablespoons of peanut butter; or an equivalent combination of these foods.
3. Vegetables and fruits: two or more to equal three-fourths cup total. Undiluted juice can be used as the equivalent of one-fourth cup of the total. The inclusion of an ascorbic-acid source daily and a vitamin A food on alternate days will help meet recognized shortages in the diets of some of the children.
4. Bread or a bread substitute, either whole-grain or made with enriched flour: one slice or its equivalent.
5. Butter or fortified margarine: two teaspoons used as a spread or in preparation of other foods.

Planning a menu that meets the preceding government specifications, contains at least 80 percent of food locally

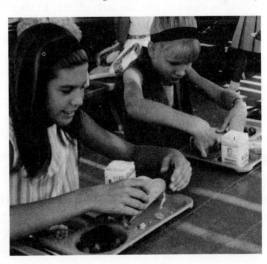

A type A school lunch and two eager consumers. The taco in the menu will be familiar fare to the children in this California school district.

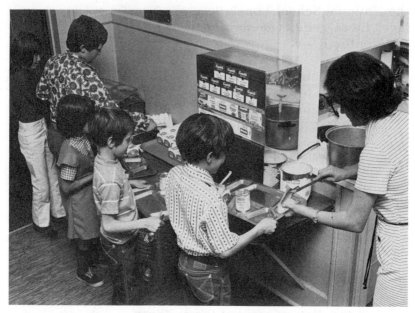

Special menus in a can have been developed for dispensing school lunches where kitchen facilities are limited.

available, fits the required cost limitations, and can be prepared within the physical setup of the school kitchen is only part of the problem. Perhaps the most difficult facet of the menu to predict is acceptance of the meal. Even when a menu meets all other criteria for a good lunch, it can be considered a failure if many children do not eat the food. Menus should be planned to include not only variety but also enough familiar foods so that they will be accepted and eaten by the children. Anyone could plan a lunch of hamburgers and potato chips day after day, and the acceptance would be relatively high, at least for a time. One purpose of the school lunch, however, is to encourage children to eat a variety of foods, and repetitious menus are not in concert with this objective. It is necessary to find other foods that children of this age will enjoy and that the cook can prepare satisfactorily.

To develop a set of menus that will be suitable for use in a particular school system, it is necessary for the school lunch supervisor to test many different recipes. She must always be on the alert to locate suitable recipes for the lunch program. The only realistic way of evaluating the new food is to see how the "judges" rate it in the lunch room. The most practical way to determine consumer acceptance is to visit the school lunch scene where it is possible to overhear children's candid comments on the food and to observe the food that is left on the plates at the end of the meal. Such a visitation is essential to correct gross errors in expected acceptance.

When planning school menus it is wise to consider the racial and cultural backgrounds of the children in the school and to include regularly some foods typical of the groups represented. Familiarity with foods helps to increase acceptance of the lunch program. Then some new, but closely related foods may be added. This approach is especially important when most of the children are from homes where a limited menu is usually served.

Physical Facilities

Once the menus have been determined, it is also necessary for the school lunch supervisor to view the setting in which the children will eat. Although the children may seem to ignore the physical arrangements for the meal, a comfortable, pleasing environment will promote acceptance. Such influences are subtle and can best be assessed by a well-trained, sensitive individual. It may seem unimportant, but children will eat a meal more eagerly when they are able to use acceptable silver. Bent fork tines or very cheap stainless steel utensils with sharp edges do not feel comfortable in the hand or in the mouth and so discourage consumption of the food. Ideally, younger elementary children will have smaller silver to use.

Food should be served neatly and carefully to make each plate attractive. Many children like to have their food arranged on the plate so that the different foods are not overlapping or running together. Distinct servings have far more appeal to children than do jumbled plates. It is also desirable to have the food hot when it is served to the children, but this factor appears to be less important to children than to adults.

Efficient service is essential because there ordinarily are many children to feed and school schedules usually allow only a short lunch period. Inefficient service will cause some children to have a long wait in line and a very short time for eating.

In addition, the tables should be comfortable for the children, of a convenient height and equipped with movable benches or chairs. If fixed benches are used, they should be close enough to the table so that the smaller youngsters can reach their plates without major difficulties. The tables should be located in a pleasant room or in a shady area outdoors. In a noisy, very hot setting the consumption of food becomes a chore to be avoided or cut to a minimum.

Scheduling

Cooperation is needed from the school administration if a really smooth-running lunch program is to be achieved. The time schedule for the school should include a reasonable time for serving and eating the food. Many schools allow such a limited lunch time that children literally have to gobble their food to finish in the allotted time. Slow eaters simply cannot consume a complete meal in ten minutes, yet this is the amount of time available if they happen to be near the end of the lunch line. This is a very real problem in many schools. It would seem far wiser to avoid such a chaotic lunch break by adding approximately ten minutes to the lunch hour.

In schools having two or more shifts for lunch service, it is advisable to serve the younger children first. An early lunch helps to keep the younger children from becoming too tired to eat.

The Lunch Room in Action

Supervision of the lunch area should be undertaken with the idea of making the lunch time as pleasant as possible for all the children. A few simple suggestions should solve most of the problems that might arise in the typical school lunch program.

One suggestion that could be used to advantage by many schools is to allow the children to sit where they wish whether they have brought their own lunch or are participating in the hot lunch programs. When "hot lunch children" and "cold lunch children" have to sit in different areas, acceptance of the hot lunch program diminishes because

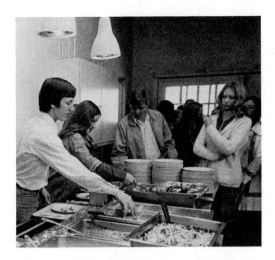

The "serve yourself" line speeds service, cuts waste, and invites participation in school lunch programs.

children who otherwise would be participating in the hot lunch program may elect to bring a cold lunch just so they can eat with their friends who regularly bring sack lunches. Certainly it is desirable to do everything possible to encourage participation in the hot lunch program. Unless parents are careful about its contents, the sack lunch is likely to be less adequate nutritionally than the hot lunch available at school.

An adult monitoring the school lunch situation can be quite effective in controlling food trading. Children in elementary school seem to thrive on the bargaining that can take place at lunch time if trading is permitted. One child may be particularly clever at this and end up with three or four desserts for which he may have bartered all the rest of his meal. Not only does he end up with a poorly balanced diet, but it is apparent that changes have taken place also in the meals of the children with whom he has been trading. Menus in the school lunch program are designed to provide an adequate meal when each child receives his share of each of the foods on the menu. Obviously, when trading occurs, lunches will bear little resemblance to the original menu.

It should also be kept in mind that older elementary school children, particularly boys, may need more food than is included in the minimum Type A lunch. Some provision should be made in the lunch program for hungry children to have additional food to satisfy appetites. As a result of government assistance, school lunches actually are quite inexpensive, and many families could and would pay for extra servings when needed.

NUTRITION EDUCATION

The elementary grades are an important time to emphasize nutrition education in the classroom as well as in the lunch room. An enthusiastic, imaginative approach is essential. The study of nutrition need not be a regimented, dull routine done entirely with a book in front of the students, but can take on many forms. After an adequate elementary introduction to nutrition has been given, this subject can be integrated very effectively with other study units throughout the school year. The program should be based on a study of the food groups and this should be carefully developed with the students.

To supplement this emphasis, various field trips might be taken. The four food groups could be given considerable emphasis if the class made four field trips, one to study some specific aspect of foods in each of the food groups. For instance, a trip to the dairy to observe the milking of cows and the subsequent pasteurization and bottling of the milk could be a very informative nutrition lesson for young elementary school children. If possible, slightly older children could be taken to watch cheese-making; many dairies make cottage cheese and some classes probably could observe the more complex manufacturing of cheddar and other cheese. In lieu of such opportunities, interest in dairy products could be stimulated by making cottage cheese or ice cream in the school room. This type of lesson can be reinforced by a summarization of the field experiences, including a discussion of the value of such foods in the diet.

Another interesting field trip is a tour to a local cannery or freezing plant to observe the processing of fruits or vegetables. An alternative for helping to emphasize the value of the fruit and vegetable group would be to plant a small vegetable garden at the school so that the children can observe the transition from seed to the mature food. The vegetables ideally would then be cooked and served to the children as a culmination of this particular project.

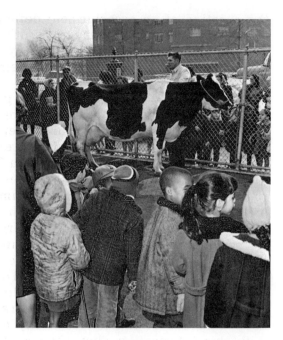

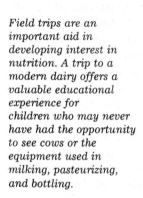

Field trips are an important aid in developing interest in nutrition. A trip to a modern dairy offers a valuable educational experience for children who may never have had the opportunity to see cows or the equipment used in milking, pasteurizing, and bottling.

The bread and cereal group gains considerable interest when a class visits a flour mill or a cereal manufacturer, but a trip to a local bakery is very suitable when the mill or manufacturing plants are not accessible. Various baking projects could be accomplished effectively in the classroom with the use of a portable electric oven or frying pan.

The meat category might be studied by visiting a farm, a large aquarium, an egg ranch, stock yards, or a fish hatchery. Students will gain a greater appreciation of the diversity of foods that are good sources of protein if more than one of these trips can be taken. If time and facilities for field trips are limited, this might be accomplished effectively by a trip to the meat market of a large grocery store.

Animal-feeding experiments hold considerable interest because most children seem to be fascinated by animals of all kinds. Guinea pigs or white rats are particularly well suited to small-scale animal-feeding experiments in the classroom. By establishing controlled experimental conditions in which the animals are fed a special diet deficient in the selected nutrient, it is possible to demonstrate graphically even to young children the importance of good nutrition. A particularly appropriate experiment of this type is the creation of an ascorbic-acid deficiency in guinea pigs. Since white rats do not need ascorbic acid, they cannot be used to demonstrate a deficiency of this vitamin, but they may be used effectively to demonstrate deficiency conditions of the other vitamins.

Children in the upper elementary grades can undertake the project of keeping a week's record of their own individual food intake. These records then can be analyzed to see whether the individual children are consuming adequate diets. The Basic Four Food Plan is a convenient standard for this evaluation. When the shortages have been assessed, suggestions can be worked out for improving the dietary habits of the children. Obviously, such an ambitious project needs to wait until the upper elementary grades.

In conjunction with a nutrition unit in the fifth or sixth grade, a dentist could talk about the roles of the various nutrients in body and tooth growth and development.

Another project for the upper elementary grades is a careful study of the school lunch program, in which students keep a record of the food actually eaten at lunch time. With this information, they have a basis to begin to consider and to appreciate the influence of food preferences and prejudices on nutrition of the individual and the group. After studying the consumption patterns at their school, the older elementary children could work with the school lunch supervisor and plan a week's menus for the school lunch program. Such a project is more educational and meaningful when it is possible to actually use these menus in the school. The class can learn a great deal from eating the meals they have planned and from observing the reactions of other children to the menus.

Nutrition can be brought very effectively into social studies units because malnutrition is commonplace in some parts of the world. For example, protein-calorie malnutrition is found in some areas of India, Africa, Central America, and South America. Some children in Malaysia are blind as a result of a severe vitamin A deficiency. United Nations films are available which will show clearly such conditions. These films carry tremendous impact because extreme cases of malnutrition are rarely observed by children in the United States. Such movies are valuable to social studies classes because they show living conditions of the people as well as their nutritional problems.

Social studies units on the locale in which school children live also may include some nutrition work. For example, a fourth-grade class in California was studying California Indians of the past. When the diets of early Indians in various sections of California were studied, nutrition began to assume greater importance in the eyes of the students. The class found that the Indians along the coast had a more prosperous, flourishing civilization than did those living in the desert regions. There were several reasons for this, but one significant contributing factor certainly was the diet of the Indians along the coast. These Indians were somewhat larger in stature and a bit more advanced in their civilization than the inland Indians, a difference that could be explained by the fact that the large amount of fish and shellfish in the diet of the coastal Indians provided considerably more protein than was available to the inland Indians who ate largely a limited vegetarian diet.

It is an interesting sidelight to note that nutrition can be drawn into an amazing variety of disciplines. For instance, nutrition knowledge was one avenue explored by archaeologists in an attempt to estimate the population of a now extinct Indian population group. By measuring the quantity of shells thrown into refuse dumps by these long-ago people after they consumed the muscle of shellfish, and then figuring the minimum amount of fish that would be needed by each person each day, a rough estimate of the population was determined. If a teacher will make the effort to ferret out such information in the library, he can bring information to the classroom which will help bring alive the study of nutrition and make it fascinating and meaningful to the elementary school child.

These examples of nutrition projects have been mentioned to stimulate thought on how nutrition can be made more interesting and meaningful to the elementary school child. To simply parrot nutrition education information to children is a waste, for no subject is interesting when it is taught in such an unimaginative manner. It is the responsibility of the teacher to plan and carry out projects that help to illustrate graphically the importance of nutrition for children in this age group.

Nutrition education programs for elementary school children have as one of their goals the development of a basic, elementary knowledge of nutrition. Studies such as the nutrition education program for fourth and fifth graders reported by Baker (1972) are being conducted by some teachers in this country. Evaluation of the effectiveness of educational programs indicates that well-planned units of study can be effective in teaching knowledge of nutrition. The difficulty is encountered in achieving a second goal: accomplishing behavioral change to modify dietary patterns consistent with the knowledge acquired. Baker (1972) found that, although her education program was effective in teaching information, it was not able to bring about behavior modification.

Gussow (1972) presented data regarding counternutritional messages contained in television ads directed at children. The frequency of nutrition messages that were counter to developing good nutrition habits was studied by monitoring children's television programs on Saturday mornings. Although the actual number of commercials varied among the three major networks, the majority of the messages was deemed to be of negative value in teaching nutrition. Ward and Wackman (1971) determined that children ages five to seven were successful in persuading their mothers to yield to their requests for food purchases of breakfast cereals, snack foods, candy, and soft drinks at least 38 percent of the time and, in the case of cereals, 88 percent of the time. When children were eight to ten years old, they were able to persuade their mothers more than 90 percent of the time. Since these children receive numerous, persuasive and reinforced food messages via television, the significance of such ads requires careful thought when considering nutrition education in its total context of behavior modification.

SUMMARY

The nutritional needs of elementary school children gradually increase as they continue to grow and prepare for the adolescent growth spurt. The needs of boys, beginning at approximately 11 years of age, increase more rapidly than do the needs of girls. The elementary school period is particularly important as a time to learn about and to develop a motivating interest in nutrition. A firm foundation in good nutrition practices at this age will greatly facilitate the achievement of good nutrition during the demanding adolescent period.

Parents need to work with their children as individuals to further improve the nutritional status of their elementary school children. Certainly it is true that the final responsibility for helping each child to be well nourished lies with the parents. The example set in the home by the father and mother will mold, to a great extent, the dietary habits of children in a family. It is important that parents recognize this exemplary influence that they exert and make every effort possible to be certain that they are helping to establish healthful dietary patterns in their children. Parents also need to be aware of the potential nutrition "education" their children receive via television.

By implementing a truly effective nutrition education program both in the classroom and in the lunch room, the school can also be an important influence on the lives of its students. Creative teachers will find ways to bring nutrition into the classroom in an interdisciplinary presentation when it seems appropriate, thus giving nutrition a broader and deeper meaning to the children. This interest aroused in school can serve as the foundation for continuing nutrition projects in the home.

BIBLIOGRAPHY

American Academy of Pediatrics, 1973. Ten-State Nutrition Survey: pediatric perspective. *Pediat.* 51: 1095.

Anonymous, 1965. *Food Intake and Nutritive Value of Diets of Men, Women, and Children in the United States, Spring, 1965.* Consumer and Food Economics Research Division. Hyattsville, Md.

Baker, M.J., 1972. Influence of nutrition education on fourth and fifth graders. *J. Nutr. Ed.* 4: 55.

Beal, V. A., 1961. Dietary intake of individuals followed through infancy and childhood. *Am. J. Pub. Health* 51, No. 8: 1107.

Bowes, A., 1955. Nutrition of children during their school years. *Amer. J. Clin. Nutr.* 3: 254.

Eppright, E.S., et al., 1963. Effect on girls of greater intake of milk, fruits, and vegetables. *Amer. Dietet. Assoc. J.* 43: 299.

Gschneidner, M.P. and C.E. Roderuck, 1960. Nutriture of school girls of different physiques. *Amer. Dietet. Assoc. J.* 36: 22.

Gussow, J.D., 1972. Counternutritional messages of TV ads aimed at children. *J. Nutr. Ed.* 4: 48.

Heald, F. and R. Hollander, 1965. The relationship between obesity in adolescence and early growth. *J. Pediat.* 67:35.

Hootman, R.H., et al., 1967. Diet practices and physical development of Iowa children from low income families. *J. Home Econ.* 59: 41.

Joint Committee on Health Problems in Education, 1962. *Health Aspects of the School Lunch Program.* American Med. Assoc., Chicago.

Kilander, H.F., 1962. *School Health Education.* Macmillan, New York.

Lavigne, M.E. and L. Siegel, 1965. Nutrition education involves total school. *Nutr. News* 28, No. 3: 10.

Lukaczer, M., 1973. National School Lunch Program in 1973. *Nutr. Reviews* 31: 385.

Miskimin, D., et al., 1974. Nutrification of frozen preplated school lunches is needed. *Food Tech.* 28, No. 2: 52.

Morgan, A.F., 1959. *Nutritional Status U.S.A.* Calif. Agricultural Experiment Station Bull. 769. Berkeley, Calif.

Nutrition Foundation, 1965. Effects of a balanced lunch program on the growth and nutritional status of school children. *Nutr. Reviews.* 23: 35.

Read, M.S., 1973. Malnutrition, hunger, and behavior. *J. Amer. Dietet. Assoc.* 63: 386.

Review, 1974. Child nutrition programs. *Dairy Council Digest* 45, No. 1: 1.

Sandstrom, M.M., 1959. School lunches, 1959. In *Food, the Yearbook of Agriculture, 1959.* p. 691. U.S. Dept. of Agriculture, Washington, D.C.

Schaefer, A.E., 1969. Malnutrition in the USA? *Nutr. News* 32, No. 4: 13.

Ward, S. and D.B. Wackman, 1971. Television advertising and intra-family influence: children's purchase influence attempts and parental yielding. *Harvard Graduate School of Business Administration.* Cambridge. Unpublished paper.

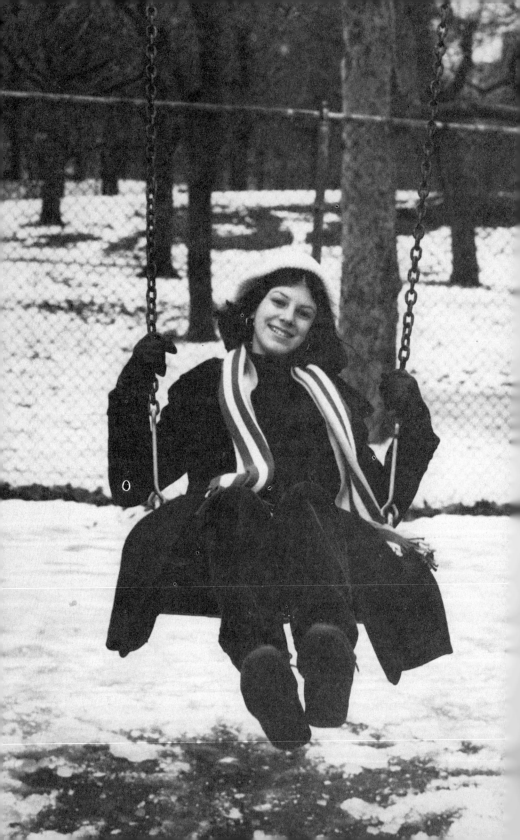

Chapter 10
Challenges of Adolescence

Study of the adolescent period in human development is not a new idea, but the role that nutrition may play in adjustments during this period is a relatively new area of research. Interdisciplinary studies are being conducted by workers from the areas of psychology and other social sciences, medicine, neurology, chemistry, endocrinology, and nutrition. A concerted effort is being made to understand the relationship between personality adjustment and nutrition. Although much of this work has centered around the problem of obesity, studies of factors influencing behavioral change in dietary practices and personal adjustment will be pursued vigorously in future research efforts.

The adolescent is viewed by psychologists and nutritionists in somewhat different ways, and yet they find certain similarities. Psychologists identify this period as a time when the individual is attempting to develop an understanding of himself and to find a way of relating to the adult world. The nutritionist views this period also as a time for significant growth, but in a physical sense rather than the psychological growth involved in development of self-identity. Adults tend to be concerned about this adolescent period because behavior patterns at this age are often different from any other time in life. The teen-age period frequently brings considerable concern with appearance and desire for a high degree of conformity to the peer group. These two aspects of development may manifest themselves in nutritional problems for a number of adolescents.

The nutritional status of the teen-ager influences his own sense of well-being and also affects his relationships with family and friends. People have long recognized that proper diet promotes a general sense of well-being, a contribution of importance to teen-agers as well as other persons of all ages. One of the general symptoms of a poor diet is irritability. Since it is also generally accepted that the adolescent period is one of additional stress in which teen-agers become more emotional than they were when they were younger, simple logic suggests that a good diet would be beneficial to a teen-ager in his attempt to cope with his emotional complications.

Various nutritional status studies have been conducted in recent years in an attempt to determine more fully the role of nutrients in the body and also to establish the extent of nutritional deficiencies in the American population. The conclusions reached regarding the nutrition of teen-agers in the United States have been a source of great concern. According to Bowes (1955), the population group with the least adequate diets is the 13- to 15-year-old girls. Everson (1960) cited the late teens as the period in which dietary deficiencies are most prominent. Nutritionists generally agree that it is the adolescent girl who is most in need of help in the United States, a conclusion borne out by the findings of the Household Food Consumption Survey of 1965, conducted by the United States Department of Agriculture.

NUTRITIONAL STATUS OF ADOLESCENTS

To better understand the scope of the nutritional problems occurring during adolescence, it is necessary to examine what is presently known regarding existing dietary practices and the effects of the resulting nutritional status on the appearance and adjustment of the individual. Pertinent studies include work done in the United States and various foreign countries during this century.

In Other Countries

Blanton (1919) has reported on the results of malnutrition in German youth during World War I. Wartime conditions prevented careful control of nutrient intake, thus the general level of nutrition toward the end of the war was distinctly inadequate. School children were notably lacking in energy and endurance. In fact, this became a problem of such magnitude that periods of physical activity were

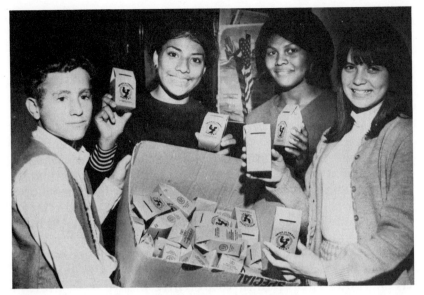

Teen-agers with a strong concern for the world's children and their need for good nutrition help by collecting funds for UNICEF.

curtailed sharply from the prewar pattern. Mental stability was reduced in cases of severe malnutrition. Misbehavior and restlessness were the pattern. Blanton felt that mental achievement was distinctly impaired, mostly through reduced memory and listlessness, but that basic intelligence was not altered.

A study of nutritional adequacy in Nigeria published by Tabrah and Hauck (1963) revealed a startlingly high incidence of reduced hemoglobin levels. In the group of children under 15 who were studied, 28 percent of the boys and 32 percent of the girls had low levels. This percentage increased slightly for women over 15, but the males over 15 had a definite improvement in their hemoglobin levels. Protein and riboflavin deficiencies also were noted in the subjects.

Although the precise relationships and influences of nutrition on menarche have not been determined, foreign studies have highlighted the correlation observed between early onset of menarche and the socioeconomic conditions, which do influence dietary adequacy. Ito (1942) reported that Japanese girls reared in California reached menarche

20 months earlier than did girls raised in Japan, despite the fact that both groups were born in California. A similar situation was reported by Wilson and Sutherland (1953) when they found that girls living in towns reached menarche at an earlier age than those living in the rural areas.

In the United States

Dietary patterns in the American adolescent. There is general agreement that boys are better nourished than girls in this country. This may be explained by the significantly larger quantity of food ingested by boys and the preoccupation of girls with the importance of a very slender figure. The tendency for teen-agers to skip breakfast has also been noted. Studies to determine seasonal variations in food intake by adolescents indicate that diets are improved in the summer and fall, a fact that may be due to increased fresh foods rather than to definite changes in dietary patterns.

Blewett and Schuck (1950) reported that male college students consumed more milk, cereal, and meat than female college students, but the women ate more fruit than their male counterparts. Both sexes reportedly had a deficiency of citrus fruits; men were also low in their total fruit and vegetable consumption.

Health problems influenced by nutritional status. In addition to deficiency diseases, poor nutrition (either undernutrition or overnutrition) encourages other complications. It has been noted that tuberculosis is rather prevalent in the teens, a fact which may be linked to lowered resistance caused by inadequate diet. Overweight places added stress on body organs, thus increasing the likelihood of malfunction and diseases. Diabetes is more prevalent in obese than non-obese individuals, a fact that is as applicable to teen-agers as it is to older people. It has also been suggested that rheumatic fever is less likely to occur and will be less severe when nutrition is optimum. Amenorrhea can be caused by poor diet. Resistance to diseases in general is optimized by adequate diet over a long period of time, and recovery is better in the well-nourished individual.

Nutritional deficiencies. Wharton (1963) depicted the nutrition of teen-agers in Illinois as being somewhat less adequate than that noted in some other areas. Boys in this study had a higher level of calcium than girls, but this mineral was still found to be inadequate in the diets of both sexes. Roth (1960) found that many teen-agers drink two to three quarts of milk a day, but Everson (1960) and Bowes (1955) both agreed that many teen-agers need more calcium, a conclusion verified by the 1965 Household Consumption Survey which found that the average calcium intake of girls throughout the teens and of boys from 9–18 was consistently below the recommended level of intake. Everson stressed this need for calcium in girls because of the possibility of early marriage and pregnancy. She emphasized the significance of this point by reporting that many of the pregnant girls from the lowest two social classes in Scotland are small and in poor physical condition and, as a result, have poor reproductive records. It is important to enter the teens in good dietary condition; adolescents may take six months to begin to overcome a calcium deficiency, and such a time lapse can be a real problem during this period of rapid growth. In addition, the teen period is noted as a time of some emotional stress which may cause calcium to be stored inefficiently.

Anderson and Sandstead (1947) studied hemoglobin levels on selected groups in Alabama and Florida. For more accurate summation of their results, it would be necessary to have a better idea of the comparative economic backgrounds of the particular white and black subjects. As the data were presented, however, there were significantly more black than white children with hemoglobin levels below 12 grams per 100 milliliters of blood. The incidence of low hemoglobin levels was reduced in subjects over the age of 13. Kaucher et al. (1948) found that 9 out of the 61 teenage boys who participated in their study were anemic. The boys tested came from poor backgrounds, both socially and economically. These same workers found that the hemoglobin level for boys rose during their teens, but no consistent changes were observed in girls of this age group. Bowes (1955) again underlined the plight of the teen-age girls by noting that this group was lower in iron than any other age group. The 1965 Household Consumption Survey documented the continuing trend of iron intake below the recommended level for girls from age nine through the teens and indeed, continuing for women until age 55. Males fell below the recommended iron intake for the period from age 12–17, but their intake was consistently higher than the intake for girls in the comparable age periods.

In 1955 Bowes found that 43 percent of the boys studied ingested diets deficient in protein. The comparable group of girls in their teens was even poorer, with 53 percent of the subjects eating diets containing inadequate levels of protein. In contrast, however, Beach et al. (1950) found very few teen-age subjects with a serum protein level outside the range of 6.0–8.6 gram percent. The figures in this study could be interpreted in a more meaningful way if unanimity could be reached on the minimum serum protein level necessary to indicate adequate protein intake. The level from 6–7 gram percent presents an area of discord for stamping a diet as good or deficient; above 7 gram percent is generally agreed to be adequate.

Assessment of the adequacy of protein intake in the 1965 Household Consumption Survey revealed that protein intake was above the 1968 recommended daily allowance for persons of all ages, including adolescent boys and girls. The adequate intake of protein is even more easily achieved in the light of the 1974 revision of the dietary allowances, which are established at a lower value than recommended in 1968. The propensity of affluent Americans for buying a diet high in meat underscores the likelihood of an adequate protein intake in prosperous periods.

Everson (1960) pointed out the low level of vitamin A consumed by teen-agers, and Robinson et al. (1948) observed that vitamin A levels were more nearly adequate in the autumn than they were in the spring. They also found that the carotenoid and vitamin A levels showed a definite rise when underprivileged children received an adequate diet during a six-week summer camp session.

McDonald (1963) did an interesting study on the ascorbic acid content of the diet of the Navajo Indians. It was found that 27 percent of the subjects between the ages of 16 and 19 had an ascorbic-acid deficiency, with the boys being slightly less deficient than the girls. Wharton (1963) listed ascorbic acid as one of the deficient nutrients in the Illinois study of nutritional adequacy but, contrary to the Navajo study, found that girls had better intakes of ascorbic acid than boys.

Surprisingly, Bowes (1955) cited vitamin D as being the nutrient most lacking in the diets of children between the ages of 4 and 20.

Nutritional status related to family income. In general, Bowes (1955) found that higher economic status of the family increased the likelihood of better diets for the children. An evaluation of a general cross section of children from the spectrum of economic backgrounds revealed that approximately 35 percent of the children had good diets. Financial security does not guarantee an adequate diet, however, for 58 percent of the children in the highest economic bracket needed to improve their diets. Stiebling (1950) noted that families in the United States who had higher incomes consumed more fruits and vegetables, especially the fresh and frozen fruits and vegetables. Other items eaten in larger quantities by the more affluent families were milk, meat, and eggs. This report was made in 1950, but it is reasonable to assume that this same general pattern exists today. Wilhelmy et al. (1950) also stated that the availability of nutrients was closely and directly related to family income. They observed that the actual amounts of the various nutrients available to each individual family member decreases in large families.

Relation of sex and nutritional status. Teen-age girls have been berated by any nutritionist who has included subjects of this age in a study. Two important motivating forces that are directly opposed to sensible nutrition in girls of this age are a desire to be slim and a desire to be independent. The motivation for slimness apparently stems, at least in part, from the desire to be attractive to boys at this time. The desire for independence may lead teen-age girls to attempt to achieve the desired slim figure by completely ignoring sound advice on nutrition.

Wharton (1963) defended girls in two categories; she found that girls had higher intakes of niacin and ascorbic acid, but indulged in snacks more often than did the boys studied. The boys, however, had more adequate levels of protein, calcium, phosphorus, iron, and riboflavin than did the girls. Bowes (1955) unequivocally concluded that teen-age boys are better nourished than teen-age girls.

Overweight in teen-agers. Since the topic of overweight is considered in some detail in Chapter 11, it is necessary only to mention the problem here. Gschneidner and Roderuck (1960) in a study of Iowa school children, found that 17 percent of the girls and 11 percent of the boys were obese. As measured by menarche, it was found that girls who were heavy matured approximately four months earlier than the thinner subjects. Girls of medium weight grew one inch more than the heavy girls over a three-year period. This study also revealed that the caloric intake of the overweight girls was lower than that of the girls of medium weight. This finding is in agreement with other studies relating food intake to the incidence of overweight. Inactivity rather than excessively large food intake frequently appears to be the primary factor in overweight.

DIETARY TRENDS OF ADOLESCENTS

Snack Patterns

Snacks are a subject of considerable interest to teenagers. Girls snack more than boys, but this in itself may not be detrimental to girls' diets. Wharton (1963) states that if snacks contribute more than 20 percent of the day's caloric intake, the diet may be more adequate in all nutrients except vitamin A and ascorbic acid than a diet eaten during the course of the three traditional meals. Obviously, it is impossible to state flatly that snacks are the answer to teen-age nutritional problems, because the quality of the snacks is certainly highly variable.

The great variability of the nutritive value and frequency of snacks in an individual's diet make it necessary to analyze a specific person's daily intake over a period of time before appropriate recommendations regarding the use of snacks might be made for him. Nutritionists frequently express concern about the increasing tendency toward snacking and the inherent problems that this pattern may generate. From a large population sample, namely black and white teenagers (12 to 14 years old, and 15 to 16) from both low and high income families participating in the Ten-State Nutrition Survey, Thomas and Call (1973) reported that inadequate levels of calcium and iron were the most frequent dietary problem among adolescents who snacked. The snacks themselves were rather low in these two nutrients, and the intake of the two minerals also was not sufficient at meals to meet the recommended allowance.

The discussions regarding the role of snacks in meeting a part of the day's nutrient needs have been concerned with the possible fortification of foods identified as common snack items. Of course, this might be an approach toward assuring adequate nutrition. However, calcium fortification is difficult to do in these types of foods, and greater stress on more use of dairy foods for snacks might be a more practical approach. Amidst the "hand wringing" of concerned nutritionists, there has been some discussion of adding protein to snack foods to fortify them. On the basis of the findings of the Ten-State Nutrition Survey, there is little justification for adding protein to the so-called "empty calorie foods". The intake of protein, riboflavin, ascorbic acid, and thiamin was found to be adequate when the total intake of snacks and meals was analyzed.

Breakfast Habits

Sidwell and Eppright (1953) found that residents of towns missed breakfast less than did either the city or rural children. Surprisingly, breakfasts were less popular on the weekend than during the week. This finding tends to contradict the common breakfast-skipping excuse that there is insufficient time to eat breakfast. These workers also found that, as children entered their teens, girls began to skip breakfast more and so did some boys. Meat and egg consumption at breakfast showed a small increase in the diets of teen-age boys. This study showed that, although it is possible for a breakfast skipper to consume an adequate daily diet, the likelihood of a good total diet is decreased. Only 20 percent of the poor breakfast eaters had good daily diets; 52 percent of the fair to good breakfast eaters had good daily diets; and 82 percent of the excellent to good breakfast eaters had good daily diets. Blewett and Schuck's data (1950) showing that twice as many men as women of college age eat breakfast corroborate Sidwell and Eppright's findings (1953). It should be pointed out that many homemakers are breakfast skippers, and it may be that some teen-age girls emulate this practice in their attempt to identify with their mothers.

Vegetarian Diets

Types. Various social movements have had an impact on the dietary patterns of some Americans in the past few

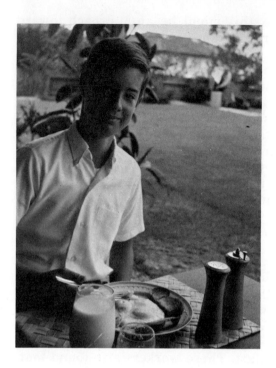

A breakfast with milk, fruit juice, eggs, and toast provides a nourishing start for an active adolescent boy.

years, and some teen-agers have been among the population adopting various forms of vegetarian diets. Lacto-ovo-vegetarian diets are rather broad in definition and provide animal foods (in the form of milk and other dairy products, as well as eggs) to round out the nutrients provided by vegetables and other plant foods. This type of vegetarian diet is potentially very adequate nutritionally. However, some persons practice vegetarianism on a much more narrowly defined dietary basis. The most extreme position is that taken by the Vegans, who are persons consuming absolutely no food of animal origin.

Motivations. The reasons for adopting a diet that contains no flesh foods of animals or fish may be religious in origin. Long established religions with specified meat avoidances include Seventh Day Adventists and Hindu. Seventh Day Adventists have conducted extensive research studies to work out adequate dietary patterns without the use of flesh foods. In contrast, extreme positions on the use of animal foods without appropriate dietary modifications have been adopted by some of the recent religious cults that characterize the late 1960s with their unrest and intense social concerns.

Other vegetarians may espouse this dietary pattern because of concern for the agricultural space required to raise the food to feed animals, space which some feel should be used for raising plants to feed people. Some gentle people refuse to include meat in their diets because of their distaste for killing any form of animal life. Others place great importance on purity of soul and hold that meats are sources of toxins and other impurities that are not compatible with their philosophy.

Vegetarianism in its intense form is not simply a dietary pattern pursued by its most ardent followers merely because of attitudes toward meats. There is an emotional value that some vegetarians place on the importance of eating these plant foods in their most natural form. This branch of vegetarians has been loud in its criticism of pesticides and chemical fertilizers. Their vegetarian foods are touted to be "organically grown" and free of any type of refinement or chemical (or nutritional) additives. (This "chemical concern" has, of course, drawn many meat eaters into a small corner of the vegetarian philosophy even though meats continue to occupy a place in their diets.)

Vegetarians in the adolescent and early adult years are described by Erhard (1973) as "usually well educated, self-reliant, socially mobile, and reflect a middle- and upper-class background that is not strongly influenced by ethnic origins." Many are living in communes which follow the vegetarian dictates.

Potential nutritional problems. Although properly planned vegetarian diets can provide adequate nutrition, nutritional consequences of the more narrowly defined vegetarian diets have been experienced by many teen-agers. If all animal products are excluded, devotees of Vegan diets may develop degenerative changes in the spinal cord due to the lack of a dietary source of vitamin B_{12} on a strict vegetarian diet. Lacto-vegetarians may develop anemia due to a deficiency of iron. Vegetarian diets that do not include milk may result in deficiencies of calcium and riboflavin. The narrow restrictions of the Zen macrobiotic diet lead to possible scurvy, anemia, lack of protein and calcium, the sum of which may be starvation and kidney failure in extreme cases. These extreme diets are particularly harmful if followed by pregnant and lactating teen-agers or their offspring.

TECHNIQUES OF ASSESSING NUTRITIONAL STATUS

Physical Evaluation

Nutritional adequacy of people can be ascertained in part through an external examination done by an experienced individual. A well-nourished individual appears vital – the eyes sparkle, the hair shines, and the skin glows. Posture is a good index of nutritional adequacy, as are stamina, skeletal development, nerves, and weight. Scales have been developed by Gastpur, Dunfermline, and Hogarth to rank varying degrees of nutritional adequacy.

Various deficiency symptoms may be evident in the individual. For example, a vitamin A deficiency might be manifested by rough dry hair, night blindness, harsh and scaly skin, or inflamed eyelids. Various signs of a shortage of thiamin include tender calf muscles, loss of tendon reflexes, muscular weakness, anorexia, and constipation. Riboflavin deficiency may cause a magenta-colored tongue with a smooth surface, angular stomatitis (fissures at the corners of the mouth), and a sore tongue; in addition, the eye capillaries may extend into the cornea and cause cloudy vision.

Although glossy hair indicates good health, a glossy tongue heralds nutritional problems. In a niacin deficiency, the papillae atrophy and cause the tongue to become slick and scarlet red, beginning at the tip and the sides. Skin rashes in symmetrical locations on areas exposed to the sun, diarrhea, and nervousness also are observed in a niacin deficiency. Ascorbic-acid deficiency may cause red and swollen gums or skin hemorrhages. An enlarged thyroid gland indicates lack of iodine. Dental caries are related to low calcium and fluoride intake as well as to inadequate dental hygiene. The edema observed in some children may be due to a protein deficiency. Caloric deficiencies or excesses are easily observed as underweight or overweight. Skinfold measurements provide a convenient means of assessing this facet of nutritional status.

Chemical Tests

Various chemical tests are useful and reliable means of measuring nutritional status. Protein adequacy is tested by serum protein levels; higher than 7 gram percent is definitely rated as satisfactory, and less than 6 gram percent is rated as an inadequate protein intake.

Hemoglobin levels are generally synonymous with iron level in the body, but it is now recognized that this same test actually indicates the adequacy of other nutrients, such as protein and copper. Hemoglobin at 13 grams per 100 milliliters of blood is considered normal, but many school children have values between 11 and 12. A value lower than 11 grams per 100 milliliters is considered to be definitely low. Ascorbic-acid levels are highly variable, but less than 0.6 milligram percent in the serum of a person who has fasted for one hour is considered low. The levels are also studied over a period of time after a large dose of ascorbic acid is administered.

Thiamin, riboflavin, and niacin are B vitamins determined in most nutritional status studies. Urinary excretion levels below 5 micrograms of thiamin are considered to be too low. For adequate thiamin levels, the hourly excretion during fasting should be more than 6 micrograms. A riboflavin excretion greater than 40 micrograms indicates good riboflavin content; less than 20 micrograms is considered deficient. Although it is assumed in establishing these values that a person with adequate stores of either of these vitamins will retain less of the vitamin (excrete larger quantities of the B vitamins) since his stores are already filled, interpretation of niacin levels of excretion has been very cautious.

There is some concern over assessing the current adequacy of dietary vitamin A, for it is efficiently utilized in the body and may be stored for some time. Therefore, measurements on vitamin A levels do not indicate the dietary intake at the time of the study, but actually measure the adequacy of the diet in the past. Both carotene and vitamin A are measured in the blood: 125 microgram percent carotene and 30 microgram percent vitamin A are normal; values of 75 and 20 microgram percent for carotene and vitamin A, respectively, are inadequate.

Alkaline phosphatase levels of 2–10 nitrophenol units indicate normal vitamin D levels. Fifteen to 30 nitrophenol units would indicate a potential rachitic (vitamin D-deficient) condition. Sex and age of the subject influence the phosphatase level and increase the problem of interpretation. X-rays provide a means of studying vitamin D adequacy by revealing bone development.

Borderline calcium deficiencies cannot be detected in laboratory analyses, but more serious deficiencies may be spotted. The normal figure for blood calcium is 10−11 milligram percent.

NUTRITIONAL NEEDS OF THE TEEN-AGER

The nutritional requirements of the body during the adolescent years are very high, as shown in Table 10.1. The allowances for energy, vitamin A, niacin, riboflavin, thiamin, iodine, and magnesium are notably higher for boys than for girls during this time. Note also that the table reflects the earlier maturation pattern of girls; the recommendations for boys continue to rise throughout the span from 11 to 18 and remain at much the same high levels (with the exception of the minerals) until age 22. In contrast, the allowances for girls reach their peak during the 11−14 range and then begin to drop gradually toward the recommendations for the adult woman. A distinct difference in protein recommendations between sexes at ages 15 to 18 is an indication of this difference in growth patterns for boys and girls.

The teen-age girl may well envy her male peers during this period for it is apparent that the number of calories a boy can consume in order to provide the recommended nutrients permits considerably more frivolous choices than are available to her. She requires considerably fewer calories than a boy of the same age, hence she must provide herself with all the nutrients she needs in this more restricted quantity of food. In order to provide the necessary calcium, iron, and vitamins in her diet, it is necessary for her to concentrate on eating a well balanced diet with only a few additional frills permitted. The teen-age boy, on the other hand, is confronted with the delightful responsibility of consuming a large number of calories, and it is likely that many boys will unconsciously meet their needs for the various nutrients simply by attempting to satisfy their ravenous appetites. Conscious planning of menus certainly is still advisable for boys, but it is slightly less critical than it is for girls at this time.

Table 10.1   Recommended daily dietary allowances for teen-agers[a]

	Males		Females	
	Age 11–14	Age 15–18	Age 11–14	Age 15–18
Weight, kg. (lb.)	44 (97)	61 (134)	44 (97)	54 (119)
Height, cm. (in.)	158 (63)	172 ((69)	155 (62)	162 (65)
Energy, kcal.	2800	3000	2400	2100
Protein, g.	44	54	44	48
Vitamin A activity, I.U.	5000	5000	4000	4000
Vitamin D, I.U.	400	400	400	400
Vitamin E activity, I.U.	12	15	12	12
Ascorbic acid, mg.	45	45	45	45
Folacin, μg.	400	400	400	400
Niacin, mg.	18	20	16	14
Riboflavin, mg.	1.5	1.8	1.3	1.4
Thiamin, mg.	1.4	1.5	1.2	1.1
Vitamin B_6, mg.	1.6	2.0	1.6	2.0
Vitamin B_{12}, μg.	3.0	3.0	3.0	3.0
Calcium, mg.	1200	1200	1200	1200
Phosphorus, mg.	1200	1200	1200	1200
Iodine, μg.	130	150	115	115
Iron, mg.	18	18	18	18
Magnesium, mg.	350	400	300	300
Zinc, mg.	15	15	15	15

[a]From 1974 revision of the table of daily dietary allowances as recommended by the Food and Nutrition Board of the National Research Council, National Academy of Sciences.

ADOLESCENT CONCERNS AND THEIR RELATION TO NUTRITION

From the preceding discussion, it is apparent that inadequate nutrition can complicate the adolescent period in a variety of ways. Evidence has been cited to prove that the nutritional status of many teen-agers, particularly girls, in the United States is less than optimum. Before it is possible to overcome the diagnosed inadequacies, however, it is necessary to identify the factors that contribute to the problem.

Development of a Satisfactory Physical Image

An important problem of adolescents is the need to achieve a desirable body size during the adolescent period. Height is perhaps of more concern to boys than to girls in the teens for, as interest in the peer group and particularly in the opposite sex increases, a certain amount of prestige is conveyed to the taller boys. Gallagher and Harris (1958) have expressed the conviction that atypical growth is a matter of grave concern for many teen-agers.

Physical growth is one way in which adolescents assess maturity of themselves and of their peers. It is true that growth patterns are somewhat variable, but proper nutrition all through childhood and adolescence is essential if an individual is to achieve his own individual growth potential. Adjustments of adolescents can be helped by proper nutrition throughout childhood and the teens so that normal physical growth occurs.

The influence that diet exerts on growth is being illustrated dramatically in Japan today. Since the late 1940s, the typical Japanese diet has been altered considerably, with the result that the average height of today's teen-ager is strikingly greater than the traditionally short height of the past generations.

It is necessary for the teen-ager not only to achieve the desired physical height, but also to succeed in attaining the appropriate weight for his height. For boys this usually means large quantities of food must be eaten daily to fill out their frames during this period of rapid growth. The problem of eating enough food is reduced for girls because of the minimal physical activity of today's adolescent female.

The common problem for the teen-age girl is usually that of fulfilling the body's nutritional requirements without consuming an excessive quantity of calories. Two factors complicate the achievement of good nutrition by the female adolescent: a penchant for snacks and a preoccupation with being thin. Teen-agers like to get together, and snacks are an important part of their parties and informal gatherings. The foods served at such times are typically high in calories and low in nutrients. Pop and potato chips are familiar examples of favorite snacks. When food is served at group gatherings, it is common for many teen-age girls to eat the snack and then reduce their intake at mealtime. The net result is that they probably are consuming close to the recommended number of calories each day, but they may not be receiving adequate amounts of the vitamins and minerals. The second obstacle to good nutrition is the teen-ager's concept of a beautiful figure. To fit the expected figure pattern of slenderness, bordering on skinniness, many teen-age girls feel that they must severely limit their caloric intake each day. Unfortunately, such a restriction usually means that important nutrients will be consumed in inadequate amounts.

Time Management

In the hectic life of the typical city teen-ager today, one of the biggest obstacles to meeting nutritional needs is the problem of finding time to eat. If an individual is active in school affairs, he may need to leave for school very early in the morning and stay until suppertime for various sports, music, and play practices. Additional time also is required for commuting to and from school. These demands may mean that the adolescent finds it difficult to have his meals with the rest of the family. All too often this leads to informal snacking rather than consumption of a good meal when he finally does find time to eat.

Financial Limitations

Some teen-agers live in families with incomes so low that good nutrition is almost an unattainable goal. Insufficient money often is coupled with inadequate knowledge of nutrition and marketing, with the result that the problems of feeding the family become even more complex than they need to be. In some areas, for example, children from low-income families may have money to purchase some food at the school lunch program, but often they use it to buy soft drinks rather than milk or other nourishing foods that are commonly available at the nutrition period and at lunch.

Limited Knowledge of Nutrition

Another problem that may lead to poor nutrition is inadequate knowledge of nutrition and lack of appreciation of the value of good nutrition habits. Teen-agers frequently have little understanding of what nutrients are contained in different foods and of the role of the various nutrients in their bodies. When a person does not understand basic nutrition principles and is unaware of the nutritional contribution of various foods, it is difficult to choose foods that supply all the body's needs, and deficiency conditions may gradually develop.

CASE STUDIES

These two case studies have been selected to illustrate the types of problems that may exist in the diets of some teen-agers. They reflect the freedom many teen-agers have in the selection of food during the day. In addition, these cases emphasize the importance of developing an appreciation of the value of good nutrition before the individual reaches this independent state.

David

This particular case is of interest because it provides actual proof that children from upper-middle and upper-class families do not automatically have adequate diets. Certainly a more comfortable income combined with the educational achievement of the parents in these social classes may influence the nutritional status of the children, but these factors do not provide a guarantee of adequacy. The boy in this study is proof of this, for he is the son of a physician.

David, a senior in high school, is 6 feet tall and weighs 152 pounds. He is slightly thin and is troubled with acne. As can be observed in the five days of menus listed in Table 10.2, several changes would need to be made in this diet to meet David's dietary needs. The intake reflects the common problems of this age group: a hurried breakfast and a snack-type dinner apparently often eaten hastily with friends rather than with the family at an organized and well-planned family meal. David needs to change his habits to include a bigger breakfast consisting of juice, a glass of milk, cereal, meat or eggs, and toast. He would probably eat a better breakfast and dinner if the family arranged to eat these meals together. Regular meals in an organized setting would help to promote increased consumption of

Table 10.2   David's dietary record for five days

Day	Breakfast	Lunch	Dinner	Snack
Monday	Oatmeal Orange juice	Roast beef sandwich Apple Potato chips	Hamburger in bun Soft drink	Chocolate ice cream
Tuesday	Oatmeal Tomato juice	Ham sandwich Orange	Toasted cheese sandwich Milk	
Wednesday	Scrambled eggs Milk	Beef sandwich Apple	Hot roast beef sandwich with gravy Mashed potatoes with gravy Soft drink	
Thursday	Oatmeal Orange juice	Roast beef sandwich Apple Potato chips	Hamburger in bun French fries Black coffee	
Friday	Orange juice Cold cereal with milk	Tuna sandwich Apple	Hamburger in bun Soft drink	

milk, fruits, and vegetables. These changes would help him gain weight and might improve his complexion.

Rosa

Rosa presents an interesting contrast to David because she is from a family with very limited income and seemingly unlimited children (twelve, to be exact). The diet of the home reflects both the Spanish-American heritage of the family and the food patterns that are fairly common among families with very limited incomes. This case emphasizes the value of a good school nutrition program at lunchtime. Rosa works in the school cafeteria and is able to have all the fruit juice and other food that she wishes at the noon meal. It is readily apparent that this opportunity is invaluable in helping to improve her food intake, although she does not adequately avail herself of the opportunity to obtain free milk. Her menus for three days are given in Table 10.3.

Table 10.3   Rosa's menus for three days

Day	Breakfast	Lunch	Dinner	Snack

Monday	Oatmeal
	Orange juice
		Hamburger in
		  bun
		Potato chips
		Orange juice
		Strawberry
		  ice cream
			1 piece of fried
			  chicken
			Refried beans
			Tortillas with
			  butter
			Milk
				Apple
				Vanilla ice
				  cream

Tuesday	No breakfast	2 fish sticks
		2 slices of
		  bread with
		  butter
		Orange juice
		Lemon pie
			3 tacos
			Soft drink
				Apple

Wednesday	Doughnut
	Cocoa
		Tamale
		Orange juice
		2 slices of
		  bread with
		  butter
		Fruit jello
			2 enchiladas
			Soft drink
				Apple
				Potato chips

FACTORS INVOLVED IN IMPROVING NUTRITION OF ADOLESCENTS

Certainly it is important not only to identify the nutrition problems of teen-agers, but also to consider some means of helping to improve the situation. A multifaceted approach toward overcoming nutritional problems in teen-agers seems to be the only means of accomplishing any observable, lasting changes. Behavioral changes in eating habits of adolescents require an approach based on education and strong personal interests.

Education

Nutrition for the teen-ager probably can be approached most effectively through education that begins in the elementary grades and continues throughout the junior and senior high school programs. Unfortunately, such a solution is difficult to implement effectively on a large scale. Elementary schools usually allot time for the study of nutrition, but many of the teachers have never had an opportunity to take a college nutrition course that would provide the background necessary to teach nutrition accurately and effectively. It is imperative that teachers in the elementary grades have at least one good nutrition course in their college program. It must be recognized that many elementary school children are teaching their parents nutrition as they learn it in school. Therefore misinformation, or inadequate information about nutrition from elementary school teachers confuses parents as well as children and greatly hinders an effective nutrition program.

Although the home economics teachers in junior and senior high school are the persons officially designated to present factual and stimulating nutrition information, the importance of nutrition should not be stressed only in home economics classes. All high school students, regardless of their sex or curriculum objectives, need to have a working knowledge of nutrition, and not all students will be enrolled in high school home economics classes. The role of nutrition also can be emphasized meaningfully in biology classes by pointing out the needs of various animals and by doing actual feeding experiments in the biology classes. Social studies teachers can add considerable interest to their subject by examining some of the nutrition problems found in other countries and determining the impact that the nutritional patterns have had on the history and development of the country. Physical education teachers are often in a unique position to make a significant contribution toward improved nutrition for the teen-ager. Certainly any coach should be concerned about the diet of each of his team members, and the close relationship that the girls' physical education teacher may have with her students also can be an effective avenue for introducing sound ideas regarding nutrition.

Obviously, if this many-pronged approach to nutrition education is to be really effective, it is imperative that the teachers cooperating in the program have an adequate understanding of basic nutrition themselves. Such an understanding should be possible through a carefully conceived college nutrition course that is effectively taught to all of the teachers in the aforementioned areas. State credential requirements for all elementary teachers, and for secondary school teachers in the fields of physical education and the biological and social sciences, should specifically include a basic nutrition course. In most states this course is presently required of home economics majors. This program needs to be extended.

Emphasis on Personal Appearance

An important reason for unhappiness in the teens is the failure to be accepted by the group, and appearance is one major criterion for acceptance. The extremely thin or heavy individual is automatically subject to rejection by the group. Not only are their bodies less attractive, but also their clothing looks less stylish. The problem of weight alone may be sufficient reason for the group to refuse admittance to a particular boy or girl.

The concern with personal appearance frequently may provide the adolescent boy with the motivation necessary for consuming the large amounts of food adequate to help fill out his frame. The large growth spurt that usually begins for boys sometime between the ages of 11 and 13 requires considerable quantities of wholesome food to meet the nutritional demands of such rapid growth. During this period, a boy's body may become rather lanky and lean. To the adolescent boy such an appearance is not pleasing, and he will attempt to eat more food to help fill out his body. To satisfy appetites and achieve the desired weight gain, boys usually eat a large quantity of food and frequently drink very adequate amounts of milk; and as a result they are likely to be eating adequately. Even with high-calorie, relatively non-nourishing snacks it is possible for a teen-age boy to meet his recommended allowances each day. This should not be construed to mean that teen-age boys are not malnourished — it is certainly possible to find adolescent boys who are poorly fed. The point is that boys are less likely to be poorly nourished than girls.

Teen-age girls need to focus their attention on the total picture they present rather than concentrating their nutritional objectives exclusively on their figures. They need to be helped to recognize the importance of regulating their choice of foods so that their entire appearance is optimum. With adequate nutrition education, they can learn how to budget their calories so that they consume the nutrients needed for healthy skin, clear eyes, shiny hair, and a general sense of physical well-being without indulging in the excess calories that lead to overweight.

The modification of snack foods to foods lower in sugar not only has the advantage of aiding the general appearance, but also is valuable because of possible dental health problems. The presence of carbohydrate materials in the mouth provides an excellent medium for tooth-decaying bacteria, and certainly it is true that few people in the United States are able to brush their teeth directly after snacking. Attention to the selection of nourishing, relatively low calorie snacks, such as fruits or raw vegetables, helps the figure as well as the smile.

Dietary Patterns of Parents

Bruch (1962) emphasizes the influence of parents on overweight in children; the tendency to imitate one's parents also may cause poor nutrition habits in children of normal weight who have only a poor example to copy.

Mothers in particular may need to examine their own dietary habits before expecting any drastic changes in their children's diets. Although mothers are usually the persons designated to plan and prepare meals, they are frequently poorly nourished themselves. This example is adopted by many teen-agers, especially girls. Mothers should be especially careful to eat a good breakfast, a practice that is healthful for them and also sets a desirable example for their children to follow.

The influence of the father's as well as the mother's example should not be underestimated. Over a period of years children will acquire many of their parents' habits and also those of their siblings.

Family Adjustments

An understanding family can be helpful in continuing good dietary patterns or in establishing good nutritional habits where poor ones existed. Parents need to be better informed about the increased nutritional needs of teen-agers, and schools may usefully extend this program by teaching adolescents about their own needs. When problems of overweight exist, a reducing regimen is more easily followed by most people if someone else is genuinely intested in the progress being made. A member of the family may well serve as the interested bystander during a period of weight reduction.

Families sometimes may be able to improve the nutrition of its teen-agers by adjusting the meal schedule to a more convenient time. If this is not possible, a hot dinner might be held in the warming oven until the tardy teen arrives.

One means of improving diets may be, surprisingly enough, in the form of snacks. This may appear to contradict the critical comments previously made about snacks, but a nutritious snack can help to meet the body's daily need for nutrients. For example, a protein food at snack time may be used very efficiently by the body. Protein is more effective when it is eaten several times a day than when the day's total protein intake is ingested in one meal.

DIETARY NEEDS OF ATHLETES

Athletic Performance and Nutrient Needs

The influence of nutritional status on athletic performance has been the subject of considerable research as well as of myths. Many teen-agers are interested in nutrition as a means of improving athletic prowess. The athletic training table has been a long-standing tradition which exemplifies the importance that coaches attach to diet for their teams. Clearly, an adequate diet is necessary for athletes, just as it is for all teen-agers, if the body is to have all nutrients present in the diet in sufficient quantities to meet physical needs. The athlete will be expending more energy in physical activity than will many of his more sedentary peers. This increased need for energy will require a larger food intake, commensurate with the total energy expended. Since thiamin, niacin, and riboflavin are required to release energy from food, the additional quantity of food will require somewhat more than the recommended intake of these B vitamins. However, the extra food that is selected for the athlete's diet can easily provide the extra nutrients related to energy needs.

On a day to day basis, it is not necessary to increase the protein intake of the athlete, for extra physical activity in a day does not increase the body's need for protein. Persons who are very active as a regular way of living will develop more muscle mass than the average person, a fact that does increase the protein need slightly. The practices of feeding athletes diets high in protein and of providing them with protein supplements are not warranted. The diet pattern recommended for athletes is the same as for nonathletes, only the total quantities need to be changed.

Meeting Energy Needs

The actual need for energy for athletic events is determined by the type of activity as well as its duration. Some sports have a comparatively low energy cost either because they require only limited muscular effort or they last for only brief periods. Examples of this type of sport activity include archery, tennis, horseback riding, and golf. Some sports require endurance and result in a higher energy expenditure. Examples of such activities are skin diving, long- and middle-distance running, and hockey. If sports in the first category are practiced for less than an hour daily, they make only a small increase in the body's need for energy. Sports classified in the category of higher energy expenditure may increase the body's need for energy to a daily total of between 4,000 and 5,000 kilocalories.

The use of food to supply energy during athletic events often is based on misconceptions and superstition rather than on demonstrated effect. If an athlete is well nourished, he will have sufficient stores of glycogen and glucose available for the immediate energy needs created in a strenuous, but short-term sports event. It is not necessary to eat some form of sugar, candy, or honey prior to participating in such events. However, for athletes participating in events requiring endurance over a long period of time, a diet contributing about half or slightly more than half of the total calories from carbohydrate is recommended. In addition, fats can be included in the diet, although the recommended level is less than the 40 percent caloric contribution typically provided by American diets.

Liquids

One of the important considerations in meeting nutritional needs of athletes is to be sure that adequate liquids are included in the diet. Milk is an appropriate beverage in athlete's diets; alcoholic beverages definitely should be avoided because of their depressant effect and their effect on coordination. Tea and coffee may be used in moderate

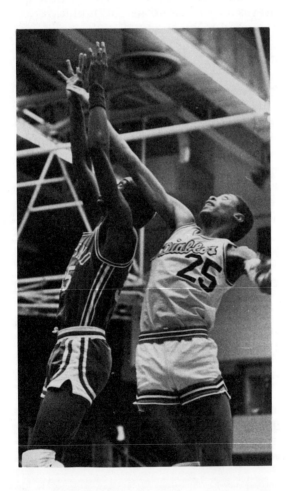

Basketball is a sport with a high energy cost; a balanced diet with large servings will supply the necessary nutrients.

quantities. In instances where perspiration has been excessive, as during practice sessions and actual events, the lost water should be replaced, partially during the activity and the remainder following the activity. Water loss can be estimated by weighing before and after the activity. A rough guide is that a quart of water is lost for approximately each 2 pounds lost. In unusually hot conditions, sodium levels may drop because of loss of salt in perspiration; this loss can be replaced by a small amount of extra salt.

In short, the dietary regimen for athletes is basically the same as for nonathletes, with larger quantities of wholesome food being consumed to provide the extra energy required. Mayer and Bullen (1959) recommend that bouillon be consumed a minimum of 3 hours before the event so that salt intake will be appropriate and the thirst factor can be satisfied before the event. The last food should be eaten about 3 hours before the activity, although some sugar can be used for additional energy, if necessary.

Educational Implications

Cho and Fryer (1974) studied the nutrition knowledge of physical education majors at the university level. As a part of the study, the sources of the students' nutrition knowledge were explored. If students rated coaches as being their primary or secondary source of nutrition information, the scores for the test of nutrition knowledge were lower than for those students who ranked the importance of their coaches' information as of lesser importance to them. On the test of nutrition knowledge, physical education majors scored significantly lower than did students from a basic nutrition class. Since coaches are viewed as an important source of nutrition information by many athletes and since evidence of lower scores of nutrition knowledge were found for students who were relying on coaches for information, there is a compelling argument for including at least a basic nutrition course in the curriculum of physical education majors at the university level so that high school athletes will have more informed coaches to aid them in meeting their dietary needs. This approach to education for coaches would be most helpful in avoiding the propagation of nutrition fallacies and myths about the need for honey, protein supplements, vitamin supplements and on ad inflnltum!

SUMMARY

The nutritional requirements of teen-agers are high because of the large growth spurt characteristic of both adolescent boys and girls. Studies have shown that the dietary habits of adolescent boys are more nearly adequate that those of the girls, but it is apparent that much work needs to be done to improve the nutrition of this age group. Suggestions for meeting the problem include: improved nutrition education programs from elementary school through high school (including required courses in nutrition for the many teachers and coaches involved in nutrition education), greater motivation through emphasis on the contribution good nutrition makes to personal appearance, and cooperation in the home to aid in making good nutrition a reality for all family members.

BIBLIOGRAPHY

American Association for Health, Physical Education, and Recreation, 1971. *Nutrition for Athletes. Handbook for Coaches.* Amer. Assoc. for Health, Physical Education, and Recreation. 1201 16th St., Washington, D.C.

Anderson, R.K. and H.R. Sandstead, 1947. Nutritional appraisal and demonstration programs of the U.S. Public Health Service. *J. Amer. Dietet. Assoc.* 23: 100.

Beach, E.F., et al., 1950. Nutritional status of children. *J. Amer. Dietet. Assoc.* 26: 681.

Beaton, G.H. and E.W. McHenry, Eds., 1966. *Nutrition − A Comprehensive Treatise. III. Nutritional Status: Assessments and Application.* Academic Press. New York.

Blanton, S., 1919. Mental and nervous changes of the Volksschulen of Trier, Germany, caused by malnutrition. *Ment. Hyg.* 3: 343.

Blewett, G.W. and C. Schuck, 1950. Comparison of food consumption of men and women college students. *J. Amer. Dietet. Assoc.* 26: 525.

Bowes, A., 1955. Nutrition of children during their school years. *Amer. J. Clin. Nutr.* 3: 254.

Bruch, H., 1957. *Importance of Overweight.* Norton. New York.

Cereal Institute, 1962. *Complete Summary of the Iowa Breakfast Studies.* Cereal Institute, Inc. Chicago, Ill.

Cho, M. and B.A. Fryer, 1974. Nutritional knowledge of collegiate physical education majors. *J. Amer. Dietet. Assoc.* 65: 30.

Cooperstock, M., et al., 1948. Nutritional status of children: III. Blood serum vitamin C. *J. Amer. Dietet. Assoc.* 24: 205.

Donovan, B.T. and J.J. Van Der Werff Ten Bosch, 1965. *Physiology of Puberty.* Williams and Wilkens Co.

Dwyer, J.T., et al., 1974. New vegetarians. *J. Amer. Dietet. Assoc.* 64: 376.

Erhard, D., 1973. New vegetarians. *Nutr. Today* 8, No. 5: 4.

Everson, G.J., 1960. Bases for concern about teenagers' diets. *J. Amer. Dietet. Assoc.* 36: 17.

Frankle, R.T. and F.K. Heussenstramm, 1974. Food zealotry and youth. *Am. J. Pub. Health* 64: 11.

Gallagher, J.R. and H.I. Harris, 1958. *Emotional Problems of Adolescents.* Oxford University Press. New York.

Gschneidner, M.P. and C.E. Roderuck, 1960. Nutriture of school girls of different physiques. *J. Amer. Dietet. Assoc.* 36: 22.

Heald, F.P., 1965. History and physiological basis of adolescent obesity. *Nutr. News* 28, No. 4: 13.

Heald, F.P., 1969. *Adolescent Nutrition and Growth.* Appleton-Century Crofts. New York.

Huenemann, R.L., 1966. A study of teenagers: body size and shape, dietary practices and physical activity. *Food Nutr. News* 37, No. 7: 1.

Ito, P.K., 1942. Comparative biometrical physique of Japanese women born and reared under different environments. *Hum. Biol.* 14: 279.

Kaucher, M., et al., 1948. Nutritional status of children: VII. Hemoglobin. *J. Amer. Dietet. Assoc.* 24: 496.

McDonald, B.S., 1963. Gingivitis – ascorbic acid deficiency in the Navajo. *J. Amer. Dietet. Assoc.* 43: 331.

Martin, E.A., 1954. *Roberts' Nutrition Work with Children.* Univ. of Chicago Press. Chicago.

Mayer, J. and B. Bullen, 1959. Nutrition and athletic performance. *Postgrad. Med.* 26, No. 6: 848.

Morgan, A.F., 1959. *Nutritional Status USA.* Calif. Agricultural Experiment Station Bull. 769. Berkeley, Calif.

Ohlson, M.A. and B.P. Hart, 1965. Influence of breakfast on total day's food intake. *J. Amer. Dietet. Assoc.* 47: 282.

Robinson, A., et al., 1948. Nutritional status of children: VI. Blood serum vitamin A and carotinoids. *J. Amer. Dietet. Assoc.* 24: 410.

Roche, A.F. and G.H. Duvilla, 1973. Growth after adolescence. *Pediat.* 50: 874.

Roth, A., 1960. The teenage clinic. *J. Amer. Dietet. Assoc.* 36: 27.

Rowe, N.H., et al., 1974. Effects of ready-to-eat breakfast cereals on dental caries experience in adolescent children: a three-year study. *J. Dent. Research* 53, No. 1: 33.

Schorr, B.C., et al., 1972. Teen-age food habits. *J. Amer. Dietet. Assoc.* 61: 415.

Sharman, I.M., et al., 1971. Effects of vitamin E and training on physiological function and athletic performance in adolescent swimmers. *Brit. J. Nutr.* 26: 265.

Sidwell, V.D. and E.S. Eppright, 1953. Food habits of Iowa children — breakfast. *J. Home Econ.* 26: 265.

Stiebling, H.K., 1950. Trends in family food consumption. *J. Amer. Dietet. Assoc.* 26: 248.

Tabrah, F.L. and H.M. Hauck, 1963. Some aspects of health and nutritional status, Awo Oinamma, Nigeria. *J. Amer. Dietet. Assoc.* 43: 321.

Thomas, J. and D.L. Call, 1973. Eating between meals — a nutrition problem among teenagers? *Nutr. Rev.* 31, No. 5: 137.

Wharton, M.A., 1963. Nutritive intake of adolescents. *J. Amer. Dietet. Assoc.* 43: 306.

Wilhelmy, O., Jr., et al., 1950. Nutritional status survey, Groton Township, New York. *J. Amer. Dietet. Assoc.* 36: 868.

Wilson, D.C. and I. Sutherland, 1953. Age of menarche in tropics. *Brit. Med. J.* 2: 607.

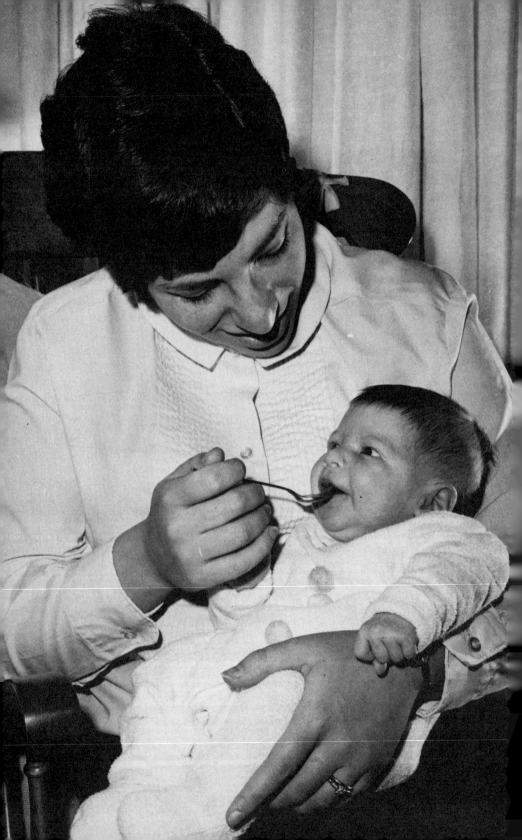

Chapter 11
Weight Control

Weight control, the apparent curse of America's adult population, should be emphasized throughout childhood, for it is during this period that lifetime dietary patterns are established. Obesity originating in childhood is more difficult to control in adulthood than is adult-onset obesity. Clearly, the original avoidance of obesity is more desirable than weight reduction programs. Children gradually can be taught about weight control as they proceed through school, but it is the parents' responsibility to help develop suitable attitudes toward food during the early, formative years. Obviously, parents need basic nutrition knowledge if they are to guide their children successfully.

This chapter provides information about achieving and maintaining weight control. Extensive research is being conducted on the causes and treatment of deviations from normal weight in both children and adults, and as these findings become available, modifications in diet therapy may evolve.

Weight control is important both for the development of a satisfactory self image in childhood and adolescence and for maintenance of optimal physical health. Activity levels may be reduced because of overweight. Children who are excessively heavy may relate to others in a different manner and others may, in turn respond differently than they would if body weight were within a normal range. Such influences are typified by the generally accepted expectation that fat people are jolly.

Children who grow up to be obese adults may find that employment practices and promotion can be influenced negatively by the burden of obesity. Mortality statistics add another dimension of concern; although obesity is not cited as the cause of death, the mortality rate for overweight patients with diabetes, cirrhosis of the liver, appendicitis, and cardiovascular disorders is significantly higher than for those within the recommended weight range.

There are several ways of determining body fatness, but perhaps the simplest and most convenient is to compare body weight with recommended desirable weights (see weight tables in Appendix and Table 4.5).

ENERGY BALANCE

When a person consumes the same amount of energy in food that he expends for basal metabolism, activity, and specific dynamic action, he will maintain a constant body weight. When more kilocalories are consumed than are expended, the individual is in positive caloric balance, and he will gain weight. Conversely, weight is lost when the energy intake is less than the energy expenditure. Thus, weight control can be considered in practical mathematical terms. Growing children and pregnant women should be in slightly positive caloric balance. Persons who wish to lose weight will need to be in negative caloric balance.

Each pound of body weight gain due to deposition of fat represents 3,500 kilocalories in excess of the energy needed for maintaining the body and its activities. This surplus of kilocalories need not occur in just one day, but ordinarily represents a gradual accumulation which becomes evident as fatty deposits. For example, the indiscretion of eating a piece of cake with icing on it each day would provide the possibility of sufficient kilocalories in a week to add one pound of body weight.

When weight loss is the goal, the food intake needs to be modified from the usual dietary pattern of the individual so that the caloric intake is somewhat less than needed for body maintenance. If the intake is reduced by approximately 500 kilocalories per day, the weight loss in a week should be approximately one pound. Such precise correlation of weight loss with energy intake may not show up immediately because of the influence of the weight of water in the body tissues and other physical adjustments. However, just about one pound is the average loss for each 3,500 kilocalorie decrement. This formula sounds simple, but the elimination of these calories should be done without reducing the nutritional adequacy of the diet.

CONCERN FOR WEIGHT CONTROL

Individual Perceptions

Weight control throughout childhood is important for both psychological and physiological reasons. By the time adolescence is reached, boys and girls generally are aware of their appearance and the importance of an appropriate weight. Interpretations of the appropriateness of a teen-ager's weight may be quite different from the viewpoint of the adolescent and from that of a nutritionist. Height-weight tables serve as a useful guide to interpretation of weight versus height data, but the teen-ager may have quite a different perception of his weight.

In 1970, the National Center for Health Statistics reported that 31 percent of the boys studied were concerned about being underweight, and 22 percent were concerned about being overweight. Girls in the same age bracket showed approximately a reverse of these interpretations, i.e., 24 percent of the girls were concerned about being underweight and 34 percent were worried about being overweight. These concerns were expressed in spite of the fact that 40 percent of the boys and girls had weighed themselves within the week prior to the interview, and 70 percent had weighed within the preceding month. Clearly, weight control is considered by many teen-agers. This concern may lead to fad diets rather than appropriate and healthful dietary measures.

Development of Fat Cells

Aside from the psychological reasons for controlling weight throughout life, the data which are being gathered regarding development of fat cells add emphasis to the need for regulating food intake in the early years. Knittle (1972) suggests that there are two significant periods in childhood when juvenile obesity is most likely to occur: between birth and age four and at the period between ages seven and eleven. Since approximately 80 percent of overweight children will carry this pattern of overweight into their adult years, the need to avoid the overweight condition in childhood is apparent. Hirsch (1972) states: "Current evidence would favor the idea that most adipose cells are laid down in the last part of gestation with some cells added in the first year of life and some in early adolescence."

In adults, there will not be an increase in the number of fat cells, but there will be an increase in the size of the existing fat cells when a person is depositing fat. Persons who were obese in childhood may have formed twice as many fat cells as those who were of normal weight in the early years. Obviously then, the individual who has developed large numbers of fat cells in childhood has significantly more potential storage sites than will the normal individual.

Preventive Measures

The child who is born to thin, ectomorphic parents is far less likely to have a problem with overweight than is the infant born of obese or endomorphic parents. The somatotype of parents is a definite key to what may be predicted for the weight pattern of children. Huenemann (1974) found mothers of "fat" babies tended to be less sure of themselves, less accepting of their babies, and from less conventional households than were mothers of "lean" babies. In instances when prediction would be for obesity in the child, careful dietary patterns in infancy and early childhood will be particularly important in preventing the development of obesity. The approach toward weight control then becomes one of prevention rather than correction. This orientation thus avoids development of the excessive numbers of fat cells that will occur in children who are eating more food than they need for an optimum rate of weight gain.

The suggestions for avoiding the development of excessive fatty depots begin in the first year for children who appear to be gaining too rapidly. Breast milk or proprietary formulas supplemented with iron can very well be fed until the infant reaches the age of a year. The infant foods that are fed should be provided in modest amounts rather than encouraging the infant to finish the jar. Pureed vegetables and fruits are relatively low in energy value and can be used with frequency. Cereals, egg yolk, and strained meats make important contributions to the diet, but can be fed in modest amounts. For infants who are predisposed toward obesity, there is a need to avoid foods high in calories, i.e., mixed dinners, wet-pack cereals, and desserts are not recommended. Overfeeding clearly is to be avoided during infancy.

Another dimension to weight control during the early period of life is that of activity level. When children begin to be mobile, they should have ample free space in which to move so that they become physically active. Playpens or prolonged periods in bed while awake curtail activity and thus limit the calories required daily.

Parents who are alert to the need for weight control can aid in promoting optimum growth through directing attention to correct feeding practices and an environment for activity. However, it is important that this concern not be developed to the point where parents become anxious and neurotic about dietary practices and activity.

In most cases children's appetites closely parallel their need for food so that weight control may largely be a self-regulating mechanism. When children tend to be sedentary or when adults attempt to force them to eat, however, some change in dietary habits is usually necessary. Problems of weight reduction are safest and most effective when undertaken with professional supervision, including continuous medical surveillance. Crash programs and fad diets pursued on one's own should be avoided.

Professional Guidance

Particularly for teen-agers, a strong word of caution is needed in the field of weight control, simply because there are so many self-styled experts and so many fad diets that persist in popping up in popular literature. Well-meaning friends and acquaintances who readily admit that they do not understand computers or other complexities of modern life will gleefully share their "authoritative knowledge" of ways to lose weight. Beware not only of this personal advice, but also beware of weight reduction suggestions in books and popular magazine articles. The appearance of a diet in print is no guarantee of its efficacy or its safety. Insist on knowing the qualifications of the person who is recommending a diet. The qualification of being a published writer simply is not sufficient to make a nutrition expert of a layman. Qualified nutritionists will have a sound academic background in organic and biochemistry, physiology, psychology, and nutrition, documented at the minimum by the appropriate B.S. or B.A. degree from an accredited university; many nutritionists have earned the M.S. or Ph.D. degrees, adding still greater depth and breadth to their understanding of weight control and other nutritional problems.

THE UNDERWEIGHT CHILD

Since the usual dietary problem in the United States today is that of overweight, little attention is being given to the problems of the underweight individual. A thin child, however, usually has lowered resistance to infection, reduced physical energy, diminished alertness, and a less attractive appearance.

Personal tastes in physical proportions may vary, but evidence indicates that health more likely will be optimum when weight is within the normal range (see Appendix). One of the problems associated with severe underweight is the increased incidence of tuberculosis. Since underweight is usually caused by a small food intake, it is likely that the thin person is receiving inadequate amounts of several of the essential nutrients needed by the body, not simply inadequate calories. These deficiencies can create health problems at any age, but they are particularly important in growing children. Therefore, when a child is underweight, it is essential to examine the dietary pattern and develop an appropriate plan for overcoming the shortages.

Causes

When a physical examination fails to reveal any physical cause for underweight, it is necessary to assess both the diet and the mealtime environment. Some changes may need to be made to increase the caloric content of the meals served each day, but usually the major changes need to be made in the home environment. Parents can play an important part in helping a child gain weight when they can understand the specific problems that have caused their child to be too thin. Often the doctor or nutritionist will be able to detect an underlying problem that needs to be corrected. Common focal points to consider are: the mother's and father's attitudes toward food, the emotional climate at the table and in the home, feelings of sibling rivalry, the mealtime schedule, and the child's activity pattern.

Frequently dietary problems encountered in underweight children have been of relatively long duration and may be traced back to the first few months of life. Some mothers are almost professional worriers when it comes to feeding their children, and they communicate this concern about appetite to their babies. When mothers regularly urge and coax their children to eat, it is not surprising that some children acquire poor appetites and resist almost anything that is fed to them. Still other children discover early in life that they can control their parents by refusing to eat the food that their parents may urge on them.

Some family tables bear a close resemblance to a battleground, at least in an emotional if not a physical sense. Sensitive children may become so tense at the table, as a result of family arguments, that eating becomes a very difficult task.

Sometimes adults have unrealistic ideas of the amount of food a small child needs to eat. Such adults may try to force children to eat more food than they need or want. One common technique employed by the adult to achieve a greater food intake is to insist that the child remain at the table until the food is gone. This grandstand play usually creates strong hostility between the two participants and only makes the likelihood of a good appetite at the next meal more remote. Sometimes parents thoughtlessly discuss their children's eating habits where their children can hear them. If a child overhears himself characterized as a picky, fussy eater, it is safe to assume that he will begin to feel that this is indeed just what he is going to be.

In some instances food problems are directly attributable to problems rooted in sibling rivalry. A child who feels he is not getting his fair share of attention may decide that refusal to eat at meals is a good way to focus family attention on himself. True, it may not be expressions of approval that he is receiving, but at least he gains some recognition as an individual. His fussy eating habits at the table then may gradually become his trademark.

Most children have better appetites for meals when they play actively and eat at reasonably regular intervals each day. A few children may become poor eaters simply because they are too tired and too hungry to eat well at the table. Children who are very tired rarely are able to eat much food. This generalization is as applicable at breakfast as it is at dinner.

Treatment

Environmental changes. The adjustments necessary in an environment to promote better appetite obviously will vary with the situation. The mother who is too concerned about her child's dietary needs will find that Johnny eats more food when she concentrates on preparing appetizing, tempting meals and refrains from reminding him that he should eat more.

It may be difficult to change the atmosphere at the table to one of pleasant congeniality, but it can be accomplished if everyone in the family makes the effort. Subtle aids in the form of soft background music, an attractive center-piece, and special preplanned topics of conversation can be used to help initiate this difficult transition. Considerable effort over a long period of time is necessary to achieve a permanent change in group behavior at the table. This change in mood, however, can be accomplished to the benefit of the entire family.

Sibling rivalry can be alleviated by conscious effort to give recognition and approval to all the children equally, or as needed, throughout the day. Genuine expressions of approval may improve the appetite when a child feels neglected or rejected, but such comments should not be centered exclusively around approval of greater food intake.

Scheduling of meals and bedtime may require special effort for some mothers whose husbands work long hours, thus necessitating a late dinner. It is usually possible, however, to arrange the daytime schedule to include a nap if young children need to stay up late in order to have some time with their father. The children's dinner could be served early and a light dessert served to them when their father has dinner. Other adjustments may need to be implemented to meet specific family scheduling problems. The important thing is to be sure that adequate rest is provided and that the food intake is spaced appropriately to ensure a hungry, interested child at meals.

Dietary modifications. Some general suggestions can be made to modify the caloric intake of thin children, but usually the most satisfactory adjustments can be made when a dietitian has the opportunity to examine the typical food pattern of the family and then make specific suggestions. The meal plan for thin children still should include a well-balanced diet rather than concentrating on a narrow selection of high-calorie foods. Whole milk definitely is preferable to skim milk or buttermilk for these children. The use of milk in soups and puddings also is recommended. Small increases in the size of the servings, particularly in the servings of meats and bread and cereal products, frequently are effective in causing modest weight gains. Snacks may be increased to provide more calories, but the quantity and the timing should be planned to avoid interfering with mealtime appetites.

Mothers may find special ways of increasing the food intake of their own children if they view the problem objectively. The important thing is to avoid making a big production of the dietary changes to increase a child's weight. Subtle changes from the kitchen are more effective than long lectures on the need for changes.

THE OVERWEIGHT CHILD

Overweight affects the very rich and the very poor, adults and children. It is the number one nutrition problem throughout the United States today. This condition in children is of particular concern because overeating is likely to become a way of life that carries on into adulthood. These cases of long duration are very difficult to treat successfully even though they represent a distinct health hazard. It is far easier to treat the problem when it begins than to wait until adulthood and then try to change the habits of a lifetime.

Overweight in Childhood and Future Health Prospects

To assess the health hazards associated with overweight in children, it is necessary to project into the future; these overweight children, in all probability, will become overweight adults. Overweight is generally detrimental to the health of adults. It should be pointed out, however, that the suicide rate in overweight individuals is lower than in the population having a normal weight, a fact that has somewhat more significance in the teen-age group than in the population as a whole. Eating apparently provides a solution of sorts for some individuals with emotional problems.

Some of the common health problems in the adult American population are conditions frequently associated with overweight. It has been shown conclusively that blood pressure increases with increasing weight and decreases with weight reduction. Hypertension is two and one-half times more likely to occur in an overweight individual than in a person of normal weight. Tendency toward atherosclerosis is twice as common in the overweight as in the underweight, with the normal individual being somewhere in between these two extremes. Nine out of ten diabetics over forty are overweight.

Studies of Norwegians during the war years when diets were highly restricted revealed some indisputable facts. A distinct drop in circulatory diseases accompanied the restriction in diet, and there was also less trouble with clotting in the veins following surgery. These trends were reversed as food once again became readily available after the war.

Insurance statistics indicate that permanent loss of excess weight can definitely enhance the chance of survival of an overweight person, but the person in the best position is the one who has never been too heavy. The percentage mortality of overweight men is 142 percent (normal weight equals 100 percent) and drops to 113 percent if the excess weight is permanently lost. Volatile weight control, that is frequent reduction and gain, is more dangerous than maintenance of a constant high weight.

With such overwhelming evidence regarding the health hazards of overweight, it should be apparent that it is an important parental responsibility to help children avoid excessive weight gain during infancy and childhood.

Causes of Overweight

Numerous specific causes of overweight may be cited, but these generally may be classified as either (1) excessive caloric intake in relation to the body's caloric expenditure, or (2) some physical malfunction. Children who have weight problems due to improper diet are of paramount interest in this chapter. Those cases caused by a physical malfunction require medical treatment if they are to be helped. Actually only a small percentage of persons weigh too much because of physical abnormalities such as metabolic disorders or glandular malfunctions.

It is easy to say that a person is overweight because he eats too much, but permanent desirable weight control can rarely be accomplished unless the reasons behind this excessive intake are understood and corrected.

Developmental overweight. Some children exhibit progressive, excessive weight gain from infancy throughout childhood. One possible explanation for this developmental overweight is that the typical activity patterns of an individual may be inborn. Since a less active individual requires fewer calories daily than does a normally active person, the less active child gradually will become overweight while eating a diet that is average for a child his age.

Perhaps a significant factor in the incidence of developmental overweight is the mother who measures her maternal prowess by the plumpness of her child. This may be a desirable criterion for farmers to use when feeding livestock, but scarcely seems an appropriate measure of successful motherhood. It is far more important to have a child within the normal weight range for his height than it is to have the fattest baby in the neighborhood.

According to Bruch (1957), food may become a comfortable form of security for some children. This attitude toward food, when maintained over a long period of time, is likely to result in excessive weight gain.

Reactive overweight. This type of weight gain may result from an adjustment to a crisis such as loss of a loved one. Some children (and adults, too) seem to derive psychological comfort from food in times of stress.

Sexual adjustment may be an underlying reason for some teen-agers being overweight. Hecht (1955) outlines the theory that a fat figure may be a defense for individuals wishing to avoid contacts with the opposite sex or secretly desiring to have physical attributes of the other sex.

The factor of disturbances in the home as a cause of overweight is apparently a difficult one to resolve. Bullen et at. (1963), reporting on a study of adolescent girls at two summer camps, found that overweight girls more frequently came from less happy family situations than did the girls of normal weight. It appeared that the insecurity felt by the overweight girls from the disturbed families was related to their fear of leaving their families.

Other less dramatic factors such as a genuine fondness for food and our sedentary society could be mentioned here also. Certainly there are many varied reasons for overweight children.

The Influence of Overweight during Adolescence

Studies directed toward gaining greater understanding of the causes of excess weight have commanded increasing attention within the past decade. Bullen et al. (1963) interviewed two groups of girls, one overweight and the other of normal weight, to attempt to determine the reasons for the difference in the size of the individuals. Forty-four percent of the overweight girls had overweight fathers; conversely only 11 percent of the girls of normal weight had overweight fathers. Mayer (1953), in a study conducted in Boston, found that 8 percent of the overweight children in his study had two obese parents.

Bullen's study (1963) revealed that overweight girls dated less, were less vigorous in their actions, participated in fewer activities, and indulged in more eating sprees than girls of normal weight. The overweight girls recognized their lack of activity, but seemed to be unaware that this inactivity contributed to their overweight condition.

Prevention of Overweight

At any age level, but particularly with children, the need for weight control before extra weight becomes a problem should be emphasized. It is far easier to maintain a normal weight than to try to remove the unnecessary pounds that have earned a child the nickname of "Fatty." By the time this point is reached, the child is faced with the dual problem of a psychological need to change his self-image as well as the physical problem of shedding the excess weight. This is a large order for anyone, and it is a task that frequently could have been avoided.

Education to fight the problem of overweight in American children is not a simple matter; the roots of overeating underlie much of our society, from the influences of family income and cultural background to the impact of technology on our physical activity patterns. Obviously no single solution can be derived to overcome a problem of such complexity. A multifaceted educational approach, however, can help people to achieve a better understanding of the underlying causes, and, with increased understanding, perhaps progress will be achieved.

A study reported by Moore et al. (1962) gives increased emphasis to the value of education in the prevention of overweight. This group of workers found that overweight was far more prevalent in the lowest group than in the highest socioeconomic group. Some of the reasons that apparently contributed to this situation were:

1. Little education on basic nutrition information
2. Limited understanding of food purchasing.
3. Habitual consumption of a diet proportionately high in cereal and other carbohydrate sources and low in fruits and vegetables.
4. Limited opportunity for interesting recreational pursuits.
5. Little emphasis on the importance of weight and its influence on personal appearance.

One effective way to help prevent overweight in children is to encourage active play and sports and to minimize the time spent viewing television. The late President Kennedy drew public attention to this national need, but there is still considerable public lethargy.

Physicians can play an important role in nutrition education geared toward prevention of undesirable weight gain. Usually doctors have sufficient contact with the preschool child and his parents to permit assessment and treatment of overweight when it first develops. If a child becomes too heavy, the physician should counsel the parents and assist in correcting the conditions that have led to the unnecessary weight gain. Advice from a doctor is particularly effective because of the high esteem most parents have for his knowledge.

The role of the physician in nutrition education need not, indeed should not, be limited to advice regarding the preschooler. Some children experience weight control problems that appear to be related to their entry into school (at the age of five or six). Other developmental crises, experienced near the beginning of puberty and again in the middle teens as emphasis begins to be placed strongly on heterosexual acceptance, may trigger weight problems. Although the doctor probably will see these children less frequently than the preschooler, it still is possible to provide the appropriate guidance when it is needed.

Perhaps the most significant and long-lasting effects in nutrition education can be accomplished by the obstetrician. A pregnant woman is usually very anxious to do whatever her doctor recommends to promote development of a healthy baby. Obstetricians can conduct classes for groups of expectant women or they can talk to them individually about the need for proper nutrition (including weight control) during pregnancy. These sessions should also include the nutritional needs of the young, and special emphasis should be given to developing attitudes within the family that will help all members achieve and maintain an appropriate weight.

Educators can play an important part in nutrition education within the school program. Home economics teachers and school nurses are in particularly favorable positions to emphasize the value of good nutrition and weight control. Other teachers, including the biology and physical education instructors, also can help to develop an interest in nutrition. It is important, however, that teachers refer students in need of special weight control assistance to appropriate medical help rather than undertaking the project themselves.

Treatment of Overweight

Pertinent research. To illustrate some of the ideas that are being explored by scientists working in the field of weight control, a few studies are briefly reported here. More extensive information is outlined in the references cited at the end of this chapter and in other technical papers.

The actual number of calories recommended in a reducing diet varies from fasting to a very slight reduction from normal intake. In 1958 Wishnofsky published a study explaining the difference in weight loss that occurred during fasting as compared with the weight loss during a low-calorie regimen. Fasting caused a loss in the body's stores of carbohydrate and protein, the loss of one pound of protein being accompanied by a loss of three pounds of water. These protein stores were automatically replaced when food was introduced once more and the appropriate amount of water was retained until the protein levels returned to normal. This result was in contrast to the loss of fat deposits accompanied by the loss of one-half pound of water when a low-calorie diet was employed. On a normal diet one pound was lost for each 3500 calories eliminated from the regular intake. Wishnofsky also noted that the basal metabolic rate drops during weight loss of significant proportions.

The percentage of calories that carbohydrates, fats, and proteins should contribute in a reducing diet has been studied at some length and with varying results. The numerout studies testing different ratios have been almost more confusing than illuminating. The biggest battles have been waged over whether a high-protein diet is better than a high-fat diet. No truce has yet been declared.

Kekwick (1960), found that, on a 1000-calorie diet composed of 90 percent of the calories from fat, the weight loss was greater than one deriving 90 percent of the calories from protein. A diet deriving 900 of its total 1000 calories from carbohydrate actually caused weight maintenance briefly before weight loss commenced. These same workers showed that four out of five obese individuals gained or maintained their weight on a 2000-calorie daily intake, whereas some people actually were able to lose weight with a 2600-calorie daily intake.

From time to time there will be reports in popular magazines of diets that are based on modification of the usual balance between protein, carbohydrate, and fat in the diet, accompanied by claims of remarkable weight loss due to such modifications. Worthington and Taylor (1974) studied the efficacy of balanced low-calorie versus high protein-low carbohydrate reducing diets. These workers found that a high protein-low carbohydrate diet did result in significantly more weight loss during the first week than did an isocaloric balanced diet. However, the weight losses in both diet groups were comparable the second week. The high protein-low carbohydrate diet was criticized because of its inadequate levels of vitamin A, ascorbic acid, iron, and calcium, as well as being criticized on the basis of limited variety.

The area of proposed weight reduction diets is vast, and the information is most meaningful in a person-to-person situation rather than in gross generalities. It does seem pertinent, however, to mention the "formula diets" that have become so much a part of the American scene. Some of the arguments favoring their use are elimination of calorie-counting guesswork, satisfactory satiety value, convenience, and weight loss results. Question has arisen, however, regarding the prolonged use of such formulas because of the body's need for more roughage to avoid alimentary tract disturbances.

Dieting guide lines.   If a child needs to lose weight, it is wise to consult with a physician and his dietitian. They will be able to analyze the problems and help work out a solution so that weight control can quickly be reestablished and then maintained.

A dietitian's help is valuable because she can provide appropriate dietary advice and encourage the child to follow the prescribed diet. Emphasis is placed on the importance of having someone who is genuinely interested in the progress of the dieter during the diet period. It appears that this interest is one reason that doctors and dietitians are reasonably effective in treating weight reduction cases. The interested observer, however, can be effective only when the individual himself desires to lose weight. It has been pointed out that the child, as he enters puberty, is likely to be particularly receptive to help in weight reduction because of the desire to be accepted by his peer group.

It is becoming increasingly apparent that a change in the physical activity patterns of a child's life may be an important factor in successfully reestablishing weight control. The argument frequently advanced is that the larger appetite resulting from the increased activity more than offsets the good accomplished by the exercise. Bullen et al. (1963) state that at a reasonable level of activity the body burns up somewhat more calories than will be ingested because of the increase in appetite.

A boon to dieting is the development of new interests during the adolescent years. When a person is busy and his mind is focused on other thoughts, food becomes secondary and less tempting. Parents can help younger children with weight problems by providing new and interesting ideas for play when food seems to be troubling them. Walks together or short trips are also helpful.

Many weight reduction diets presently are circulating and many more will come into existence in the future. Some diets are good, some are ineffectual, and some are harmful. A doctor should be consulted before undertaking a weight reduction regimen of significant proportions.

The purposes of any good diet designed for weight loss are twofold: (1) to permit weight loss at a reasonable rate, and (2) to\ retrain the appetite so that the lost weight will not be regained. To lose weight, it is necessary to eat fewer calories than were being eaten when the child was gaining the extra weight. Most children and adults are often most successful in keeping off the weight if the diet is similar to the diet ordinarily eaten in the home.

Young et al. (1971) explored the merits of various frequencies of feeding in relation to weight reduction and body composition. These researchers, using a carefully constructed experimental design, tested the effect of dividing the day's intake into six, three, and one meal daily. Results indicated that frequency of eating had no significant effect on weight loss or on fat losses (skinfold thickness or body circumference). Reaction to the various frequencies of feeding favored three meals. Some subjects felt that six meals daily were a nuisance, while one meal created a strain.

The following suggestions are appropriate guide lines to observe during any weight reduction program:

1. Weight reduction is best undertaken when the patient first begins to gain too much weight.
2. The decision to reduce must be internalized within the patient; that is, another person cannot provide the primary motivating force for reduction.
3. Moderate activity will help to modify the normal physical activity pattern and assist in developing actual physical need for more calories.
4. Acquisition of new hobbies or interests will help to prevent the boredom that often leads to overeating.

5. An attempt should be made to understand and modify the psychologic factors that may have caused the weight problem.
6. The assistance of an interested person—layman, dietitian, or physician—can help to provide the extra boost needed occasionally to persist in the reduction program.
7. The diet plan itself should provide sufficient satiety value to keep the patient from feeling like a martyr, but it must still reduce the caloric intake sufficiently to provide the necessary weight loss.
8. The dieter should be prepared to expect slow weight loss, but the loss must not be so slow that he loses interest and motivation.
9. Emphasis must be given constantly to the importance of keeping the weight off once it is lost. Volatile weight losses and gains definitely are harmful to health.
10. The diet should be patterned as closely as is practical after the customary diet of the individual. This makes it easier to follow the diet and it also makes the retraining of diet habits to maintain the lower weight a simple process, for the retraining occurs during the diet period itself.
11. A good weight reduction diet will provide the necessary good nutrients, but will restrict the calories. Particular attention should be given to the inclusion of the nutrients needed by children for growth.
12. For the person with only modest weight problems, weight control probably can be achieved by simply reducing the size of the servings and avoiding second helpings.
13. Parents can help children with weight control by avoiding giving undue emphasis to food. Food should not be used as a threat or as a reward.
14. Simple changes in the diets of children can be very effective in avoiding excess pounds. After the first year of life, skim milk can be substituted very satisfactorily for whole milk and it provides far fewer calories. Raw carrots, celery sticks, and other raw vegetables provide the desired crunchiness and bulk children often seek in a snack. If these items are available and ice cream, cookies, and crackers

virtually vanish from the kitchen, weight control problems often depart, too.

SUMMARY

Weight control is a component of good nutrition which needs to be monitored and corrected as necessary. When the body's need for energy (calories for basal metabolism, physical activity, and specific dynamic effect of food) is in concert with the calories in the food consumed, a person will not gain weight. However, if he is eating a diet providing more energy than needed, he will gain weight. Conversely, weight is lost when the body's energy needs exceed the energy provided in the diet.

Excess deposition of fat is undesirable even in infancy for adipose cells are formed during infancy. An increased number of adipose cells affords more potential sites for subsequent fat deposition. The reasons for failing to achieve weight control are varied, ranging from physical to sociological, psychological, and economic factors. If weight control is to be achieved and maintained, the original cause(s) of the weight abnormality should be identified and corrected. Ideally, appropriate dietary patterns and attitudes toward food will be established in early childhood, thus eliminating the frustration of the need to concern oneself with constant attention to weight control throughout life.

BIBLIOGRAPHY

Bruch, H., 1957. *Importance of Overweight.* Norton. New York.

Bruch, H., 1958. Psychological aspects of obesity in adolescence. *Amer. J. Pub. Health* 48: 1349.

Bullen, B.A., et al., 1963. Attitudes towards physical activity, food and family in obese and nonobese adolescent girls. *Amer. J. Clin. Nutr.* 12: 1:

Heald, F.P., 1965. History and physiological basis of adolescent obesity. *Nutr. News* 28, No. 4: 13.

Hecht, M.B., 1955. Obesity in women: a psychiatric study. *Psychiat. Quart.* 29: 203.

Hood, C., et al., 1970. Observations on obese patients eating isocaloric reducing diets with varying proportions of carbohydrate. *Brit. J. Nutr.* 24: 39.

Huenemann, R.L., 1974. Environmental factors associated with preschool obesity. *J. Amer. Dietet. Assoc.* 64: 480.

Kekwick, A., 1960. On adiposity. *Brit. Med. J.* 5196: 407.

Knittle, J.L., 1972. Obesity in childhood: problem in adipose tissue cellular development. *J. Pediat.* 81: 1048.

Leverton, R., 1970. *Girl and Her Figure.* National Dairy Council. Chicago.

Lowrey, G.H., 1958. Obesity in the adolescent. *Amer. J. Pub. Health* 48: 1354.

Maxfield, E. and F. Konishi, 1966. Patterns of food intake and physical activity in obesity. *J. Amer. Dietet. Assoc.* 49: 406.

Mayer, J., 1953. Genetic, traumatic and environmental factors in the etiology of obesity. *Physiol. Rev.* 33: 472.

Mayer, J., 1966. Why people get hungry. *Nutr. Today* 1, No. 2: 2.

Moore, M.E., et al., 1962. Obesity, social class and mental illness. *J. Amer. Med. Assoc.* 181: 926.

Moore, M.E., et al., 1966. Energy expenditure of preadolescent girls. *J. Amer. Dietet. Assoc.* 49: 409.

National Center for Health Statistics, 1970. *Height and weight of children, U.S. Vital and Health Statistics.* P.H.S. Pub. No. 1000 – Series 11 – No. 104. Public Health Service. Washington, D.C.

Peckos, P.S., 1971. Teenage obesity problem – why? *Food and Nutr. News* 42, No. 5-6: 1.

Prugh, D.E., 1961. Some psychologic considerations concerned with the problem of overnutrition. *Amer. J. Clin. Nutr.* 9: 538.

Schacter, S., 1971. Eat, eat. *Psych. Today* 5, No. 5: 45.

Seltzer, C.C. and J. Mayer, 1970. Effective weight control program in public school system. *Amer. J. Pub. Health* 60: 679.

Shutter, Z. and D.C. Garell, 1966. Obesity in children and adolescents. *J. School Health* 36: 273.

Smith, N.J., 1972. *Challenge of Obesity.* Ross Laboratories. Columbus, Ohio.

Sohar, E. and E. Sneh, 1973. Follow-up of obese patients: 14 years after a successful reducing diet. *Amer. J. Clin. Nutr.* 26: 845.

Thomas, D.W. and J. Mayer, 1973. Search for secret of fat. *Psych. Today* 7, No. 4: 74.

Winick, M., 1974. Childhood obesity. *Nutr. Today* 9, No. 3:6.

Wishnofsky, M., 1958. Caloric equivalents of gained or lost weight. *Amer. J. Clin. Nutr.* 6: 542.

Worthington, B.S. and L.E. Taylor, 1974. Balanced low-calorie vs. high-protein-low-carbohydrate reducing diets. *J. Amer. Dietet. Assoc.* 64: 47.

Wyden, P., 1965. *The Overweight Society.* Morrow. New York.

Young, C.M., 1964. The prevention of obesity. *Med. Clin. N. Amer.* 48, No. 5: 1317.

Young, C.M., 1964. Some comments on the obesities. *J. Amer. Dietet. Assoc.* 45, No. 2: 134.

Young, C.M., 1966. Measurements of caloric overnutrition. *Rev. Nutr. Food Sci.* 3: 2.

Young, C.M., et al., 1971. Frequency of feeding, weight reduction, and body composition. *J. Amer. Dietet. Assoc.* 59: 466.

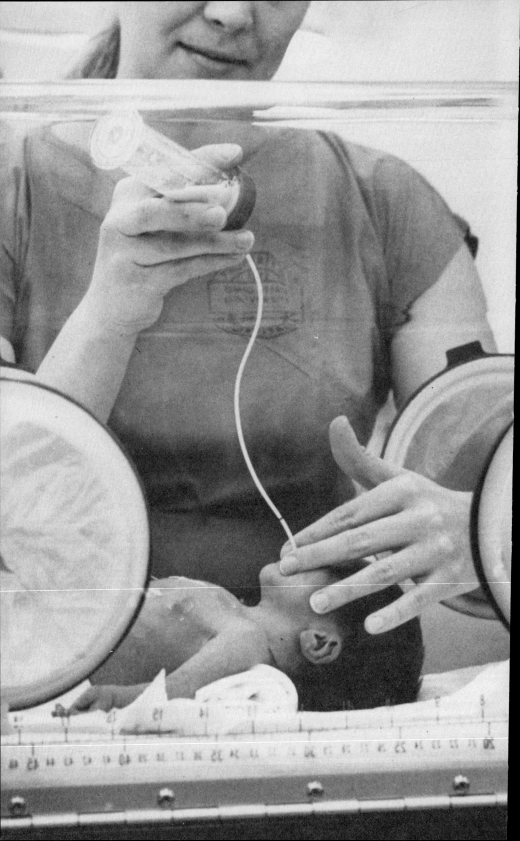

Chapter 12
Managing Special Needs

Dietary care of a sick child differs distinctly from the day-to-day feeding of an active, healthy child with a good appetite. The body needs are somewhat altered during sickness, and the appetite frequently becomes poor or nonexistent. For the usual childhood diseases a few dietary changes of short duration will suffice. In certain chronic conditions the body may fail to metabolize particular substances in the usual manner, thus necessitating specific changes from the usual diet pattern. When a child has a chronic condition the physician will make any necessary dietary recommendations for long-term dietary changes.

THE SICK CHILD

When a child is sick the doctor will diagnose the problem and prescribe the appropriate treatment. Frequently he will suggest specific dietary changes designed to assist in a rapid recovery. The following discussion outlines some practical suggestions to help parents provide the general nutritional requirements of sick children. Specific dietary needs will be prescribed and explained by the doctor.

General Guide Lines

Although the specific dietary treatment of sick children varies according to the illness and its severity, a few generalizations may provide a helpful guide when children contract some of the more routine childhood diseases.

1. It is normal for children to lose their appetites when they are ill. Even though food is important during

convalescence, it is unwise to urge children to eat during an illness. If a poor appetite persists for a day or two, many parents become most anxious about the small quantity of food eaten and worry about possible weight losses. Even though a child actually is losing weight during an illness, it is usually not advisable to urge him to eat more than he actually wants. His appetite is quite a reliable indicator of what his body can manage. Extra food may only serve to once again irritate the gastrointestinal system and cause further disturbances. When the infection has subsided sufficiently the patient will begin to respond with a marked increase in appetite, and he may soon be eating more food than he does when he is healthy.

If parents coax a child to eat when his system rebels against food, they may unwittingly establish psychological blocks that result in a pattern of continued urging by the parents countered by rebellion on the part of the child. It is far more difficult to break such a behavior pattern than it is to establish it; common sense and medical opinion dictate that parents avoid attempting to coerce children to eat more than they want during an illness.

2. Particular attention should be given during convalescence to serving tempting foods that invite a child to eat them. Once recovery has progressed to the point where the appetite begins to return, food intake will be improved when special touches are added to the meal. A small decoration on the tray or a surprise of a particularly well-liked food may help reawaken the appetite. Colored straws, bright napkins, and paper plates with perky designs aid in breaking the monotony of being a temporary invalid.

3. During the acute first stages of an illness, it is often appropriate to serve no solid foods, even to preschoolers, and school children. As the appetite begins to improve, it is usually best to begin the return to normal meals gradually by first offering small servings of easily digested solid foods. Large servings may cause complete rejection of the meal, whereas small servings encourage a child to try at least a bite or two.

4. Plain foods, low in fat and delicately seasoned, almost always have more appeal to sick children than do

fried or highly seasoned foods. Foods containing little fat or spice are also likely to be well tolerated by the digestive system. Particularly suitable foods for the early convalescent period are skim milk, plain gelatin or gelatin with ripe banana, baked custard, toast, and plain puddings.

5. When possible, someone should sit and talk with the patient while he is having his meal. Meals are dreary affairs for a child if he is left alone in his room with a tray of food which he did not really want in the first place. When parents or siblings read to him, chat, or even listen to a ball game with the patient, they help to make the meal more attractive and tempting. A happy mealtime atmosphere is as important for a sick child as for a healthy one. If circumstances permit, it might be wise to take a tray in and eat with the patient. The convalescing child may appreciate such sociability even more than he would when he is well.

6. Frequent small meals, rather than three larger meals, are often preferred by convalescing children. The timing of the meals actually is best determined by the desires of the patient.

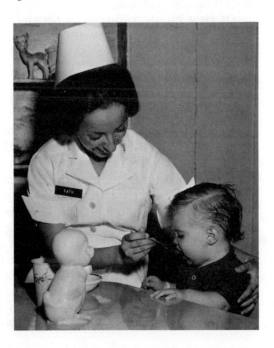

Whether in a hospital or at home, sick children usually are more interested in eating when they have pleasant companionship.

7. A small bit of pampering is appreciated by most sick children. Many young children relish the opportunity to decide what they want prepared. Food intake is usually greater when the patient suggests the menu. During convalescence the appearance of his favorite food may help to spur the desire to eat. It seems that familiar foods help to restore a child's sense of security after the upset of an illness. On the other hand, acceptance of new foods is likely to be nil when a child is sick. Because of the suspicion with which unfamiliar foods are greeted at this time, it is wise to avoid introducing new foods unless the doctor specifically requests a particular food.

Food and Fever

The recommendations for diet during a fever are based on the fact that basal metabolic rate is increased in proportion to the rise in body temperature, thus necessitating a marked rise in the number of calories needed by the body. The need for calories increases still more when the patient is extremely restless.

Of first concern during a fever is fluid intake. It may be necessary to give only water at first, but as soon as possible it is desirable to give liquids that also provide calories. Carbonated beverages, containing sugar rather than artificial sweeteners, provide useful calories and are generally well tolerated by sick children. Bouillon is a useful addition because it provides a palatable source of salt and liquid. Some fruit juices also may be enjoyed at this time. Skim milk may then be added to the diet to provide the much-needed protein for the sick child; it is not uncommon for whole milk, because of the fat content, to be more difficult to digest during the early stages of an illness. After skim milk at full strength is accepted and retained in the body in a normal manner, whole milk may be used in preference to skim milk. This substitution is useful in increasing the caloric content of the diet. Soups, ice cream, and sherbet are very useful means of providing the liquid needed by a child with a fever.

When the fever continues over a prolonged period, the doctor will usually provide special dietary instructions which include a high proportion of protein in the diet. This emphasis on providing a diet high in protein is important because a fever increases the body's protein need.

Dietary Treatment for Diarrhea

Diarrhea is frequently a problem when children, especially young babies, are sick. This condition should be corrected in all children, but it is of particular concern in the young infant because dehydration can occur very quickly. Severe diarrhea requires medical treatment immediately and, possibly, hospitalization. The first step in treating mild diarrhea is to remove food, including milk, and give water or weak tea frequently until the diarrhea lessens. For breast fed infants, nursing usually can be resumed in 12 hours. Bottle fed infants may require 1 to 2 days of water, tea, or 5 percent glucose solution before the diarrhea is controlled sufficiently to warrant adding milk and other foods.

When feeding is begun, it is common practice to feed skim milk diluted to half strength first. This type of milk is chosen because it is more easily digested than fat-containing whole milk and sugar. As the condition begins to improve, gelatin, toast, and cooked cereals may be added gradually to the diet. After the diarrhea has stopped, whole milk or the usual formula with sugar may be fed, along with a gradual expansion into the normal diet of the child. If the diarrhea begins to return when other foods are added to the diet, it is necessary to backtrack to the skim milk treatment and gradually build back to the regular diet. Fats and foods high in roughage should be added only after the diarrhea is controlled.

Dietary Management during Vomiting

It is not uncommon for a child to desire a drink of water immediately after vomiting, but it is best that he wait for about two hours before drinking anything at all. Older children may rinse their mouths with water if they will avoid swallowing any. The resting period seems to make it easier for the stomach to tolerate a small amount of liquid. After the next period a small drink of water may be offered, followed in twenty minutes by a little more water if the first drink has been tolerated successfully. Many children can satisfactorily sip ginger ale and other lightly flavored, carbonated drinks during this stage of convalescence.

A cracker is usually the first solid food that will be tolerated well by the stomach. Dry toast also may be used. Gradually other foods may be reintroduced into the diet. Skim milk may be added about four hours after the crackers have been accepted. Whole milk, however, may trigger the vomiting again because of the fat content; it is not recommended until foods are being retained satisfactorily.

Feeding in the Hospital Setting

The premature infant. Dietary management for the premature infant is but one of the special aspects of care required during the critical period from delivery until a satisfactory weight has been achieved. Although sterile conditions for formula preparation are always important, even more critical attention is needed for these high risk infants. All persons in contact with the infant also must be free of any infectious disease and be very careful not to introduce microbiological contaminants to the nursery environment.

Feeding of the premature infant begins approximately 12 hours after birth, at which time four or five milliliters of either sterile water or five percent glucose water will be given at approximately two-hour intervals for the next 12 hours. This pattern of limited intake and frequent feedings is necessitated by the premature infant's very limited capacity. A few of the larger premature infants may be able to suck satisfactorily for feeding purposes, but the smaller and weaker ones may be either unable to suck or too weak to suck long enough for adequate intake. In such instances, feeding may need to be done with a medicine dropper or by gavage. With feeding using a medicine dropper or a bottle, careful attention must be given to avoiding aspiration. A semisitting position for the infant is recommended.

When the infant is able to tolerate the glucose solution, he is ready to begin special formula feeding. This change in feeding can usually begin when the infant is about 36 hours old. The amount of formula at a feeding generally will be six milliliters for infants 2½ pounds or less, ten milliliters for three pounds, and 15 milliliters for four pound infants. The formula (see Table 12.1) to be fed is mixed with equal amounts of five per cent glucose solution for feeding during the period from 36 hours to two days of age. Then the formula is diluted with decreasing amounts of the glucose solution until the full strength formula (55 kilocalories per pound of body weight) is being given by the third day of life. The ultimate goal in regulating the intake of the premature infant during the next week is to achieve a formula providing about 60 kilocalories per pound and a fluid level of between 60 and 75 milliliters per pound of body weight. Dietary supplementation with ascorbic acid and vitamin D in drop form is added by the end of the second week.

The older child. Hospitalization is a strange experience to many children. The situation may be well accepted by some children, but many may be distracted by the routines or find it difficult to accept the food served them in these strange surroundings. The consumption of a diet appropriate to the reason for hospitalization is an important part of the treatment for the patient. When possible, the presence of

Table 12.1   Feeding formulas for premature infants[a]

Type of Milk	Amount per Kilogram Body Weight	Grams/Kilogram Body Weight			Percentage of Total Kilocalories		
		Protein	Fat	Carbo-hydrate	Protein	Fat	Carbo-hydrate
Human	180 ml.	2.2	6.7	12.9	7	50	43
Evaporated	70 ml.	4.8	5.5	12.9	16	41	43
Carbohydrate	6 g.						
Water to make	150 ml.						
Half skim milk							
powder	18 g.	6.0	2.2	19.4	20	16	64
Carbohydrate	11 g.						
Water to make	150 ml.						

[a]From Gordon, H.H., et al. Feeding of premature infants. Comparison of human and cow's milk. Am. J. Dis. Child 73: 442. 1947.

a parent at mealtime is recommended. Parents help to provide a more familiar context for eating and add to the psychological support the child needs for adaptation to the hospital.

If a special diet is required for the particular condition begin treated, this will need to be followed in feeding the child. However, this food should be served in as attractive a manner as possible to help encourage the child to eat. When a general diet can be given, the older child may wish to make some selections from the menu. For younger children, one of the parents can help in identifying the types of foods that likely will be well accepted by the patient. The foods on the tray should be prepared in a manner which will allow children to feed themselves as much as possible. In particular, meats may need to be cut into bite size pieces.

SPECIAL DIETARY PROBLEMS OF CHILDREN

A minority of children have specific physical problems that require special diets at all times. Such cases should be handled under a doctor's supervision and with the careful cooperation of the parent. The regimen of diet therapy appropriate for the many conditions known to present particular problems in childhood will only be mentioned here. It is necessary, however, to underline and emphasize the importance of parental effort to carefully control the food intake of children who need restricted diets.

Some of the conditions of children that require such careful dietary attention include diabetes, celiac disease, ulcers, hypercalcemia, allergies, and kidney, liver, and heart diseases. While children are preschoolers, their parents can supervise their intake to conform with the modifications needed for good nutrition. However, these children need to be educated about their diets before they are eating in a regular school situation. Dietitians can be very helpful in aiding families to adjust to special diets and suggesting appropriate special recipes.

The problems associated with inborn errors of metabolism have been receiving considerable attention among researchers, and the contribution that diet control can make to control of these problems has been noted. Detection at the earliest possible moment permits dietary restrictions to be implemented before irreversible changes such as mental retardation become too extensive. Restriction of the amino acid phenylalanine in the diets of children with phenylketonuria is one illustration of the importance of diet control at a very early age. Galactosemia, another inborn metabolic disorder, also requires very careful dietary controls to minimize physical and mental changes in affected children. As other metabolic errors are studied, necessary dietary changes can be implemented as needed.

HANDICAPPED CHILDREN

The dietary requirements of handicapped children may be the same as for children without physical limitations, but the problems associated with meeting these needs are often quite different. Of course, the approaches to feeding handicapped children will vary, depending upon the nature of the handicap.

Children who are mentally retarded or who have handicaps which tend to make the development of self feeding techniques difficult need to experience the varieties of flavors and textures that are available in the diet of the normal infant, However, the difficulties associated with the feeding of these babies may lead parents to keep them on the bottle and on strained foods for a prolonged period of time. Such a delay in introducing textures may make the initial presentations of textures more difficult than would have been the case earlier. Transitions in texture can be provided by changing from the strained products to the use of finely ground meats, eggs, and small strips of very tender cooked meats and poultry. Cooked vegetables can be boiled until quite tender and then chopped coarsely. Even the device of preparing cooked cereals with some lumps in them can be a useful point of transition.

Handicapped children will need special patience and help in learning to feed themselves, and yet this is a most important step. The first step toward self feeding can be self-drinking training. It may be necessary to use a modified cup with a small spout for drinking, double handles for easier grasping, a weighted base to make tipping less of a problem, and perhaps a transparent cup so that the child can see the liquid more easily. After self-drinking from a cup has been mastered, some handicapped children may benefit from being trained to use a drinking straw. A plastic or paper straw can be used for this. The value of learning to use a straw is the opportunity this provides for using the lips and sucking strongly.

The next step can be learning to feed with the fingers. One approach to finger feeding is to provide opportunities for the child to learn to grasp small objects, such as toys. When he is able to pick up these objects without too much frustration, he can begin to feed himself with his fingers. Self-feeding is an important step forward, a step that needs to focus on pride in his accomplishment and not one that is accompanied at first by chiding comments about the messiness of the operation. The cleaning up operation can be much less frustrating to the adult present if the child's chair is placed on a large sheet of newspaper, which can be discarded after the meal.

The choice of dishes and equipment for self-feeding can make significant differences in the level of accomplishment in feeding as well as in the general atmosphere of the meal. Plastic dishes reduce the concern that is present when breakable dishes are used. A table that is cut out to allow the child's chair to be positioned in a way that permits the table to help support the handicapped child can be a very useful piece of equipment for children who have some difficulty in maintaining a correct sitting position in the chair. The chair should be a good height to permit the child's feet to rest firmly on the floor or on a sturdy foot rest.

Silverware may need to have modified handles for easier grasping. Padding the handles of a spoon by the use of foam rubber or a rubber handle may be the difference between successful feeding and frustration for the handicapped child who has difficulty grasping objects.

Until he is able to swallow liquids and solids without choking, sit in a balanced position and control his head, and lift his hand from the plate to his mouth, the child has not mastered the tasks which will be essential to self-feeding. The use of silverware is a difficult manipulation for severely handicapped children, and is certainly fraught with frustration at the beginning of the learning stage. It is wise to pick times when the child is rested and not distracted to begin to try to teach him the use of a spoon. At first, it may be necessary to help him grasp the spoon, move it to the bowl, and then transport the food to the mouth. A calm approach and constant, encouraging reinforcement will help to foster successful learning. The use of rather thick foods or mashed foods is recommended as the type of food which is easiest for the handicapped child to feed himself at first. Small servings will also help him to feel more successful as his efforts begin to reduce the amount of material remaining on the plate.

There is a need for careful attention to the actual quantity that a handicapped child is eating. In some instances handicapped children may have such limited physical activity that there will be a tendency to become too heavy. In other cases, underweight may be a problem. Since the feeding situation for handicapped children clearly is more complex than is true for normal children, assesssment of actual intake is appropriate to be certain that adequate amounts of the total nutrients needed for good nutrition actually are being consumed and not merely being presented. Parents with handicapped children will need careful guidance and counseling to be able to help their children meet this very important aspect of living, that is, of learning to feed one's self independently and adequately.

Children with handicaps may develop eating behaviors that are detrimental to themselves and those who are caring for them. When meals are served in the midst of highly emotional outbursts and food is being spit out or thrown, good nutrition simply will not be achieved. In such cases, professional help in behavior modification may be required. Thompson and Palmer (1974) have outlined the use of positive reinforcement to modify behavior. In professional settings the use of video tape recordings permits careful analysis of specific situations to allow a review and program planning for working with handicapped children.

Nutrition education for handicapped children is certainly as important as it is for normal children, but the approaches will need to be modified to meet the problems created by the handicap. Garton and Bass (1974) found that deaf children have less nutrition education being provided from external sources than is true of normal children who are able to hear comments people make regarding food. The knowledge that deaf children will have about nutrition will need to be presented through visual cues and conscious presentations of material. Similarly, blind children will not receive the usual visual cues regarding the appearance of food. The educational materials will need to be developed with this handicap in mind. For example, to teach a blind child that dark green, leafy and yellow vegetables are good sources of vitamin A is meaningless. Nutrition educators must develop the ability to project themselves into the total context of the handicap and modify educational materials and information accordingly.

SUMMARY

Even when it is of short duration, illness modifies dietary patterns and nutritional needs. A fever causes a significant increase in caloric need and also raises the requirement for fluids. Vomiting and diarrhea greatly limit the body's ability to digest and absorb the nutrients in food. Usually, childhood illnesses are of brief duration and require only a short time on a modified dietary pattern. Dehydration and mineral imbalances are potential hazards to be avoided. The dietary management of premature infants and the feeding of young children who are hospitalized require special attention if nutrition is to be optimum.

Some children are born with congenital errors of metabolism which require special dietary practices. For example, the child with phenylketonuria must be fed a diet with a very low level of phenylalanine.

Handicapped children have unique needs which must be met if adequate nutrition is to be the final result. With considerable patience and ingenuity, it is possible to aid many handicapped children to reach the point where they can feed themselves. Several suggestions for promoting food acceptance and developing motor skills have been presented.

BIBLIOGRAPHY

Acosta, P., et al., Undated. *Nutritional Management of Galactosemia.* Child Development Clinic and Metabolic Division of the Los Angeles Children's Hospital and the Department of Pediatrics, Univ. of S. Calif., Los Angeles.

Bandura, A., 1969. *Principles of Behavior Modification.* Holt, Rinehart, and Winston. New York.

Blanchard, I., 1966. Developing motor control for self-feeding. *Cerebral Palsy J.* 27: 9.

Buehler, P.A., 1966. Blanchard method of feeding the cerebral palsied child. *Amer. J. Occup. Ther.* 20: 1.

Bureau of Public Health Nutrition of the California State Department of Public Health, Undated. *The Low Phenylalanine Diet.* Berkeley, Calif.

Coffey, K.R. and J. Crawford, 1971. Nutrition problems commonly encountered in developmentally handicapped. In *Feeding the Handicapped Child.* Smith, M.A., ed. Child Development Center. Memphis, Tenn. p. 64.

Dixon, D.J.W., 1965. *Diets for Sick Children.* Blackwell Scientific Publ., Oxford, England.

Donnell, G.N., et al., 1961. Growth and development of children with galactosemia. *J. Pediat.* 58, No. 6: 836.

Francis, D.E.M., 1966. Recent advances in paediatric dietetics. *Nutrition* 20 (Summer): 64.

Garton, N.B. and M.A. Bass, 1974. Food preferences and nutrition knowledge of deaf children. *J. Nutr. Ed.* 6: 60.

Ireton, C.L. and H.A. Guthrie, 1972. Modification of vegetable-eating behavior in preschool children. *J. Nutr. Ed.* 4: 100.

Krause, M.V., 1966. *Food, Nutrition, and Diet Therapy,* 4th ed. Saunders. Philadelphia.

Redmond, A., 1973. *Premature Infant.* Ross Laboratories. Columbus, Ohio.

Smith, M.A., ed., 1971. *Feeding the Handicapped Child.* Child Development Center. Memphis, Tenn.

Sofka, D., Undated. *Nutrition and Feeding Techniques for Handicapped Children Series.* Developmental Disabilities Program, Room 892. California State Department of Health. Sacramento, Calif. 95814.

Thompson, R.J. and S. Palmer, 1974. Treatment of feeding problems – a behavioral approach. *J. Nutr. Ed.* 6: 63.

U.S. Dept. of Health, Education, and Welfare. *Surveys of Phenylketonuria High Risk Groups.* Children's Bureau Washington, D.C. 1961.

Waisman, H.A. and G.R. Kerr. Advantages and disadvantages in use of restricted diets in treatment of inborn errors of metabolism. In *Amino Acid Metabolism and Genetic Variation.* Ed., W.L. Nyhan. McGraw-Hill. New York.

Wright, L.D., 1965. An inborn error of metabolism associated with deficiency of enzyme cystathionine synthetase leading to hemocystinuria. *N.Y. State J. Med.* 65, No. 4: 559.

Wright, S.W., 1965. *Phenylketonuria.* Report to the Council on Foods and Nutrition. American Medical Association. Chicago.

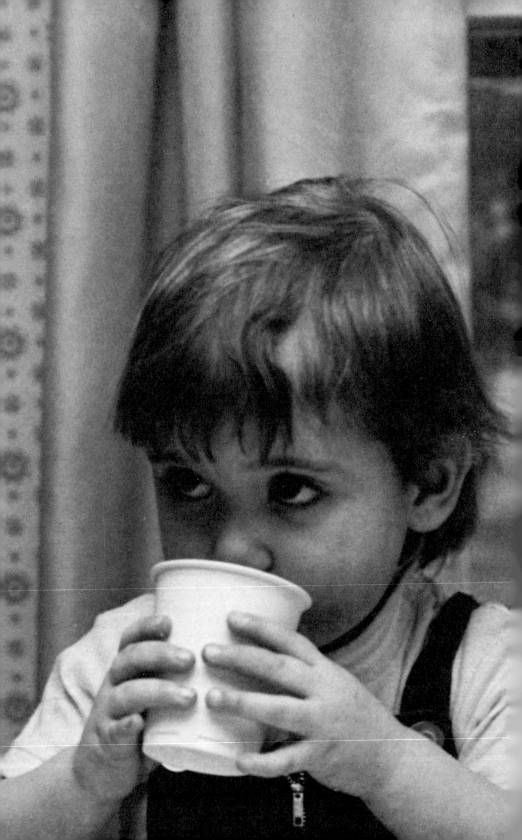

Chapter 13
Questions Often Asked

In any gathering of mothers, regardless of economic level or educational background, there is a good possibility that some aspect of child feeding will be discussed. Today's parents are becoming increasingly aware of the influence nutrition has on the physical and mental development of their children. Therefore it is not surprising that they seek additional information on this very important aspect of child development.

Certainly it is impossible to outline the ABC's of nutrition and expect that parents will be 100 percent effective in feeding their children, for children have distinct personalities and preferences that make each one an individual case. Parents need to have an understanding of basic nutrition which can be applied thoughtfully to each child. It is apparent that pat answers will not necessarily provide solutions for individuals, but they can provide a basis on which to work out individual solutions. This chapter is a compilation of questions parents have asked the author in class, at lectures, and over a cup of coffee at home.

Should I give my child a vitamin supplement?

In most instances, the practical answer is no, but a better answer requires some explanation. To explore this question on an individual basis, it would be necessary to know first what kind of diet the child is eating. If a normal, healthy child is eating a varied and well-balanced diet in adequate amounts, he will be receiving an adequate supply of vitamins (as well as protein and minerals), and there is no need for an additional vitamin supplement. The pills are an unnecessary expense for the family.

If children are eating very inadequate diets, vitamin pills may be one means of helping to improve their diets. Vitamin pills are not, however, the panacea many people think they are. Unfortunately, vitamin pills have become overrated in the minds of the general public. Most vitamin capsules supply only vitamins; they never supply protein and they seldom supply the minerals that are needed by the body. They were never intended by the manufacturers to take the place of a good diet. All too often the mother who gives her child vitamin pills is lulled into a false sense of security and feels that she has adequately cared for her child's nutritional needs simply by giving the vitamin supplement. Obviously, the vitamin pills will eliminate only the vitamin shortages in a diet; any deficiencies of minerals and protein will continue.

With these ideas in mind, let us now examine more carefully the question of vitamin supplements for children. First of all, the newborn or very young infant has a limited diet and will benefit from the addition of a daily vitamin supplement, particularly until a quart of milk is being consumed each day. A more thorough look at the vitamin needs of the young infant is included in Chapter 6 and should be referred to there.

It is simple to agree on paper that it is preferable to modify a child's dietary habits so that his diet is adequate in all respects, rather than relying on vitamin pills. It is unrealistic, however, to assume that all families will be successful in training their children to eat an adequate diet. From the practical viewpoint it may be necessary to give vitamin pills to supplement inadequate diets that defy improvement. Nevertheless the goal of an adequate diet should always be maintained.

A word of caution must be included here. It appears that large amounts of most vitamins are a waste of money, but will not cause physical harm. The hazards of excess quantities of vitamins A and D, discussed previously, should be borne in mind. Certainly it is unwise to administer large doses of either vitamin A or vitamin D because overdoses unquestionably can cause physical damage.

Should children eat iodized salt, or is plain salt better?

Adults and children alike benefit from iodized salt because it provides the iodide necessary to make the hormone, thyroxine, in the thyroid gland. If a person does not consume enough iodide, the thyroid gland gradually begins to enlarge in a futile attempt to produce the normal quantity of thyroxine. This enlargement of the thyroid gland is termed goiter. Iodide was so limited in the natural diets of many people in the United States that it seemed advisable to add this mineral to an inexpensive, commonly used foodstuff. Salt was selected, but it was also decided that some salt should be marketed without iodide for those persons who did not wish to take advantage of the new product. As a result both products are marketed side by side on the shelf, and many consumers buy the plain salt because they are unaware of the value of the iodization program. Thanks to the use of iodized salt by a reasonable segment of the population, the prevalence of goiter in this country has been greatly reduced, but the hazard still exists. In fact, people recently seemed to be forgetting about the importance of iodized salt. Failure on the part of many consumers to use iodized salt was causing the incidence of goiter to begin to rise again. Legislation now requires a labeling reminder of the need for this mineral. Wise consumers will buy iodized salt whether they live in the Midwest goiter belt or in other areas of the country.

Is fluoridation of water beneficial for children's teeth?

The answer to this question is a resounding yes; fluoridated water definitely aids in maintaining the integrity of children's teeth. It has been proven in study after study that, when the fluoride content in water is maintained at the level of one part fluorine per million parts water (1 ppm), the incidence of dental caries is dramatically reduced and no harmful effects have been observed. In the few towns with excess fluorides naturally present in the water supply, it is necessary to remove some fluorides to attain the desired one part per million, but, far more commonly, fluorides need to be added to raise the fluoride content to the tooth-protecting level (1 ppm).

Many emotional arguments regarding the hazards of fluoridation and the reasons why city water supplies should

not be fluoridated have been expounded from time to time
by well-meaning, but poorly informed citizens. Their charges
that fluorides will cause mottling and chalkiness of the
teeth are only partial truths, for such results have been
observed only when the amount of fluorine is considerably
in excess of the one ppm recommended for fluoridation. It
is true that a few natural water supplies contain toxic levels
of fluoride, but most areas have natural amounts of fluoride
in the water appreciably below the recommended level.
Since modern water plants can very efficiently and
accurately control the desired level of fluoride, there is
no reason to fear that harmful amounts of fluorine will
occur in the city water.

Some citizens are concerned about the cost of fluoridating
the city water supply and feel that the cost is not justified
because the fluorides only benefit children through their
teens. This argument can be countered by a 1966 report
stating that the estimated cost of fluoridation for each
citizen in Los Angeles would be approximately ten cents a
year. Certainly for most individuals this could not be viewed
as an excessive cost. Even though all costs have risen since
that year, fluoridation is still very inexpensive, certainly
far less costly than numerous dental bills for filling teeth.

There has been increasing evidence that fluorides also
benefit older people by reducing the demineralization that
commonly occurs in bones due to aging. The increased
hardness of the bones that results when fluoridated water
is available may help to decrease the incidence of broken
bones in this population group.

In the face of such evidence, it is difficult to understand
how anyone could be opposed to fluoridation. Certainly it
should be apparent that fluoridation is a very important
health measure for the children of this country.

If the city water supply is not fluoridated, it frequently is
possible to buy bottled fluoridated water. Such a solution
is reasonably effective for preschoolers who are at home
almost all of the time. Unfortunately, however, school-age
children receive much less benefit from the bottled water
because they must drink unfluoridated water during the
large part of the day when they are at school. There is the
additional disadvantage that it is far less convenient to
get drinking water from a water dispenser than it is to simply
turn on the nearest water faucet. Therefore school children

usually get less than the recommended amount of fluoride when it is available only in bottled water, but they do receive full benefit when the city water, which is available to them anyplace in town, is fluoridated. Fluoridated bottled water is definitely better than nothing, but city-wide water fluoridation is the best answer.

In areas where fluoridation has not yet been accepted, it would be wise for public-spirited parents to join with local dentists in launching an aggressive program that would lead toward fluoridation of the local water supply.

Is it possible for a child to drink too much milk?

Yes, some children will drink too much milk. The problem here is that children who drink large quantities of milk usually are too full to eat the other foods necessary to supply the nutrients not available in milk. Since milk is notably low in ascorbic acid and iron, the intake of both of these nutrients probably will be inadequate when milk intake is excessive. If an individual habitually drinks considerably more than a quart of milk a day—perhaps as much as eight or more glasses—it would be wise to reduce the quantity to one quart and then increase the intake of other foods.

What can be done to increase milk consumption when a child doesn't like milk?

Invariably in parents' groups the question of ways to encourage children to drink more milk is raised. The first thing parents need to do when they have this problem is to examine their own attitudes. They may find that they have been pushing milk with such desperate enthusiasm that the child has become apprehensive about drinking milk. He may even use milk refusal as a weapon against parents to get his own way. In this situation the mother (or father) should deliberately relax the pressure being exerted. It should be apparent, even to the emotionally involved parent, that force and pressure have only magnified the problem. In such a case the milk intake will frequently be improved if milk simply is made easily available without comment at each meal.

Sometimes a child who has become reluctant to drink milk may enjoy a change in the way his milk is served. A smaller glass, but one that is regularly refilled, may encourage him to try some milk. He might also enjoy the chance to pour his own milk. Sometimes children seem to think milk tastes better when it is served in a gaily colored glass or a mug painted with an appealing design. Such changes should be tried without comment or false enthusiasm; simply quietly make the substitution in glassware. Occasionally it is fun to vary the routine by serving a brightly colored straw with the milk.

Another factor that influences the milk-drinking habits of some children is directly traceable to the parents. When the parents do not drink milk, the children frequently will drink less than the recommended amount of milk. Parents who drink milk along with the children seldom have a problem with milk consumption among their youngsters. Immediately, some people will say that they cannot drink milk because it makes them fat. This is an excuse that they are hiding behind; they could very well drink skim milk while still setting the example that their children seem to need.

Many children prefer the taste of milk when it is quite cold. When a child is known to have this preference, it is desirable to keep the milk chilled in the refrigerator until just before the family comes to the table rather than having it on the table getting warm while the rest of the meal is being prepared and served.

What can be done when all these suggestions have been tried and a child still does not drink the necessary amount of milk each day? This is the time to exercise a bit of ingenuity in the kitchen in order to prepare foods that contain large amounts of milk. Many homemade soups like cream of potato and cream of tomato are delicious ways of serving milk. Vegetable, tomato, mushroom, and several other canned, concentrated commercial soups may be diluted to their proper strength with milk. Main dishes such as chicken a la king or creamed tuna add variety to family meals and increase milk consumption. Various flavors of cream puddings, stirred or baked custards, and ice cream are other milk-containing foods that children enjoy.

How much candy should my child eat?

Ideally, the answer to this question is none, for candy supplies many calories and little else of nutritional value. Unfortunately, it is far easier to say that a child should not eat candy than it is to achieve and maintain this goal. The easiest and most practical way to control the amount of candy a child eats is to limit the availability. In families this naturally means limiting the amount of candy available to parents, too, but this is one of the keys to success. How can children possibly be expected to understand that they should not eat candy when they see adults eating it? If adults set the example of eating almost no candy, it is easier for children to understand that they also do not need to eat it. This stratagem has the additional advantage of helping adults avoid the empty calories of candy, which can create a weight problem at any age.

Even when a family does not keep candy at home, there still will be times when candy will be available to the child. These isolated instances are not a cause for alarm because they are not establishing firm habits in the young child. Grandparents still should be granted a few privileges, and one that many of them enjoy is giving some candy to their grandchildren. If this happens only occasionally, there is no reason to be concerned about it. It is better to let the grandparents enjoy their privilege and role than it is to take a completely rigid stand on this matter. If grandparents live nearby and persist in giving candy frequently, perhaps as often as every day or every other day, it would be wise to suggest that they might bestow their favors in different ways rather than always offering candy.

Another regular source of candy is a lollipop from the doctor's office. It is true that most children do not visit the doctor frequently enough for this source to be a cause of concern to parents. Still, one might wish that doctors, who certainly are aware of nutrition, would emphasize the importance of good diet by substituting a small box of raisins for the candy.

This may be summarized by saying that candy does not need to become a problem unless the parents make it one. No issue needs to be made about candy; simply avoid keeping candy in the home to tempt the parents and the children.

Do children need carbonated drinks and artifically flavored fruit drinks?

Carbonated drinks are essentially in a class with candy. They are a source of calories, unless made with artificial sweeteners, but they have little else to offer nutritionally. Artificially flavored fruit drinks also are in this category. They are very high in sugar and again have no nutritional assets.

Not only do these drinks tend to contribute to obesity, but the sugar in these products has been indicted as a factor in the development of dental caries. Therefore most dentists strongly recommend that these soft drinks ordinarily should be omitted from the diet.

One of the important problems regarding consumption of these drinks is that they are often bought in fairly large quantities by low-income families who really need to spend this money to buy milk and other nourishing foods. An informal inquiry in a local high school revealed that it was not unusual for families who ate only small amounts of meat, fruit, and vegetables to buy large quantities of carbonated drinks. At nutrition time in school, children from these families often spent their money on an artifically flavored fruit punch rather than on milk, which was also available. The milk intake of these children was almost universally inadequate in their daily diets.

On warm days when children desire something refreshing and cold to drink, what might be substituted for carbonated or artificially flavored fruit drinks? Milk, of course, is one substitute that immediately comes to mind; colorful and nutritious beverages may also suitably fulfill the need for something cold to drink. Most children thoroughly enjoy refrigerated fruit juices of various kinds. Such fruit juices could be either fresh, canned, or frozen. These juices can be served either in their regular form or they can be frozen into popsicles or ice cubes of juice in the refrigerator. These are particularly enjoyed by children on hot days.

Is butter better for children than margarine?

Butter is naturally an excellent source of vitamin A, which is necessary in human nutrition. Margarine does not naturally contain either this vitamin or a precursor of the vitamin, but most margarines today are fortified with

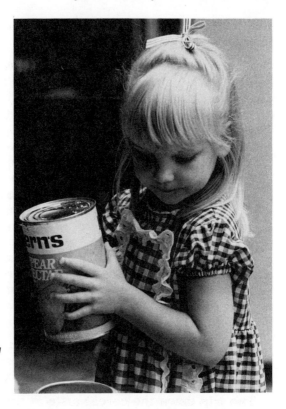

Chilled fruit juice is a refreshing and nourishing beverage which even young children enjoy preparing.

vitamin A at the level of 35,000 International Units (I.U.) per pound of margarine. This level of the vitamin corresponds approximately to the vitamin A level in butter, and is as available to the body as the vitamin A in butter. Hence fortified margarine and butter are comparable in their vitamin A content.

There is a difference in the fatty-acid composition of margarine and butter. Butter has a higher proportion of the more highly saturated fatty acids, as evidenced by its firmness when removed from the refrigerator; margarine is somewhat more plastic or spreadable when it comes from the refrigerator because it has a high percentage of the polyunsaturated fatty acids. The question of the value to children of the more fluid polyunsaturated fatty acids in the diet—that is, the vegetable oils versus the animal fats—has not been definitely resolved as of this writing. At this point it seems reasonable to say that either margarine or butter may be eaten by most children.

Will children be poorly nourished if they eat white bread instead of whole-wheat bread?

Frequently one hears that white bread is almost totally lacking in vitamins and consequently has no place in the diet. At one time this criticism was justified because milling of the wheat into white flour removed almost all of the B vitamins. Products made from this white flour were, as a result, a poor source of the B vitamins.

Vitamins lost during the milling process are now added to enriched white flour according to the standards specified by the federal enrichment program. The addition of thiamin, riboflavin, niacin, and iron to the flour at the mill makes it nutritionally practical to serve enriched white bread when desired. If people prefer white bread to whole-wheat products, there is now little reason why they need to be denied their preference. The only precaution is to read the label to be sure that the white bread was made with enriched flour.

How can I hope to make an intelligent selection from the potpourri of ready-to-eat cereals presently available, or is is necessary to serve only cooked cereal products?

The trip down the cereal aisle at the supermarket today can be a very time-consuming process, especially when children are along. Surely in no other food category has so much television advertising been used to extol a mixture of nutritional virtues and give-away prizes.

An examination of labels reveals that many of the cereal products available now are enriched according to the federal enrichment program. Again, as with the enrichment of white bread and flour, such enrichment will always be stated on the package.

It is necessary not only to determine that a cereal is enriched, but also to ascertain what quantities of the nutrients are present in a bowl-sized serving. Close scrutiny frequently will reveal that a considerable volume of cereal must be eaten to obtain reasonable amounts of the B vitamins, which are the prime reason for eating the cereal products. The increased volume, of course, is due to the processing techniques, such as puffing, that are employed in the manufacture of the cereals. The swelling that occurs during the production of some cereals may present space limitations for a child with a small stomach capacity.

It is easy to be critical of their bulkiness, but it is also necessary to appreciate that the wide variety of cereal products frequently provides considerable breakfast appeal to the various family members, and these cereals are often quite a boon to appetites at breakfast.

Decisions in the cereal aisle are not governed entirely by vitamin enrichment and prizes. There has also been an increasing interest in the protein content of cereal, an interest that has led to the development and production of some very satisfactory high-protein cereals. These cereals are of greater value for the person who has no other source of protein at breakfast time than to the individual who eats bacon and eggs. The extra protein in these cereals is unnecessary when eggs, milk, or meat are in the breakfast menu.

The need for protein at breakfast is emphasized by studies showing that protein is utilized more effectively by the body when it is available at several times during the day rather than in one meal. On this basis there might be some merit in selecting a cereal that is high in protein if cereal is the chief source of protein for breakfast.

The preceding remarks have been based strictly on the nutritional assessment of cereals, without regard for cost. A brief time in a grocery store is sufficient to remind one that it is also necessary to carefully consider price. Some of the sugar-coated and high-protein cereals are more expensive than the products that are only enriched. The sugar-coated cereals should be used only when the teeth will be brushed right away because the frequent presence of sugar in the mouth predisposes toward increased incidence of dental caries. Cereals containing freeze-dried fruits are generally well liked, but their cost is significantly higher than other cereals. The final decision must be made by the individual homemaker on the basis of the nutritional qualifications of the cereal and the condition of her pocketbook.

Is rice a nourishing food?

Rice has long been the staple cereal grain in Oriental countries, but it has only recently gained favor with

in several different forms. From a nutritional viewpoint, brown rice is a good source of the B vitamins, but some people object to its brown color, rough texture, and long cooking time. These characteristics of brown rice long ago led to the practice of polishing the rice grains. When the coarse bran layer is removed by polishing, the pleasing white endosperm of the cereal emerges and the B vitamins disappear (into the bran waste that is fed to the animals). This polished rice often is served even though it offers little nutritional value except the calories provided by the starch.

It is possible to buy two types of rice that are very similar in appearance to plain polished rice, yet considerably richer in thiamin, niacin, and iron. Enriched rice, available in some places in this country, has been coated with a premix of these nutrients. Riboflavin can also be added via the premix, but the slight yellow color it imparts may create resistance to product acceptance. Parboiled rice has been subjected first to a steam treatment under pressure to cause migration of the vitamins from the bran layers into the endosperm; second, the grain is polished to produce a rice with the desired white color and high nutritive value. This is an excellent product, but is more expensive than plain polished rice.

On the basis of nutritive value, it is necessary to recommend avoidance of polished rice and purchase of brown enriched polished, or parboiled polished rice. Wild rice, which is actually a wild grass, is a very nourishing food with an unfortunately high price tag.

Are there ways to retain vitamins during food preparation?

The vitamins most susceptible to destruction before consumption are ascorbic acid and the B vitamins. Since the B vitamins and ascorbic acid are water soluble, they have a tendency to leach out into cooking or soaking water rather than remaining in the food. To minimize the loss of vitamins into water that will be discarded, it is desirable to avoid soaking periods and to cook in as little water as possible. When only a small amount of water is used for cooking, there will be almost no water left and the food itself will contain most of the water-soluble vitamins at the end of the cooking period. This applies to rice, legumes, vegetables, and any other foods that are good sources of the water-soluble vitamins.

Ascorbic acid unfortunately is easily destroyed by oxidation. This means that foods that are good sources of ascorbic acid should be exposed to air as briefly as possible and that cut surfaces should be kept to a minimum. Since oxidation occurs gradually when this vitamin is exposed to air, it is advisable to slice ascorbic-acid-rich foods just before serving rather than leaving cut surfaces exposed to air for long periods of time. For instance, sliced oranges can be peeled somewhat ahead of the meal, but cut into slices immediately before they are served. With this technique, very little ascorbic acid will be lost through oxidation.

The addition of soda to the water used in cooking green vegetables or legumes is nutritionally wasteful. It is true that the alkaline cooking medium created with the addition of soda does cause the vegetable to become a bright green, but thiamin is readily destroyed by alkali. Sometimes soda is added to the water used to soak or simmer legumes, because soda shortens the long time required to soften the cellulose. Unfortunately, this practical advantage is outweighed by the increased destruction of thiamin.

It is wise always to cook foods the shortest possible time compatible with palatability if vitamin content of foods is to be maximized. Long cooking periods only decrease vitamin content; they do not increase vitamin values.

Are nutritional needs different in hot weather?

When children are playing hard in hot weather, the need for salt and liquids increases because of perspiration losses. Occasionally it may be necessary in hot climates for active children to eat a very small amount of salt in addition to that used regularly on their foods. This intake should be very carefully controlled, because salt regularly consumed in excess will result eventually in elevated blood pressure.

How can children be encouraged to eat breakfast?

The key to this problem usually lies with the mother. Informal surveys to determine whether or not children have had breakfast before going to school (and if not, why they have not had breakfast) frequently reveal that the mother has had little to do with getting the child ready for school.

Mothers can help by preparing breakfast rather than expecting the children to prepare it themselves.

Another important contribution mothers can make is to organize the family's morning so that there is time to eat breakfast before the family members scatter to school and jobs. Some families may be able to eat a formal breakfast together. In other families this arrangement is not practical because of varying schedules among the family members. Then it is more practical to serve an informal but nourishing breakfast at the convenience of the family members. Many breakfast items such as bacon, sausage, and hot breads may be prepared for the entire family when the first person has breakfast and these hot foods can then be held in the warming oven until the others are ready to eat. This arrangement makes a little more work, but it also means an increased likelihood of a good breakfast for everyone.

As children get older they are more likely to observe their mother's habits at meals, particularly at breakfast. Mothers who skip breakfast may find that their children in the elementary grades and high school begin to skip breakfast. Usually this situation can be corrected simply by having the mother eat breakfast with the children.

Breakfast is often poorly planned and hastily prepared in comparison with the other meals of the day. Mothers who are troubled about the amount of breakfast their children are eating would do well to examine their planning habits for breakfast and see whether changes might be appropriate. Some children seem to enjoy the routine of eating the same breakfast every morning; others may find breakfast more tempting if they have a variety of menus from day to day.

Sometimes breakfast appetites can be improved when adults manage to discard their preconceived notions about what is appropriate food for breakfast. There is no rule sacred to the human body that says only cereal, toast, bacon, and eggs may be consumed for breakfast. Sometimes adults are shocked that children may enjoy a wiener or perhaps even a taco for breakfast. There is no reason, from a nutritional standpoint, why these individual but unconventional preferences cannot be permitted at breakfast. Certainly a frankfurter is a useful food at this time of day because of its protein content. Any mother no doubt could add some amazing food requests to a list of foods not ordinarily considered on the breakfast menu.

The menu and the service of breakfast can well be tailored to the desires of the individual. The important thing is that breakfast be eaten and that it provide a reasonable proportion of the nutrients needed during the day. Breakfast ideally should supply between one-fourth and one-third of the day's recommended allowances, with particular attention being given to the inclusion of protein in the meal. By improving the morning organization of the family, by setting a good example, and by providing nutritious foods that appeal to the family members regardless of the preconceived prejudices of the adults, the consumption of breakfast in a home can usually become very satisfactory.

How can I "get" my child to eat vegetables?

Often the tone of voice or manner in which this question is asked gives a clue to the root of this problem. For some reason parents often feel apprehensive and overconcerned about vegetables even when they start to feed strained vegetables to their babies. This attitude is quickly communicated to the baby and the problem with vegetables is initiated. When parents continue to have a defensive, yet aggressive attitude about promoting vegetable consumption in their families, they may only intensify the problem.

It is not unusual to find that the parents who ask this question frequently do not like vegetables themselves. Here again, as is true with other foods, the key to vegetable acceptance is the attitude of the parents themselves. The foods that are accepted and enjoyed by the parents usually are popular also with the children.

Vegetable rejection by children will be helped if parents can learn to like the vegetables. Mothers profitably could seek to find attractive, appetizing ways to prepare and serve vegetables since vegetable palatability is greatly influenced by the quality of preparation. Poor preparation is the root of vegetable consumption problems in many instances. The author informally tested this theory with her own family. When Brussels sprouts, a favorite vegetable in her family, were overcooked until they were strong in flavor and poor in color, they soon were not consumed at all by her children and were just dutifully eaten by the adults. As soon as the sprouts were once again prepared in the preferred manner—that is, cooked as short a time as possible to retain the bright green color and to keep the flavor mild—the vegetable was again well received and enjoyed. This illustration can serve as a guide to mothers who are concerned with this problem.

One of the greatest problems with vegetable preparation is that they are so frequently overcooked. They do not need to be cooked until they beg for mercy, but rather should be boiled until they are just tender. A slight trace of crispness adds interest to the texture.

Overcooking becomes a particularly important factor in acceptance of vegetables when strong-flavored or green vegetables are being cooked. Cabbage-like flavors grow stronger with increased cooking. If such vegetables are cooked until they are just barely tender, the flavor and aroma will be far more pleasing than if they are boiled an extra fifteen minutes just to be sure that they are done. Strong odors in foods may be an important factor in their rejection by children.

Not only does the flavor change with prolonged cooking, but also the green chlorophyll changes color. This can easily be demonstrated in your own kitchen. When green vegetables are first boiled without a cover, they will be a beautiful green; but as cooking is extended longer and longer, the green slowly changes to a much less attractive, less appetizing olive-green color. Retention of an attractive color in green vegetables can be partially controlled by cooking these vegetables without a cover; use of a lid traps volatile, organic acids in the pan which hastens the breakdown of the green chlorophyll to a less desirable olive-green color.

Although boiling is probably the most common way of cooking vegetables, mothers would do well to explore a variety of ways to cook vegetables. Some vegetables are particularly pleasing when they are broiled or fried, and others are tempting when they are stewed or baked. The important thing is to approach vegetables in a creative mood. Strive for vegetable variety in menu planning, and follow through with careful preparation and attractive service of all vegetables. When such measures have been taken, they pay a double dividend: children will begin to consume vegetables with much more enthusiasm, and adults will also enjoy the benefits of these efforts.

Vegetables do not always need to be cooked. Strips and slices of raw vegetables make excellent finger foods for both children and adults. Flowerets of raw cauliflower are effective either in a salad or served with a cheese dip. One other suggestion that sometimes is of particular pleasure to preschool children is the use of frozen unthawed vegetables as a snack food. These cold vegetables have considerable appeal to the preschooler and they certainly are more nourishing than a piece of candy or a cracker. Vegetables do not need to be a "duty" food at the table; they can and should provide positive pleasure in a meal.

How much emphasis should be given to developing good table manners?

The primary purpose of a meal, the consumption of a nourishing diet, is most easily achieved in a happy family environment. On this basis it is highly desirable to maintain an accepting attitude so that children feel comfortable at the table. Constant nagging about table manners is more likely to result in problem eaters than in model children. On the other hand parents also need to be able to enjoy their meals and there certainly is less enjoyment for adults when children have untidy and extremely noisy eating habits. A balance can be achieved gradually between the needs of the very young and the adults.

One of the most effective means of improving the table manners of children is through adult example at the table. Since children are such excellent imitators, example can provide a firm basis for manners in much the same way that good speech habits in the family help a child to learn correct grammar. Example, however, will not make a perfect eater of a preschooler. Adults should adjust their expectations to the age of the child and then help him to master behavioral tasks appropriate to his abilities. An 18-month-old child who is doing well not to tip over his milk certainly cannot be expected to always chew with his mouth closed or even to always put food neatly into his mouth. The refinements of manners that are desired at the table must be expected to come gradually. Pleasant suggestions by the parents, patiently repeated from time to time, will be the most effective and rapid way of helping children to become more mannerly at the table.

How can teen-agers be helped to improve their nutrition?

This question is discussed in some depth in Chapter 10, but some salient points may be reiterated here to help parents better understand the problems that influence nutrition of adolescents. Some teen-agers have very full schedules that may conflict with the normal family mealtimes. When a mother appreciates these scheduling problems and is willing to help serve adequate meals even at times that may be inconvenient for her, she may find that the nutrition of her teen-ager is definitely better than when he is left to fend for himself in the kitchen. With today's ovens that can maintain low temperatures of 150 – 175°F, it is a very simple matter to serve all the dinner plates at one time and place the plates (loosely covered with aluminum foil) of absent family members in the oven at the low setting until late diners arrive.

Breakfast skipping is another problem with teen-agers, again often because of time limitations. Although it is true that teen-agers are old enough to prepare their own breakfasts, it is also true that many of them will not bother or take the time to prepare their own food. Mothers again can solve this problem by preparing breakfast for the children.

Despite the fact that elementary school children have had several exposures to information about nutrition, it is unfortunately true that these same children will often select a poor lunch at school when they become teen-agers. If parents were to actively seek a more effective school nutrition program, the junior and senior high schools could perhaps be encouraged to strengthen the curricula at both levels by increasing the emphasis on nutrition.

Both within the family and the school, nutrition can gain interest and acceptance among teen-agers if the relationship between appearance and nutrition is emphasized to this age group. Teen-agers are very much aware of themselves as individuals and are concerned with their own image, and nutrition certainly affects the image they present to the world. If teen-agers are aware that good nutrition helps to promote a healthy skin and a well-proportioned figure, they will view nutrition as an important part of life rather than as a subject to be ignored.

How can my preschooler be encouraged to eat more?

This concern, which many mothers share, becomes worrisome when a mother has an idea of what the "normal" preschooler eats. One characteristic of the young child is that his intake is a highly variable and individual matter. Some days the preschooler may eat very large amounts and on other days he may not be very hungry. This is a typical pattern and need not be of concern to mothers. The knowledgeable mother will base her concern for nutrition on the appearance and general health of her child rather than worrying about the total amount eaten in a particular day.

Feeding problems with preschoolers are frequently the result of overanxious mothers pushing food at their children rather than letting the children determine for themselves the amounts they feel they want to eat. The mother's role can best be described by saying that she should be sure that she provides well-prepared, well-balanced meals in a pleasant, happy setting to a well-rested, relaxed child.

Is it all right to serve skim milk to my children?

Skim milk is an excellent food for children at least 2 years old, and, in some cases, may actually be more desirable than whole milk. Skim milk has had the fat, along with the fat-soluble vitamins, removed from it. The vitamin A and vitamin D content of skim milk would be nil, but fortified skim milk is often available and one quart of this fortified milk contains the 400 International Units of vitamin D needed daily by a child. Vitamin A will need to be supplied from other dietary sources when skim milk is used regularly. The protein content of the two milks is comparable, although skim milk actually has a little more protein than whole milk. The other vitamins, since they are water soluble, are not removed when the milk is separated.

When children tend to be overweight, the use of skim milk, in preference to whole milk, is often recommended because skim milk that is fortified with vitamin D provides all the nutrients contained in whole milk (except vitamin A) and contributes only approximately half the calories. If a child tends to be a bit thin, however, whole milk definitely is preferable because of its greater caloric content for an equal volume.

Are health foods such as wheat germ necessary for children?

When foods have been carefully prepared and the meals planned to include a well-balanced diet, there is absolutely no need to purchase various products classified as "health foods." Whole-grain cereals or enriched cereal products supply the B vitamins in adequate amounts; high-quality, complete proteins can be obtained readily from milk, meats, poultry, and fish; and additional minerals and vitamins are readily available in the wide variety of fruits and vegetables in grocery stores. Certainly it is apparent that no problem needs to exist in supplying the body's needs through foods that are readily available in the grocery store. Health foods simply add an unnecessary expense. The money could be used far more effectively in the grocery store where prices are competitive, rather than in the health food store where excessive charges frequently are made for inferior or equivalent products.

Is it possible to help children learn to like a food?

Everyone, whether adult or child, has some foods that he likes better than others. Such preferences are natural, but it is important that children learn to eat a wide variety of foods. Acceptance of many different foods increases the likelihood of being well nourished. The ability to appreciate new foods becomes still more valuable when children begin to eat away from home socially or at school.

One of the important keys to accepting new foods is cultivation of a positive, curious attitude. This example, when set by parents, will usually be followed by children.

If a child is regularly exposed to new foods as a preschooler, he will be accustomed to experiencing new odors, tastes, and textures and will not be hesitant to approach something new. It is helpful if new recipes are tried frequently at home. Experience is also broadened by eating in restaurants and in friends' homes.

When a new food is served, everyone should be expected to try it. Even if a child does not particularly like the new food, he can taste it. Many times children will gradually learn to like a food as they become more accustomed to it. The new food does not need to be served regularly, but it should be served occasionally to increase familiarity and gradually increase its acceptance. Do not be discouraged if a new food is not accepted immediately. Sometimes acceptance of a new food requires considerable perseverance. Keep in mind that children will adapt to new meal situations much more readily if they have learned to accept and enjoy a wide variety of foods.

Is is all right for children to go on food "jags"?

Whenever a child narrows his food intake to just one or two foods, he will not be receiving all the nutrients his body needs. Children will go through periods when they want some particular food. It is fun for a child to have a part in planning meals, and his wish for a particular food may be included in a meal. He should understand, however, that others in the family also have special likes and these desires also need to be considered in planning meals. This approach gives a child some status in the family and yet encourages him to think of other foods that would be good in a meal, thus helping to expand his intake from just one food to several in the meal.

SUMMARY

The development of healthy attitudes toward food is an important responsibility of parents. Parental example is an important way of helping to develop dietary patterns that will form the basis for a lifetime of good nutrition. To be effective in this role, parents need to review their own food preferences and practices as well as to review their children's patterns and attitudes. The important point is to establish appropriate dietary practices early in life without placing undue pressures on children. If parents are successful in achieving good dietary practices for themselves, they will have made a major step toward helping their children be well nourished. Rational, moderate approaches to child nutrition are well suited to developing practical patterns that will suit children well throughout their childhood and adult years. Several common concerns in achieving adequate nutrition for children have been discussed and practical suggestions have been offered.

Appendix

Table A.1 *Weight and Length of Boys from Birth to 2 Years*

Age	Measurement		Percentile						
			3	10	25	50	75	90	97
Birth	Weight	pounds	5.8	6.3	6.9	7.5	8.3	9.1	10.1
		kilograms	2.63	2.86	3.13	3.4	3.76	4.13	4.58
	Length	inches	18.2	18.9	19.4	19.9	20.5	21.0	21.5
		centimeters	46.3	48.1	49.3	50.6	52.0	53.3	54.6
3 months	Weight	pounds	10.6	11.1	11.8	12.6	13.6	14.5	16.4
		kilograms	4.81	5.03	5.35	5.72	6.17	6.58	7.44
	Length	inches	22.4	22.8	23.3	23.8	24.3	24.7	25.1
		centimeters	56.8	57.8	59.3	60.4	61.8	62.8	63.7
6 months	Weight	pounds	14.0	14.8	15.6	16.7	18.0	19.2	20.8
		kilograms	6.35	6.71	7.08	7.58	8.16	8.71	9.43
	Length	inches	24.8	25.2	25.7	26.1	26.7	27.3	27.7
		centimeters	63.0	63.9	65.2	66.4	67.8	69.3	70.4
9 months	Weight	pounds	16.6	17.8	18.7	20.0	21.5	22.9	24.4
		kilograms	7.53	8.07	8.48	9.07	9.75	10.39	11.07
	Length	inches	26.6	27.0	27.5	28.0	28.7	29.2	29.9
		centimeters	67.7	68.6	69.8	71.2	72.9	74.2	75.9
12 months	Weight	pounds	18.5	19.6	20.9	22.2	23.8	25.4	27.3
		kilograms	8.39	8.89	9.48	10.07	10.8	11.52	12.38
	Length	inches	28.1	28.5	29.0	29.6	30.3	30.7	31.6
		centimeters	71.3	72.4	73.7	75.2	76.9	78.1	80.3
15 months	Weight	pounds	19.8	21.0	22.4	23.7	25.4	27.2	29.4
		kilograms	8.98	9.53	10.16	10.75	11.52	12.34	13.33
	Length	inches	29.3	29.8	30.3	30.9	31.6	32.1	33.1
		centimeters	74.4	75.6	77.0	78.5	80.3	81.5	84.2
18 months	Weight	pounds	21.1	22.3	23.8	25.2	26.9	29.0	31.5
		kilograms	9.57	10.12	10.8	11.43	12.2	13.15	14.29
	Length	inches	30.5	31.0	31.6	32.2	32.9	33.5	34.7
		centimeters	77.5	78.8	80.3	81.8	83.7	85.0	88.2
2 years	Weight	pounds	23.3	24.7	26.3	27.7	29.7	31.9	34.9
		kilograms	10.57	11.2	11.93	12.56	13.47	14.47	15.83
	Length	inches	32.6	33.1	33.8	34.4	35.2	35.9	37.2
		centimeters	82.7	84.2	85.8	87.5	89.4	91.1	94.6

Source: H. C. Stuart, in Nelson, *Textbook of Pediatrics*, 8th ed., Saunders, Philadelphia, 1964.

Table A.2   *Weight and Height of Boys from 2 to 5 Years*

Age	Measurement		Percentile						
			3	10	25	50	75	90	97
2 years	Weight	pounds	23.3	24.7	26.3	27.7	29.7	31.9	34.9
		kilograms	10.57	11.2	11.93	12.56	13.47	14.47	15.83
	Height	inches	32.6	33.1	33.8	34.4	35.2	35.9	37.2
		centimeters	82.7	84.2	85.8	87.5	89.4	91.1	94.6
2½ years	Weight	pounds	25.2	26.6	28.4	30.0	32.2	34.5	37.0
		kilograms	11.43	12.07	12.88	13.61	14.61	15.65	16.78
	Height	inches	34.2	34.8	35.5	36.3	37.0	37.9	39.2
		centimeters	86.9	88.5	90.2	92.1	94.1	96.2	99.5
3 years	Weight	pounds	27.0	28.7	30.3	32.2	34.5	36.8	39.2
		kilograms	12.25	13.02	13.74	14.61	15.65	16.69	17.78
	Height	inches	35.7	36.3	37.0	37.9	38.8	39.6	40.5
		centimeters	90.6	92.3	93.9	96.2	98.5	100.5	102.8
3½ years	Weight	pounds	28.5	30.4	32.3	34.3	36.7	39.1	41.5
		kilograms	12.93	13.79	14.65	15.56	16.65	17.74	18.82
	Height	inches	37.1	37.8	38.4	39.3	40.3	41.1	41.9
		centimeters	94.3	96.0	97.5	99.8	102.5	104.5	106.5
4 years	Weight	pounds	30.1	32.1	34.0	36.4	39.0	41.4	44.3
		kilograms	13.65	14.56	15.42	16.51	17.69	18.78	20.09
	Height	inches	38.4	39.1	39.7	40.7	41.9	42.7	43.5
		centimeters	97.5	99.3	100.8	103.4	106.5	108.5	110.4
4½ years	Weight	pounds	31.6	33.8	35.7	38.4	41.4	43.9	47.4
		kilograms	14.33	15.33	16.19	17.42	18.78	19.91	21.5
	Height	inches	39.6	40.3	40.9	42.0	43.3	44.2	45.0
		centimeters	100.6	102.4	104.0	106.7	109.9	112.3	114.3
5 years	Weight	pounds	33.6	35.5	37.5	40.5	44.1	46.7	50.4
		kilograms	15.24	16.1	17.01	18.37	20.0	21.18	22.86
	Height	inches	40.2	40.8	41.7	42.8	44.2	45.2	46.1
		centimeters	102.0	103.7	105.9	108.7	112.3	114.7	117.1

Source: H. C. Stuart, in Nelson, *Textbook of Pediatrics*, 8th ed., Saunders, Philadelphia, 1964.

Table A.3   *Weight and Height of Boys from 5 to 18 Years*

Age	Measurement		Percentile						
			3	10	25	50	75	90	97
5 years[a]	Weight	pounds	34.5	36.6	39.6	42.8	46.5	49.7	53.2
		kilograms	15.65	16.6	17.96	19.41	21.09	22.54	24.13
	Height	inches	40.2	41.5	42.6	43.8	45.0	45.9	47.0
		centimeters	102.1	105.3	108.3	111.3	114.2	116.7	119.5
6 years	Weight	pounds	38.5	40.9	44.4	48.3	52.1	56.4	61.1
		kilograms	17.46	18.55	20.14	21.91	23.63	25.58	27.71
	Height	inches	42.7	43.8	44.9	46.3	47.6	48.6	49.7
		centimeters	108.5	111.2	114.1	117.5	120.8	123.5	126.2
7 years	Weight	pounds	43.0	45.8	49.7	54.1	58.7	64.4	69.9
		kilograms	19.5	20.77	22.54	24.54	26.63	29.21	31.71
	Height	inches	44.9	46.0	47.4	48.9	50.2	51.4	52.5
		centimeters	114.0	116.9	120.3	124.1	127.6	130.5	133.4
8 years	Weight	pounds	48.0	51.2	55.5	60.1	65.5	73.0	79.4
		kilograms	21.77	23.22	25.17	27.26	29.71	33.11	36.02
	Height	inches	47.1	48.5	49.8	51.2	52.8	54.0	55.2
		centimeters	119.6	123.1	126.6	130.0	134.2	137.3	140.2
9 years	Weight	pounds	52.5	56.3	61.1	66.0	72.3	81.0	89.8
		kilograms	23.81	25.54	27.71	29.94	32.8	36.74	40.73
	Height	inches	48.9	50.5	51.8	53.3	55.0	56.1	57.2
		centimeters	124.2	128.3	131.6	135.5	139.8	142.6	145.3
10 years	Weight	pounds	56.8	61.1	66.3	71.9	79.6	89.9	100.0
		kilograms	25.76	27.71	30.07	32.61	36.11	40.78	45.36
	Height	inches	50.7	52.3	53.7	55.2	56.8	58.1	59.2
		centimeters	128.7	132.8	136.3	140.3	144.4	147.5	150.3
11 years	Weight	pounds	61.8	66.3	71.6	77.6	87.2	99.3	111.7
		kilograms	28.03	30.07	32.48	35.2	39.55	45.04	50.67
	Height	inches	52.5	54.0	55.3	56.8	58.7	59.8	60.8
		centimeters	133.4	137.3	140.5	144.2	149.2	151.8	154.4
12 years	Weight	pounds	67.2	72.0	77.5	84.4	96.0	109.6	124.2
		kilograms	30.48	32.66	35.15	38.28	43.55	49.71	56.34
	Height	inches	54.4	56.1	57.2	58.9	60.4	62.2	63.7
		centimeters	138.1	142.4	145.2	149.6	153.5	157.9	161.9

Table A.3 *(Continued)*

Age	Measurement		Percentile						
			3	10	25	50	75	90	97
13 years	Weight	pounds	72.0	77.1	83.7	93.0	107.9	123.2	138.0
		kilograms	32.66	34.97	37.97	42.18	48.94	55.88	62.6
	Height	inches	56.0	57.7	58.9	61.0	63.3	65.1	66.7
		centimeters	142.2	146.6	149.7	155.0	160.8	165.3	169.5
14 years	Weight	pounds	79.8	87.2	95.5	107.6	123.1	136.9	150.6
		kilograms	36.2	39.55	43.32	48.81	55.84	62.1	68.31
	Height	inches	57.6	59.9	61.6	64.0	66.3	67.9	69.7
		centimeters	146.4	152.1	156.5	162.7	168.4	172.4	177.1
15 years	Weight	pounds	91.3	99.4	108.2	120.1	135.0	147.8	161.6
		kilograms	41.41	45.09	49.08	54.48	61.23	67.04	73.3
	Height	inches	59.7	62.1	63.9	66.1	68.1	69.6	71.6
		centimeters	151.7	157.8	162.3	167.8	173.0	176.7	181.8
16 years	Weight	pounds	103.4	111.0	118.7	129.7	144.4	157.3	170.5
		kilograms	46.9	50.35	53.84	58.83	65.5	71.35	77.34
	Height	inches	61.6	64.1	65.8	67.8	69.5	70.7	73.1
		centimeters	156.5	162.8	167.1	171.6	176.6	179.7	185.6
17 years	Weight	pounds	110.5	117.5	124.5	136.2	151.4	164.6	175.6
		kilograms	50.12	53.3	56.47	61.78	68.67	74.66	79.65
	Height	inches	62.6	65.2	66.8	68.4	70.1	71.5	73.5
		centimeters	159.0	165.5	169.7	173.7	178.1	181.6	186.6
18 years	Weight	pounds	113.0	120.0	127.1	139.0	155.7	169.0	179.0
		kilograms	51.26	54.43	57.65	63.05	70.62	76.66	81.19
	Height	inches	62.8	65.5	67.0	68.7	70.4	71.8	73.9
		centimeters	159.6	166.3	170.5	174.5	178.9	182.4	187.6

[a]Several measurements at 5 years differ slightly from their counterparts in Table A.2 because they were obtained from a different population of children.
Source: The data in this table are from studies by and are reproduced by courtesy of Howard V. Meredith, Ph.D., Professor of Child Somatology, Institute of Child Behavior and Development, University of Iowa.

Table A.4 *Weight and Length of Girls from Birth to 2 Years*

Age	Measurement		3	10	25	50	75	90	97
						Percentile			
Birth	Weight	pounds	5.8	6.2	6.9	7.4	8.1	8.6	9.4
		kilograms	2.63	2.81	3.13	3.36	3.67	3.9	4.26
	Length	inches	18.5	18.8	19.3	19.8	20.1	20.4	21.1
		centimeters	47.1	47.8	49.0	50.2	51.0	51.9	53.6
3 months	Weight	pounds	9.8	10.7	11.4	12.4	13.2	14.0	14.9
		kilograms	4.45	4.85	5.17	5.62	5.99	6.35	6.76
	Length	inches	22.0	22.4	22.8	23.4	23.9	24.3	24.8
		centimeters	55.8	56.9	57.9	59.5	60.7	61.7	63.1
6 months	Weight	pounds	12.7	14.1	15.0	16.0	17.5	18.6	20.0
		kilograms	5.76	6.4	6.8	7.26	7.94	8.44	9.07
	Length	inches	24.0	24.6	25.1	25.7	26.2	26.7	27.1
		centimeters	61.1	62.5	63.7	65.2	66.6	67.8	68.8
9 months	Weight	pounds	15.1	16.6	17.8	19.2	20.8	22.4	24.2
		kilograms	6.85	7.53	8.03	8.71	9.43	10.16	10.98
	Length	inches	25.7	26.4	26.9	27.6	28.2	28.7	29.2
		centimeters	65.4	67.0	68.4	70.1	71.7	72.9	74.1
12 months	Weight	pounds	16.8	18.4	19.8	21.5	23.0	24.8	27.1
		kilograms	7.62	8.35	8.98	9.75	10.43	11.25	12.29
	Length	inches	27.1	27.8	28.5	29.2	29.9	30.3	31.0
		centimeters	68.9	70.6	72.3	74.2	75.9	77.1	78.8
15 months	Weight	pounds	18.1	19.8	21.3	23.0	24.6	26.6	29.0
		kilograms	8.21	8.98	9.66	10.43	11.16	12.07	13.15
	Length	inches	28.3	29.0	29.8	30.5	31.3	31.8	32.6
		centimeters	71.9	73.7	75.6	77.6	79.4	80.8	82.8
18 months	Weight	pounds	19.4	21.2	22.7	24.5	26.2	28.3	30.9
		kilograms	8.8	9.62	10.3	11.11	11.88	12.84	14.02
	Length	inches	29.5	30.2	31.1	31.8	32.6	33.3	34.1
		centimeters	74.9	76.8	79.0	80.9	82.9	84.5	86.7
2 years	Weight	pounds	21.6	23.5	25.3	27.1	29.2	31.7	34.4
		kilograms	9.8	10.66	11.48	12.29	13.25	14.38	15.6
	Length	inches	31.5	32.3	33.3	34.1	35.0	35.8	36.7
		centimeters	80.1	82.0	84.7	86.6	88.9	91.0	93.3

Source: H. C. Stuart, in Nelson, *Textbook of Pediatrics*, 8th ed., Saunders, Philadelphia, 1964.

Table A.5   *Weight and Height of Girls from 2 to 5 Years*

Age	Measurement		Percentile						
			3	10	25	50	75	90	97
2 years	Weight { pounds		21.6	23.5	25.3	27.1	29.2	31.7	34.4
	kilograms		9.8	10.66	11.48	12.29	13.25	14.38	15.6
	Height { inches		31.5	32.3	33.3	34.1	35.0	35.8	36.7
	centimeters		80.1	82.0	84.7	86.6	88.9	91.0	93.3
2½ years	Weight { pounds		23.6	25.5	27.4	29.6	31.9	34.6	38.2
	kilograms		10.7	11.57	12.43	13.43	14.47	15.69	17.33
	Height { inches		33.3	34.0	35.2	36.0	36.9	37.9	38.9
	centimeters		84.5	86.3	89.3	91.4	93.8	96.4	98.7
3 years	Weight { pounds		25.6	27.6	29.6	31.8	34.6	37.4	41.8
	kilograms		11.61	12.52	13.43	14.42	15.69	16.96	18.96
	Height { inches		34.8	35.6	36.8	37.7	38.6	39.8	40.7
	centimeters		88.4	90.5	93.4	95.7	98.1	101.1	103.5
3½ years	Weight { pounds		27.5	29.5	31.5	33.9	37.0	40.4	45.3
	kilograms		12.47	13.38	14.29	15.38	16.78	18.33	20.55
	Height { inches		36.2	37.1	38.1	39.2	40.2	41.5	42.5
	centimeters		92.0	94.2	96.9	99.5	102.0	105.4	108.0
4 years	Weight { pounds		29.2	31.2	33.5	36.2	39.6	43.5	48.2
	kilograms		13.25	14.15	15.2	16.42	17.96	19.73	21.86
	Height { inches		37.5	38.4	39.5	40.6	41.6	43.1	44.2
	centimeters		95.2	97.6	100.3	103.2	105.8	109.6	112.3
4½ years	Weight { pounds		30.7	32.9	35.3	38.5	42.1	46.7	50.9
	kilograms		13.93	14.92	16.01	17.46	19.1	21.18	23.09
	Height { inches		38.6	39.7	40.8	42.0	43.0	44.7	45.7
	centimeters		98.1	100.9	103.6	106.8	109.3	113.5	116.2
5 years	Weight { pounds		32.1	34.8	37.4	40.5	44.8	49.2	52.8
	kilograms		14.56	15.79	16.96	18.37	20.32	22.32	23.95
	Height { inches		39.4	40.5	41.6	42.9	44.0	45.4	46.8
	centimeters		100.0	103.0	105.7	109.1	111.7	115.4	118.8

Source: H. C. Stuart, in Nelson, *Textbook of Pediatrics*, 8th ed., Saunders, Philadelphia, 1964.

Table A.6 *Weight and Height of Girls from 5 to 18 Years*

Age	Measurement		Percentile						
			3	10	25	50	75	90	97
5 years[a]	Weight	pounds	33.7	36.1	38.6	41.4	44.2	48.2	51.8
		kilograms	15.29	16.37	17.51	18.78	20.05	21.86	23.5
	Height	inches	40.4	41.3	42.2	43.2	44.4	45.4	46.5
		centimeters	102.6	105.0	107.2	109.7	112.9	115.4	118.0
6 years	Weight	pounds	37.2	39.6	42.9	46.5	50.2	54.2	58.7
		kilograms	16.87	17.96	19.46	21.09	22.77	24.58	26.63
	Height	inches	42.5	43.5	44.6	45.6	47.0	48.1	49.4
		centimeters	108.0	110.6	113.2	115.9	119.3	122.3	125.4
7 years	Weight	pounds	41.3	44.5	48.1	52.2	56.3	61.2	67.3
		kilograms	18.73	20.19	21.82	23.68	25.54	27.76	30.53
	Height	inches	44.9	46.0	46.9	48.1	49.6	50.7	51.9
		centimeters	114.0	116.8	119.2	122.3	125.9	128.9	131.7
8 years	Weight	pounds	45.3	48.6	53.1	58.1	63.3	69.9	78.9
		kilograms	20.55	22.04	24.09	26.35	28.71	31.71	35.79
	Height	inches	46.9	48.1	49.1	50.4	51.8	53.0	54.1
		centimeters	119.1	122.1	124.8	128.0	131.6	134.6	137.4
9 years	Weight	pounds	49.1	52.6	57.9	63.8	70.5	79.1	89.9
		kilograms	22.27	23.86	26.26	28.94	31.98	35.88	40.78
	Height	inches	48.7	50.0	51.1	52.3	54.0	55.3	56.5
		centimeters	123.6	127.0	129.7	132.9	137.1	140.4	143.4
10 years	Weight	pounds	53.2	57.1	62.8	70.3	79.1	89.7	101.9
		kilograms	24.13	25.9	28.49	31.89	35.88	40.69	46.22
	Height	inches	50.3	51.8	53.0	54.6	56.1	57.5	58.8
		centimeters	127.7	131.7	134.6	138.6	142.6	146.0	149.3
11 years	Weight	pounds	57.9	62.6	69.9	78.8	89.1	100.4	112.9
		kilograms	26.26	28.4	31.71	35.74	40.42	45.54	51.21
	Height	inches	52.1	53.9	55.2	57.0	58.7	60.4	62.0
		centimeters	132.3	137.0	140.3	144.7	149.2	153.4	157.4
12 years	Weight	pounds	63.6	69.5	78.0	87.6	98.8	111.5	127.7
		kilograms	28.85	31.52	35.38	39.74	44.82	50.58	57.92
	Height	inches	54.3	56.1	57.4	59.8	61.6	63.2	64.8
		centimeters	137.8	142.6	145.9	151.9	156.6	160.6	164.6

Table A.6   *(Continued)*

Age	Measurement		Percentile						
			3	10	25	50	75	90	97
13 years	Weight	pounds	72.2	79.9	89.4	99.1	111.0	124.5	142.3
		kilograms	32.75	36.24	40.55	44.95	50.35	56.47	64.55
	Height	inches	56.6	58.7	60.1	61.8	63.6	64.9	66.3
		centimeters	143.7	149.1	152.6	157.1	161.5	164.8	168.4
14 years	Weight	pounds	83.1	91.0	99.8	108.4	119.7	133.3	150.8
		kilograms	37.69	41.28	45.27	49.17	54.29	60.46	68.4
	Height	inches	58.3	60.2	61.5	62.8	64.4	65.7	67.2
		centimeters	148.2	153.0	156.1	159.6	163.7	167.0	170.7
15 years	Weight	pounds	89.0	97.4	105.1	113.5	123.9	138.1	155.2
		kilograms	40.37	44.18	47.67	51.48	56.2	62.64	70.4
	Height	inches	59.1	61.1	62.1	63.4	64.9	66.2	67.6
		centimeters	150.2	155.2	157.7	161.1	164.9	168.1	171.6
16 years	Weight	pounds	91.8	100.9	108.4	117.0	127.2	141.1	157.7
		kilograms	41.64	45.77	49.17	53.07	57.7	64.0	71.53
	Height	inches	59.4	61.5	62.4	63.9	65.2	66.5	67.7
		centimeters	150.8	156.1	158.6	162.2	165.7	169.0	172.0
17 years	Weight	pounds	93.9	102.8	110.4	119.1	129.6	143.3	159.5
		kilograms	42.59	46.63	50.08	54.02	58.79	65.0	72.35
	Height	inches	59.4	61.5	62.6	64.0	65.4	66.7	67.8
		centimeters	151.0	156.3	159.0	162.5	166.1	169.4	172.2
18 years	Weight	pounds	94.5	103.5	111.2	119.9	130.8	144.5	160.7
		kilograms	42.87	46.95	50.44	54.39	59.33	65.54	72.89
	Height	inches	59.4	61.5	62.6	64.0	65.4	66.7	67.8
		centimeters	151.0	156.3	159.0	162.5	166.1	169.4	172.2

[a]Several measurements at 5 years differ slightly from their counterparts in Table A.5 because they were obtained from a different population of children.

Source: The data in this table are from studies by and are reproduced by courtesy of Howard V. Meredith, Ph.D., Professor of Child Somatology, Institute of Child Behavior and Development, University of Iowa.

Tables A.7–A.25 reproduced by permission of Gerber Products Co.

Table A.7 INFANT FORMULA
Average Nutrient Values per 100 Grams and of Amounts Commonly Purchased or Used

PRODUCT	MEASURE*	WEIGHT gm.	oz.	CALORIES	PROTEIN gm.	FAT gm.	CARBOHYDRATE gm.	ASH gm.	TOTAL SOLIDS gm.	CALCIUM mg.	PHOSPHORUS mg.	IRON mg.	COPPER mg.	SODIUM mg.	POTASSIUM mg.	CHLORIDE mg.	MAGNESIUM mg.
MBF™ (Meat Base Formula) AS PURCHASED, CONCENTRATED	3.2 fl. oz.	100	3.5	137	6.8	7.8	9.9	1.5	26.0	240	160	3.70	0.14	43	91	61	10
	1 fl. oz. or 2 tbsp.	32	1.2	43	2.2	2.5	3.2	0.5	8.3	77	51	1.20	0.05	14	29	20	3
	13 fl. oz. or 1 can	407	14.4	558	27.7	31.8	40.3	6.0	105.8	975	650	15.00	0.57	175	370	248	41
SUGGESTED (1:1½) DILUTION	3.3 fl. oz.	100	3.5	58	2.9	3.3	4.2	0.6	10.9	101	67	1.50	0.06	18	38	26	4
	1 fl. oz. or 1 tbsp.	30	1.1	17	0.9	1.0	1.3	0.2	3.3	30	20	0.50	0.02	5	11	8	1
	32 fl. oz. or 1 qt.	970	34.2	558	27.7	31.8	40.3	6.0	105.8	975	650	15.00	0.57	175	370	248	41

PRODUCT continued	MEASURE*	WEIGHT gm.	oz.	SULFUR mg.	IODINE µg.	VITAMIN A I.U.	THIAMIN mg.	RIBOFLAVIN mg.	NIACIN mg.	VITAMIN B6 mg.	VITAMIN B12 µg.	FOLACIN µg.	PANTOTHENIC ACID mg.	ASCORBIC ACID mg.	VITAMIN D I.U.	VITAMIN E I.U.
MBF™ (Meat Base Formula) AS PURCHASED, CONCENTRATED	3.2 fl. oz.	100	3.5	40	7	369	0.12	0.32	2.46	0.17	1.8	5.4	0.7	12.3	98	1.2
	1 fl. oz. or 1 tbsp.	32	1.2	13	2	118	0.04	0.10	0.79	0.05	0.6	0.2	0.2	3.7	31	0.4
	13 fl. oz. or 1 can	407	14.4	163	29	1500	0.50	1.30	10.00	0.70	7.3	22.0	2.7	50.0	400	5.0
SUGGESTED (1:1½) DILUTION	3.3 fl. oz.	100	3.5	17	3	155	0.05	0.13	1.03	0.07	0.8	2.0	0.3	5.2	41	0.5
	1 fl. oz. or 1 tbsp.	30	1.1	5	1	47	0.02	0.04	0.31	0.02	0.2	0.6	0.1	1.6	12	0.2
	32 fl. oz. or 1 qt.	970	34.2	163	29	1500	0.50	1.30	10.00	0.70	7.3	22.0	2.7	50.0	400	5.0

AMINO ACID CONTENT PER 100 GRAMS AND PER QUART AS FED

PRODUCT	MEASURE*	WEIGHT gm.	oz.	TRYPTOPHAN mg.	THREONINE mg.	ISOLEUCINE mg.	LEUCINE mg.	LYSINE mg.	METHIONINE mg.	CYSTINE mg.	PHENYLALANINE mg.	TYROSINE mg.
MBF™ (Meat Base Formula)	3.3 fl. oz.	100	3.5	33.9	159.3	86.0	227.6	204.7	76.7	22.5	121.7	90.0
SUGGESTED (1:1½) DILUTION	32 fl. oz. or 1 qt.	970	34.2	328.8	1545.2	834.2	2207.7	1985.6	744.0	218.3	1180.5	873.0

PRODUCT continued	MEASURE*	WEIGHT gm.	oz.	VALINE mg.	ARGININE mg.	HISTIDINE mg.	ALANINE mg.	ASPARTIC ACID mg.	GLUTAMIC ACID mg.	GLYCINE mg.	PROLINE mg.	SERINE mg.
MBF™ (Meat Base Formula)	3.3 fl. oz.	100	3.5	135.9	70.6	90.0	175.2	288.1	558.9	142.9	205.2	138.6
SUGGESTED (1:1½) DILUTION	32 fl. oz. or 1 qt.	970	34.2	1318.2	684.8	873.0	1699.4	2794.6	5421.3	1386.1	1990.4	1344.4

ELECTROLYTE CONTENT PER 100 GRAMS AND PER QUART AS FED

PRODUCT	MEASURE*	WEIGHT gm.	oz.	SODIUM mEq.	POTASSIUM mEq.	CALCIUM mEq.	PHOSPHORUS mEq.	CHLORIDE mEq.	MAGNESIUM mEq.	SULFUR mEq.	TOTAL mEq.
MBF™ (Meat Base Formula)	3.3 fl. oz.	100	3.5	0.8	1.0	5.0	3.9	0.7	0.4	1.0	12.8
SUGGESTED (1:1½) DILUTION	32 fl. oz. or 1 qt.	970	34.2	7.6	9.5	48.6	37.7	7.0	3.4	10.0	123.8

*All measures level

tbsp. = tablespoon   oz. = ounce   gm. = gram   mEq. = milliequivalent   mg. = milligram   µg. = microgram   I.U. = International Unit

Table A.8 STRAINED JUICES
Average Nutrient Values per 100 Grams and per Can

PRODUCT	MEASURE*	WEIGHT gm.	WEIGHT oz.	CALORIES	PROTEIN gm.	FAT gm.	CARBO-HYDRATE gm.	ASH gm.	CRUDE FIBER gm.	TOTAL SOLIDS gm.	CALCIUM mg.	PHOSPHORUS mg.	IRON mg.	SODIUM mg.	POTASSIUM mg.	VITAMIN A I.U.	THIAMIN mg.	RIBOFLAVIN mg.	NIACIN mg.	VITAMIN B mg.	ASCORBIC ACID mg.
APPLE	3.2 fl. oz.	100	3.5	49	0.1	—	12.2	0.2	0.1	12.6	3	5	0.65	2	73	—	0.005	0.006	0.08	0.03	40.0
	1 can (4.2 fl. oz.)	131	4.6	65	0.2	0.1	15.9	0.3	0.1	16.6	4	7	0.85	3	96	—	0.007	0.008	0.10	0.04	52.4
APPLE-CHERRY	3.2 fl. oz.	100	3.5	45	0.2	0.1	10.9	0.4	—	11.6	4	6	0.95	2	79	—	0.007	0.012	0.09	0.03	40.0
	1 can (4.2 fl. oz.)	131	4.6	59	0.3	0.1	14.1	0.6	0.1	15.2	6	8	1.24	2	104	—	0.010	0.016	0.12	0.04	52.4
APPLE-GRAPE	3.2 fl. oz.	100	3.5	65	0.2	—	16.0	0.2	0.1	16.5	5	8	1.20	3	113	—	0.040	0.040	0.14	0.05	40.0
	1 can (4.2 fl. oz.)	131	4.6	85	0.3	—	21.0	0.3	0.1	21.6	7	10	1.57	4	148	—	0.052	0.052	0.18	0.07	52.4
MIXED FRUIT	3.2 fl. oz.	100	3.5	59	0.3	0.3	13.8	0.3	0.1	14.8	6	7	0.45	2	100	7	0.025	0.010	0.13	0.04	40.0
	1 can (4.2 fl. oz.)	131	4.6	77	0.3	0.3	18.2	0.4	0.1	19.3	8	9	0.59	3	131	9	0.033	0.013	0.17	0.05	52.4
ORANGE	3.2 fl. oz.	100	3.5	50	0.5	0.4	11.0	0.3	0.1	12.3	6	9	0.29	2	163	30	0.042	0.015	0.20	0.03	40.0
	1 can (4.2 fl. oz.)	131	4.6	65	0.7	0.5	14.4	0.4	0.1	16.1	8	12	0.38	3	213	39	0.055	0.020	0.26	0.04	52.4
ORANGE-APPLE	3.2 fl. oz.	100	3.5	54	0.3	0.4	12.3	0.3	0.1	13.4	6	9	0.45	2	130	23	0.030	0.010	0.14	0.06	40.0
	1 can (4.2 fl. oz.)	131	4.6	71	0.4	0.5	16.2	0.4	0.1	17.6	7	11	0.60	3	170	31	0.039	0.013	0.19	0.08	52.4
ORANGE-APPLE-BANANA	3.2 fl. oz.	100	3.5	65	0.5	0.2	15.2	0.3	0.1	16.3	8	16	0.86	3	160	—	0.024	0.020	0.19	0.08	40.0
	1 can (4.2 fl. oz.)	131	4.6	86	0.6	0.3	20.1	0.3	0.1	21.4	10	20	1.13	4	210	—	0.032	0.026	0.25	0.10	52.4
ORANGE-APRICOT	3.2 fl. oz.	100	3.5	61	0.6	0.2	14.2	0.4	0.1	15.5	8	12	0.45	2	207	150	0.054	0.024	0.18	0.05	40.0
	1 can (4.2 fl. oz.)	131	4.6	79	0.8	0.2	18.6	0.5	0.2	20.3	10	16	0.59	2	271	196	0.071	0.031	0.24	0.07	52.4
ORANGE-PINEAPPLE	3.2 fl. oz.	100	3.5	59	0.5	0.1	14.1	0.4	0.1	15.2	7	10	0.30	1	142	12	0.062	0.010	0.18	0.03	40.0
	1 can (4.2 fl. oz.)	131	4.6	78	0.7	0.2	18.4	0.5	0.2	20.0	9	13	0.39	2	186	15	0.081	0.014	0.23	0.04	52.4
PINEAPPLE-GRAPE-FRUIT JUICE DRINK	3.2 fl. oz.	100	3.5	58	0.3	0.1	13.9	0.2	0.1	14.6	7	4	0.38	2	68	2	0.023	0.007	0.09	0.03	40.0
	1 can (4.2 fl. oz.)	131	4.6	76	0.3	0.1	18.5	0.2	0.1	19.2	9	5	0.49	3	89	2	0.031	0.010	0.12	0.04	52.4
PRUNE-ORANGE	3.2 fl. oz.	100	3.5	75	0.5	0.2	17.9	0.4	0.1	19.1	10	16	0.51	4	164	17	0.045	0.012	0.32	0.06	40.0
	1 can (4.2 fl. oz.)	131	4.6	99	0.7	0.2	23.5	0.6	0.1	25.1	14	21	0.66	5	214	22	0.059	0.016	0.42	0.08	52.4
SUMMARY OF STRAINED JUICES	Average Values per Can			76	0.5	0.2	18.1	0.2	0.1	19.3	8	12	0.77	3	167	28	0.043	0.020	0.21	0.06	52.4
	% RDA (6-12 mo. infant)			8.4	2.2						1.3	2.4	5.1			1.9	8.6	3.3	2.6	15.0	149.7
	% RDA (1-2 year child)			6.9	2.0						1.1	1.7	5.1			1.4	7.2	3.3	2.6	12.0	131.0
	% Calories				2.6	2.4	95.1														

*All measures level   oz. = ounce   gm. = gram   mg. = milligram   I.U. = International Unit   —— = quantity insignificant

Table A.9   READY-TO-SERVE DRY CEREALS
Average Nutrient Values per 100 Grams and per Common Servings

PRODUCT	MEASURE*	WEIGHT gm.	WEIGHT oz.	CALORIES	PROTEIN gm.	FAT gm.	CARBOHYDRATE gm.	CRUDE FIBER gm.	ASH gm.	TOTAL SOLIDS gm.	CALCIUM mg.	PHOSPHORUS mg.	IRON mg.	SODIUM mg.	POTASSIUM mg.	THIAMIN mg.	RIBOFLAVIN mg.	NIACIN mg.	VITAMIN B_6 mg.
BARLEY CEREAL	2.6 cups	100	3.5	375	11.3	3.9	73.7	1.3	2.8	93.0	660	751	100.2	10	308	2.82	2.12	14.1	0.46
	6 tbsp.	14.2	0.5	54	1.6	0.6	10.5	0.2	0.4	13.2	94	107	14.2	1	44	0.40	0.30	2.0	0.07
	3 tbsp.	7.1	0.25	27	0.8	0.3	5.2	0.1	0.2	6.6	47	53	7.1	1	22	0.20	0.15	1.0	0.03
HIGH PROTEIN CEREAL	2.6 cups	100	3.5	372	35.0	6.2	44.0	2.3	5.5	93.0	660	751	100.2	10	1492	2.82	2.12	14.1	0.56
	6 tbsp.	14.2	0.5	53	5.0	0.9	6.2	0.3	0.8	13.2	94	107	14.2	1	212	0.40	0.30	2.0	0.08
	3 tbsp.	7.1	0.25	26	2.5	0.4	3.1	0.2	0.4	6.6	47	53	7.1	1	106	0.20	0.15	1.0	0.04
MIXED CEREAL	2.6 cups	100	3.5	379	11.7	4.5	73.0	1.1	2.7	93.0	660	698	100.2	10	281	2.82	2.12	14.1	0.24
	6 tbsp.	14.2	0.5	54	1.7	0.6	10.3	0.2	0.4	13.2	94	99	14.2	1	40	0.40	0.30	2.0	0.03
	3 tbsp.	7.1	0.25	27	0.8	0.3	5.2	0.1	0.2	6.6	47	50	7.1	1	20	0.20	0.15	1.0	0.02
MIXED CEREAL WITH BANANAS	2.6 cups	100	3.5	387	10.6	4.8	75.4	1.0	4.2	96.0	660	801	100.2	171	549	2.82	2.12	14.1	0.52
	6 tbsp.	14.2	0.5	55	1.5	0.7	10.7	0.1	0.6	13.6	94	114	14.2	24	78	0.40	0.30	2.0	0.07
	3 tbsp.	7.1	0.25	28	0.8	0.3	5.4	0.1	0.3	6.8	47	57	7.1	12	39	0.20	0.15	1.0	0.04
OATMEAL	2.6 cups	100	3.5	393	15.1	8.0	65.2	1.4	3.3	93.0	660	751	100.2	10	362	2.82	2.12	14.1	0.24
	6 tbsp.	14.2	0.5	56	2.1	1.1	9.3	0.2	0.5	13.2	94	105	14.2	1	51	0.40	0.30	2.0	0.03
	3 tbsp.	7.1	0.25	28	1.1	0.6	4.6	0.1	0.2	6.6	47	53	7.1	1	26	0.20	0.15	1.0	0.02
OATMEAL WITH BANANAS	2.6 cups	100	3.5	393	12.6	6.2	71.6	1.1	4.5	96.0	660	801	100.2	189	623	2.82	2.12	14.1	0.52
	6 tbsp.	14.2	0.5	56	1.8	0.9	10.2	0.2	0.6	13.6	94	114	14.2	27	88	0.40	0.30	2.0	0.07
	3 tbsp.	7.1	0.25	28	0.9	0.4	5.1	0.1	0.3	6.8	47	57	7.1	13	44	0.20	0.15	1.0	0.04
RICE CEREAL	2.6 cups	100	3.5	376	6.7	4.9	76.2	0.9	3.8	92.5	660	829	100.2	10	316	2.82	2.12	14.1	0.55
	6 tbsp.	14.2	0.5	54	1.0	0.7	10.8	0.1	0.5	13.1	94	118	14.2	1	45	0.40	0.30	2.0	0.08
	3 tbsp.	7.1	0.25	26	0.5	0.3	5.4	0.1	0.3	6.6	47	59	7.1	1	22	0.20	0.15	1.0	0.04
RICE CEREAL WITH STRAWBERRIES	2.6 cups	100	3.5	387	7.2	5.0	78.4	1.0	3.9	95.5	660	720	100.2	75	355	2.82	2.12	14.1	0.16
	6 tbsp.	14.2	0.5	55	1.0	0.7	11.1	0.1	0.6	13.6	94	102	14.2	11	50	0.40	0.30	2.0	0.02
	3 tbsp.	7.1	0.25	28	0.5	0.4	5.6	0.1	0.3	6.8	47	51	7.1	5	25	0.20	0.15	1.0	0.01
SUMMARY OF DRY CEREALS	Average Values per 0.5 oz.			55	2.0	0.8	9.9	0.2	0.6	13.3	94	108	14.2	8	76	0.40	0.30	2.0	0.06
	% RDA (6-12 mos. infant)			6.1	8.7	13.1					15.7	21.6	94.7			80.0	50.0	25.0	14.0
	% RDA (1-2 year child)			5.0	8.0						13.4	15.4	94.7			66.7	50.0	25.0	11.2
	% Calories				14.6	13.1	72.3												

*All measures level   tbsp. = tablespoon   oz. = ounce   gm. = gram   mg. = milligram

Table A 10 STRAINED FRUITS
Average Nutrient Values per 100 Grams and per Jar

PRODUCT	MEASURE*	WEIGHT gm.	WEIGHT oz.	CAL-ORIES	PRO-TEIN gm.	FAT gm.	CARBO-HY-DRATE gm.	CRUDE FIBER gm.	ASH gm.	TOTAL SOLIDS gm.	CAL-CIUM mg.	PHOS-PHORUS mg.	IRON mg.	SODIUM mg.	POTAS-SIUM mg.	VITA-MIN A I.U.	THIA-MIN mg.	RIBO-FLAVIN mg.	NIACIN mg.	VITA-MIN B₆ mg.	ASCOR-BIC ACID † mg.
APPLESAUCE	7 tbsp.	100	3.5	81	0.2	0.1	19.7	0.7	0.2	20.9	3	6	0.39	2	63	—	0.013	0.012	0.07	0.03	30.0
	1 jar	134	4.7	109	0.2	0.2	26.5	0.9	0.2	28.0	4	8	0.53	2	84	—	0.018	0.016	0.09	0.04	40.2
APPLESAUCE AND APRICOTS	7 tbsp.	100	3.5	87	0.3	0.1	21.2	0.7	0.3	22.6	4	7	0.32	2	84	245	0.012	0.011	0.16	0.03	13.1
	1 jar	134	4.7	116	0.4	0.2	28.2	1.0	0.4	30.2	6	10	0.43	2	113	328	0.017	0.015	0.21	0.04	17.5
APPLESAUCE WITH PINEAPPLE	7 tbsp.	100	3.5	79	0.2	0.2	19.1	0.6	0.2	20.3	4	6	0.31	1	74	14	0.031	0.009	0.08	0.04	13.1
	1 jar	134	4.7	106	0.3	0.3	25.6	0.8	0.2	27.2	5	8	0.41	2	99	19	0.042	0.013	0.11	0.05	17.5
APRICOTS WITH TAPIOCA	7 tbsp.	100	3.5	80	0.4	0.1	19.3	0.3	0.3	20.4	6	10	0.31	31	107	681	0.005	0.012	0.25	0.03	13.1
	1 jar	134	4.7	107	0.5	0.1	26.0	0.4	0.4	27.4	9	13	0.41	42	143	912	0.007	0.017	0.33	0.04	17.5
BANANAS WITH TAPIOCA	7 tbsp.	100	3.5	88	0.5	0.1	21.2	0.2	0.3	22.3	4	9	0.42	29	117	54	0.016	0.019	0.23	0.16	13.1
	1 jar	134	4.7	117	0.6	0.1	28.5	0.3	0.4	29.9	5	12	0.56	39	156	72	0.021	0.026	0.30	0.21	17.5
BANANAS WITH PINEAPPLE AND TAPIOCA	7 tbsp.	100	3.5	84	0.3	0.2	20.3	0.2	0.2	21.2	4	5	0.23	30	71	31	0.011	0.012	0.14	0.09	7.5
	1 jar	134	4.7	113	0.4	0.3	27.1	0.3	0.3	28.4	6	7	0.31	40	96	42	0.014	0.017	0.19	0.12	10.0
PEACHES	7 tbsp.	100	3.5	81	0.6	0.1	19.3	0.8	0.4	21.9	3	11	0.40	3	125	209	0.007	0.019	0.65	0.03	13.1
	1 jar	134	4.7	107	0.8	0.1	25.8	1.1	0.5	29.3	4	15	0.54	3	168	281	0.010	0.025	0.89	0.04	17.5
PEARS	7 tbsp.	100	3.5	69	0.4	0.1	16.6	1.5	0.2	18.8	8	9	0.28	2	87	—	0.011	0.015	0.20	0.02	13.1
	1 jar	134	4.7	92	0.5	0.1	22.3	2.0	0.3	25.2	11	12	0.38	3	117	—	0.014	0.021	0.27	0.03	17.5
PEARS AND PINEAPPLE	7 tbsp.	100	3.5	71	0.4	0.2	17.0	1.3	0.3	19.2	9	10	0.43	2	92	15	0.025	0.028	0.18	0.03	13.1
	1 jar	134	4.7	95	0.5	0.2	22.9	1.7	0.4	25.7	12	13	0.57	3	129	20	0.033	0.038	0.24	0.04	17.5
PLUMS WITH TAPIOCA	7 tbsp.	100	3.5	98	0.3	0.1	24.0	0.4	0.2	25.0	6	7	0.29	4	70	106	0.009	0.013	0.27	0.05	2.2
	1 jar	134	4.7	132	0.4	0.2	32.2	0.5	0.2	33.5	8	10	0.39	6	94	141	0.013	0.018	0.36	0.07	3.0
PRUNES WITH TAPIOCA	7 tbsp.	100	3.5	88	0.6	0.1	21.1	0.6	0.4	22.8	14	17	0.76	19	153	209	0.014	0.014	0.44	0.07	4.5
	1 jar	134	4.7	118	0.8	0.2	28.3	1.0	0.5	31.2	19	23	1.02	26	205	280	0.019	0.018	0.59	0.09	6.0
SUMMARY OF STRAINED FRUITS	Average Values per Jar			110	0.5	0.2	26.7	0.9	0.3	28.7	8	12	0.50	15	128	190	0.019	0.020	0.32	0.07	16.5
	% RDA (2-6 mos. infant)			14.3	2.5						1.6	3.0	5.0			12.7	4.7	4.0	4.6	23.3	47.1
	% RDA (6-12 mo. infant)			12.2	2.2						1.3	2.4	3.3			12.7	3.8	3.3	4.0	17.5	47.1
	% Calories				1.8	1.6	96.6														

*All measures level   tbsp. = tablespoon   oz. = ounce   gm. = gram   mg. = milligram   I.U. = International Unit   —— = quantity insignificant   † = quantity insignificant

Table A.11 *STRAINED CEREALS WITH FRUIT*
Average Nutrient Values per 100 Grams and per Jar

PRODUCT	MEASURE*	WEIGHT gm.	WEIGHT oz.	CAL-ORIES	PRO-TEIN gm.	FAT gm.	CARBO-HY-DRATE gm.	CRUDE FIBER gm.	ASH gm.	TOTAL SOLIDS gm.	CAL-CIUM mg.	PHOS-PHORUS mg.	IRON mg.	SODIUM mg.	POTAS-SIUM mg.	VITA-MIN A I.U.	THIA-MIN mg.	RIBO-FLAVIN mg.	NIACIN mg.	VITA-MIN B, mg.	ASCOR-BIC ACID mg.
HIGH PROTEIN CEREAL WITH APPLESAUCE AND BANANAS	7 tbsp.	100	3.5	93	4.6	0.5	17.6	0.3	0.8	23.8	30	83	7.46	121	181	—	0.187	0.448	2.99	0.19	20.0
	1 jar	134	4.7	125	6.2	0.7	23.5	0.4	1.1	31.9	40	111	10.00	162	243	—	0.250	0.600	4.00	0.25	26.8
MIXED CEREAL WITH APPLESAUCE AND BANANAS	7 tbsp.	100	3.5	83	1.2	0.7	17.9	0.3	0.3	20.4	4	55	3.73	100	25	2	0.187	0.448	2.99	0.19	4.3
	1 jar	134	4.7	111	1.6	0.9	24.0	0.4	0.5	27.4	5	74	5.00	134	33	2	0.250	0.600	4.00	0.25	5.8
OATMEAL WITH APPLESAUCE AND BANANAS	7 tbsp.	100	3.5	75	1.4	0.9	15.2	0.3	0.5	18.3	6	74	3.73	146	33	—	0.187	0.448	2.99	0.19	4.3
	1 jar	134	4.7	99	1.9	1.2	20.2	0.5	0.7	24.5	8	99	5.00	196	44	—	0.250	0.600	4.00	0.25	5.8
RICE CEREAL WITH APPLESAUCE AND BANANAS	7 tbsp.	100	3.5	69	0.3	0.6	15.7	0.2	0.3	17.1	8	12	0.18	122	10	2	0.187	0.448	2.99	0.19	20.0
	1 jar	134	4.7	93	0.5	0.8	21.0	0.3	0.4	23.0	11	16	0.24	163	13	2	0.250	0.600	4.00	0.25	26.8
SUMMARY OF STRAINED CEREALS WITH FRUIT	Average Values per Jar			107	2.6	0.9	22.2	0.4	0.7	26.7	16	75	5.06	164	83	1	0.250	0.600	4.00	0.25	16.3
	% RDA (2-6 mos. infant)			13.9	13.0						3.2	16.3	50.6			0.1	62.5	120.0	57.1	83.3	46.6
	% RDA (6-12 mo. infant)			11.9	11.3						2.7	15.0	33.7			0.1	50.0	100.0	50.0	62.5	46.6
	% Calories				9.7	7.5	82.9														

Table A.12 *STRAINED VEGETABLES*
Average Nutrient Values per 100 Grams and per Jar

PRODUCT	MEASURE*	WEIGHT gm.	WEIGHT oz.	CAL-ORIES	PRO-TEIN gm.	FAT gm.	CARBO-HY-DRATE gm.	CRUDE FIBER gm.	ASH gm.	TOTAL SOLIDS gm.	CAL-CIUM mg.	PHOS-PHORUS mg.	IRON mg.	SODIUM mg.	POTAS-SIUM mg.	VITA-MIN A I.U.	THIA-MIN mg.	RIBO-FLAVIN mg.	NIACIN mg.	VITA-MIN B₆ mg.	ASCOR-BIC ACID mg.
BEETS	7 tbsp.	100	3.5	38	1.3	0.1	7.9	0.7	1.1	11.1	13	22	0.46	160	236	—	0.016	0.017	0.12	0.04	1.7
	1 jar	128	4.5	48	1.7	0.1	10.1	0.9	1.4	14.2	17	28	0.60	205	302	—	0.020	0.022	0.16	0.05	2.2
CARROTS	7 tbsp.	100	3.5	29	0.7	0.1	6.3	0.8	0.9	8.8	21	21	0.29	122	187	11833	0.023	0.029	0.34	0.09	4.7
	1 jar	128	4.5	37	0.9	0.2	8.0	1.0	1.1	11.2	27	26	0.37	156	239	15147	0.030	0.037	0.43	0.12	6.0
CREAMED CORN	7 tbsp.	100	3.5	63	1.5	0.2	13.8	0.3	0.9	16.7	31	33	0.24	101	69	21	0.016	0.060	0.31	0.04	2.4
	1 jar	128	4.5	82	1.9	0.3	17.8	0.3	1.1	21.4	40	42	0.31	129	88	26	0.021	0.077	0.39	0.05	3.1
CREAMED SPINACH	7 tbsp.	100	3.5	42	2.7	0.8	6.0	0.5	1.3	11.3	96†	53	0.88	117	178	2578	0.041	0.092	0.25	0.07	8.9
	1 jar	128	4.5	53	3.5	1.0	7.6	0.7	1.7	14.5	123†	68	1.13	150	228	3300	0.052	0.118	0.32	0.09	11.4
GARDEN VEGETABLES	7 tbsp.	100	3.5	32	2.2	0.3	5.2	1.0	1.0	9.7	35	42	0.97	111	143	4156	0.072	0.050	0.68	0.08	7.0
	1 jar	128	4.5	41	2.9	0.3	6.7	1.2	1.3	12.4	45	54	1.25	142	183	5319	0.092	0.064	0.88	0.10	9.0
GREEN BEANS	7 tbsp.	100	3.5	29	1.3	0.1	5.6	1.1	0.9	9.0	38	26	0.88	114	137	325	0.043	0.062	0.34	0.03	6.2
	1 jar	128	4.5	36	1.7	0.1	7.1	1.4	1.2	11.5	48	33	1.13	146	175	416	0.055	0.079	0.43	0.04	7.9
MIXED VEGETABLES	7 tbsp.	100	3.5	39	1.2	0.1	8.2	0.4	0.9	10.8	13	26	0.36	170	93	4050	0.041	0.020	0.31	0.07	3.7
	1 jar	128	4.5	49	1.6	0.1	10.4	0.5	1.2	13.8	17	33	0.47	218	118	5184	0.053	0.026	0.39	0.09	4.7
PEAS	7 tbsp.	100	3.5	44	3.5	0.3	6.8	1.2	0.7	12.5	14	57	1.32	101	94	319	0.113	0.054	1.10	0.10	6.7
	1 jar	128	4.5	56	4.5	0.4	8.5	1.6	1.0	16.0	19	73	1.69	129	120	409	0.145	0.070	1.41	0.13	8.6
SQUASH	7 tbsp.	100	3.5	27	0.8	0.2	5.6	0.8	0.8	8.2	24	19	0.37	101	152	1322	0.025	0.027	0.41	0.06	8.4
	1 jar.	128	4.5	35	1.1	0.2	7.1	1.1	1.0	10.5	31	24	0.47	129	194	1692	0.032	0.034	0.52	0.08	10.7
SWEET POTATOES	7 tbsp.	100	3.5	69	1.4	0.1	15.5	0.6	1.0	18.6	19	33	0.38	101	234	5033	0.048	0.027	0.42	0.13	10.7
	1 jar	134	4.7	92	1.8	0.1	20.9	0.8	1.3	24.9	26	44	0.51	135	314	6745	0.064	0.037	0.56	0.17	14.3
SUMMARY OF STRAINED VEGETABLES	Average Values per Jar			53	2.2	0.3	10.4	1.0	1.2	15.0	39	42	0.79	154	196	3824	0.056	0.056	0.55	0.09	7.8
	% RDA (2-6 mos. infant)			6.9	11.0						7.8	10.5	7.9			254.9	14.0	11.2	7.9	30.0	22.3
	% RDA (6-12 mos. infant)			5.9	9.6						6.5	8.4	5.3			254.9	11.2	9.3	6.9	22.5	22.3
	% Calories				16.6	5.1	78.3														

*All measures level   tbsp. = tablespoon   oz. = ounce   gm. = gram   mg. = milligram   I.U. = International Unit   —— = quantity insignificant   † = partially unavailable

Table A.13 *STRAINED MEATS AND EGG YOLKS*
Average Nutrient Values per 100 Grams and per Jar

PRODUCT	MEASURE*	WEIGHT gm.	WEIGHT oz.	CAL-ORIES	PRO-TEIN gm.	FAT gm.	CARBO-HY-DRATE gm.	CRUDE FIBER gm.	ASH gm.	TOTAL SOLIDS gm.	CAL-CIUM mg.	PHOS-PHORUS mg.	IRON mg.	SODIUM mg.	POTAS-SIUM mg.	VITA-MIN A I.U.	THIA-MIN mg.	RIBO-FLAVIN mg.	NIACIN mg.	VITA-MIN B_6 mg.	ASCOR-BIC ACID mg.
BEEF	7 tbsp.	100	3.5	91	13.6	4.1	—	—	1.1	18.8	7	107	1.82	182	195	—	0.012	0.149	2.60	0.20	3.9
	1 jar	99	3.5	90	13.4	4.1	—	—	1.1	18.6	7	106	1.80	180	193	—	0.012	0.147	2.57	0.20	3.8
BEEF WITH BEEF HEART	7 tbsp.	100	3.5	86	12.5	3.7	0.7	—	1.0	17.9	6	109	2.12	151	159	—	0.048	0.388	3.19	0.26	3.2
	1 jar	99	3.5	85	12.3	3.7	0.7	—	1.0	17.7	6	108	2.10	149	157	—	0.048	0.384	3.16	0.26	3.2
BEEF LIVER	7 tbsp.	100	3.5	93	14.1	3.2	2.0	—	1.2	20.5	4	204	4.43	162	205	25655	0.102	2.283	8.42	0.81	19.2
	1 jar	99	3.5	92	14.0	3.2	2.0	—	1.2	20.4	4	201	4.38	160	203	25398	0.101	2.260	8.33	0.80	19.0
CHICKEN	7 tbsp.	100	3.5	132	13.6	8.6	0.1	—	1.2	23.5	38	127	1.34	170	119	—	0.022	0.189	2.98	0.29	3.2
	1 jar	99	3.5	131	13.5	8.5	0.1	—	1.2	23.3	37	125	1.32	168	118	—	0.022	0.187	2.95	0.29	3.2
EGG YOLKS	7 tbsp.	100	3.5	199	9.8	17.8	—	—	1.5	29.1	82	291	3.18	176	68	620	0.182	0.397	0.02	0.03	3.8
	1 jar	94	3.3	187	9.2	16.7	—	—	1.4	27.3	77	274	2.99	165	64	614	0.171	0.373	0.02	0.03	3.5
EGG YOLKS AND HAM	7 tbsp.	100	3.5	194	9.9	17.1	—	—	1.4	28.4	59	250	2.45	332	91	273	0.306	0.365	0.69	0.53	2.7
	1 jar	94	3.3	182	9.3	16.1	—	—	1.3	26.7	55	235	2.31	312	86	270	0.287	0.343	0.65	0.52	2.6
HAM	7 tbsp.	100	3.5	115	13.9	6.3	0.7	—	1.2	22.1	5	121	0.94	202	206	—	0.226	0.203	2.56	0.80	4.0
	1 jar	99	3.5	113	13.7	6.2	0.7	—	1.1	21.7	5	120	0.93	200	204	—	0.224	0.201	2.53	0.79	4.0
LAMB	7 tbsp.	100	3.5	97	15.2	4.0	—	—	1.3	20.5	6	117	1.38	166	193	—	0.088	0.181	3.16	0.35	2.8
	1 jar	99	3.5	96	15.1	4.0	—	—	1.3	20.4	6	116	1.37	164	191	—	0.087	0.179	3.13	0.35	2.8
PORK	7 tbsp.	100	3.5	111	13.9	6.1	—	—	1.1	21.1	6	119	1.09	220	227	—	0.216	0.219	2.68	0.49	3.6
	1 jar	99	3.5	109	13.7	6.0	—	—	1.1	20.8	6	118	1.08	218	224	—	0.214	0.217	2.65	0.49	3.6
TURKEY	7 tbsp.	100	3.5	130	13.8	8.2	0.3	—	0.9	23.2	20	109	1.63	182	126	—	0.025	0.265	3.01	0.14	4.0
	1 jar	99	3.5	129	13.7	8.1	0.3	—	0.9	23.0	20	108	1.61	180	125	—	0.025	0.262	2.98	0.14	3.9
VEAL	7 tbsp.	100	3.5	90	13.5	4.0	—	—	1.1	18.6	6	108	1.01	179	215	—	0.022	0.180	3.19	0.27	4.5
	1 jar	99	3.5	89	13.4	4.0	—	—	1.1	18.5	6	107	1.00	177	213	—	0.021	0.179	3.16	0.27	4.4
SUMMARY OF STRAINED MEATS AND EGG YOLKS	Average Values per Jar			118	12.8	7.3	0.4	—	1.2	21.7	20.8	147	1.10	188	162	2389	0.110	0.430	2.92	0.38	4.9
	% RDA (2-6 mo. infant)			15.3	64.0						4.2	36.7	19.0			159.3	27.5	86.0	41.7	126.7	14.0
	% RDA (6-12 mo. infant)			13.1	55.7						3.5	29.4	12.7			159.3	22.0	71.7	36.5	95.0	14.0
	% Calories				43.2	55.4	1.3														

Table A-4 *STRAINED HIGH MEAT DINNERS*
Average Nutrient Values per 100 Grams and per Jar

PRODUCT	MEASURE*	WEIGHT gm.	WEIGHT oz.	CAL-ORIES	PRO-TEIN gm.	FAT gm.	CARBO-HY-DRATE gm.	CRUDE FIBER gm.	ASH gm.	TOTAL SOLIDS gm.	CAL-CIUM mg.	PHOS-PHORUS mg.	IRON mg.	SODIUM mg.	POTAS-SIUM mg.	VITA-MIN A I.U.	THIA-MIN mg.	RIBO-FLAVIN mg.	NIACIN mg.	VITA-MIN B₆ mg.	ASCOR-BIC ACID mg.
BEEF WITH VEGETABLES	7 tbsp.	100	3.5	82	6.1	3.7	6.0	0.3	1.1	17.2	7	52	0.95	152	104	456	0.014	0.062	1.47	0.20	2.8
	1 jar	128	4.5	104	7.8	4.7	7.6	0.4	1.5	22.0	8	66	1.22	194	133	583	0.018	0.080	1.88	0.26	3.6
CHICKEN WITH VEGETABLES	7 tbsp.	100	3.5	86	6.2	4.2	5.8	0.2	1.1	17.5	36	57	1.71	134	58	444	0.009	0.060	0.98	0.14	2.3
	1 jar	128	4.5	110	8.0	5.3	7.5	0.2	1.4	22.4	47	73	2.18	172	74	569	0.011	0.077	1.26	0.18	3.0
CREAMED COTTAGE CHEESE WITH PINEAPPLE	7 tbsp.	100	3.5	136	6.2	4.7	17.3	0.9	0.9	30.0	67	91	0.37	153	97	17	0.055	0.160	0.11	0.04	2.8
	1 jar	134	4.7	174	8.0	6.0	22.1	1.2	1.1	38.4	86	116	0.47	195	125	22	0.070	0.205	0.14	0.05	3.6
HAM WITH VEGETABLES	7 tbsp.	100	3.5	79	6.5	2.9	6.6	0.2	1.1	17.3	6	66	0.77	175	135	39	0.111	0.050	2.10	0.63	2.8
	1 jar	128	4.5	101	8.4	3.8	8.2	0.3	1.4	22.1	8	85	0.98	224	173	50	0.142	0.064	2.69	0.81	3.6
TURKEY WITH VEGETABLES	7 tbsp.	100	3.5	75	5.5	3.2	6.1	0.1	1.0	15.9	14	42	0.82	152	65	22	0.010	0.068	1.16	0.21	2.5
	1 jar	128	4.5	96	7.1	4.1	7.6	0.2	1.3	20.3	17	54	1.05	195	84	28	0.012	0.087	1.49	0.27	3.1
VEAL WITH VEGETABLES	7 tbsp.	100	3.5	63	6.3	1.4	6.4	0.3	1.2	15.6	6	60	1.02	126	127	44	0.025	0.066	1.65	0.13	2.6
	1 jar	128	4.5	82	8.1	1.8	8.3	0.3	1.5	20.0	8	77	1.31	161	162	57	0.032	0.084	2.11	0.17	3.4
SUMMARY OF STRAINED HIGH MEAT DINNERS	Average Values per Jar			111	7.9	4.3	10.2	0.4	1.4	24.2	29	78	1.20	190	125	218	0.048	0.100	1.60	0.29	3.4
	% RDA (2-6 mos. infant)			14.4	39.5						5.8	19.5	12.0			14.5	12.0	20.0	22.9	96.7	9.7
	% RDA (6-12 mo. infant)			12.3	34.3						4.8	15.6	8.0			14.5	9.6	16.7	20.0	72.5	9.7
	% Calories				28.4	34.8	36.7														

Table A.15 STRAINED VEGETABLES AND MEATS
Average Nutrient Values per 100 Grams and per Jar

PRODUCT	MEASURE*	WEIGHT gm.	WEIGHT oz.	CALORIES	PROTEIN gm.	FAT gm.	CARBOHYDRATE gm.	CRUDE FIBER gm.	ASH gm.	TOTAL SOLIDS gm.	CALCIUM mg.	PHOSPHORUS mg.	IRON mg.	SODIUM mg.	POTASSIUM mg.	VITAMIN A I.U.	THIAMIN mg.	RIBOFLAVIN mg.	NIACIN mg.	VITAMIN B, mg.	ASCORBIC ACID mg.
BEEF AND EGG NOODLES	7 tbsp.	100	3.5	48	2.8	0.9	7.2	0.3	0.9	12.1	7	29	0.66	127	57	672	0.054	0.046	0.08	0.05	1.9
	1 jar	128	4.5	61	3.6	1.1	9.2	0.4	1.2	15.5	9	37	0.84	163	73	860	0.070	0.059	1.06	0.06	2.4
CEREAL, EGG YOLKS AND BACON	7 tbsp.	100	3.5	72	2.2	3.9	6.9	0.1	1.0	14.0	23	42	0.47	134	36	6	0.035	0.071	0.16	0.12	1.3
	1 jar	128	4.5	92	2.8	5.0	8.9	0.1	1.1	17.9	29	54	0.61	172	46	7	0.044	0.091	0.21	0.15	1.7
CHICKEN NOODLE DINNER	7 tbsp.	100	3.5	47	2.3	0.7	7.8	0.3	1.0	12.1	24	37	0.51	115	61	514	0.051	0.042	0.48	0.06	1.9
	1 jar	128	4.5	60	2.9	0.9	10.0	0.4	1.3	15.5	30	48	0.66	147	78	658	0.065	0.054	0.61	0.08	2.4
CREAM OF CHICKEN SOUP	7 tbsp.	100	3.5	57	2.5	1.0	9.4	0.3	1.0	14.2	32	36	0.38	138	63	413	0.019	0.043	0.35	0.06	1.7
	1 jar	128	4.5	73	3.2	1.3	12.1	0.3	1.3	18.2	41	47	0.49	177	81	528	0.024	0.055	0.45	0.08	2.2
MACARONI, TOMATO, BEEF AND BACON	7 tbsp.	100	3.5	61	2.1	1.9	8.9	0.4	1.0	14.3	17	33	0.60	107	79	350	0.060	0.047	0.66	0.05	2.4
	1 jar	128	4.5	78	2.7	2.4	11.3	0.6	1.3	18.3	22	43	0.76	137	101	448	0.077	0.060	0.85	0.06	3.1
TURKEY RICE DINNER	7 tbsp.	100	3.5	46	2.1	0.9	7.4	0.1	0.9	11.4	12	20	0.35	101	41	496	0.009	0.027	0.29	0.05	2.0
	1 jar	128	4.5	59	2.6	1.2	9.5	0.2	1.1	14.6	16	25	0.47	129	52	635	0.011	0.035	0.37	0.06	2.6
VEGETABLES & BACON	7 tbsp.	100	3.5	73	1.7	3.1	9.6	0.4	0.8	15.6	10	31	0.38	143	114	2167	0.041	0.029	0.61	0.08	2.4
	1 jar	128	4.5	94	2.1	3.9	12.5	0.5	1.0	20.0	13	39	0.49	183	145	2773	0.052	0.037	0.78	0.10	3.0
VEGETABLES & BEEF	7 tbsp.	100	3.5	52	1.9	2.0	6.6	0.2	1.0	11.7	6	22	0.46	135	60	1004	0.028	0.029	0.49	0.07	1.6
	1 jar	128	4.5	67	2.5	2.6	8.4	0.2	1.3	15.0	8	28	0.59	173	77	1285	0.036	0.038	0.63	0.09	2.1
VEGETABLES & CHICKEN	7 tbsp.	100	3.5	41	2.0	0.6	6.9	0.2	0.8	10.5	13	25	0.33	107	26	779	0.023	0.026	0.21	0.06	2.7
	1 jar	128	4.5	53	2.6	0.8	8.8	0.2	1.0	13.4	17	32	0.42	137	33	997	0.030	0.034	0.27	0.08	3.4
VEGETABLES & HAM WITH BACON	7 tbsp.	100	3.5	54	1.7	2.0	7.4	0.2	0.9	12.2	5	23	0.47	233	39	383	0.066	0.024	0.46	0.07	2.1
	1 jar	128	4.5	70	2.1	2.6	9.5	0.3	1.1	15.6	7	29	0.60	298	50	491	0.084	0.031	0.59	0.09	2.7
VEGETABLES & LAMB	7 tbsp.	100	3.5	49	2.0	1.3	7.4	0.3	1.0	12.0	7	23	0.32	144	77	1425	0.022	0.025	0.45	0.08	1.6
	1 jar	128	4.5	64	2.6	1.7	9.5	0.4	1.2	15.4	9	29	0.42	184	98	1824	0.029	0.033	0.58	0.10	2.1
VEGETABLES & LIVER WITH BACON	7 tbsp.	100	3.5	60	2.2	2.8	6.4	0.2	1.1	12.7	7	40	2.13	205	78	1050	0.030	0.252	1.22	0.13	3.2
	1 jar	128	4.5	77	2.9	3.6	8.2	0.2	1.4	16.3	9	51	2.73	262	100	1344	0.038	0.323	1.57	0.17	4.1
VEGETABLES & TURKEY	7 tbsp.	100	3.5	44	1.8	0.4	8.3	0.2	0.9	11.6	9	19	0.42	123	44	500	0.009	0.021	0.38	0.06	2.4
	1 jar	128	4.5	57	2.3	0.5	10.7	0.3	1.1	14.9	11	24	0.53	157	57	640	0.012	0.027	0.49	0.08	3.1
SUMMARY OF STR. VEGETABLES & MEAT COMBINATIONS	Average Values per Jar			70	2.7	2.1	9.9	0.3	1.2	16.2	17	37	0.74	178	76	961	0.044	0.068	0.65	0.09	2.7
	% RDA (2-6 mos. infant)			9.1	13.5						3.4	9.3	7.4			64.1	11.0	13.6	9.3	30.0	7.7
	% RDA (6-12 mo. infant)			7.8	11.7						2.8	7.4	4.9			64.1	8.8	11.3	8.1	22.5	7.7
	% Calories				15.6	27.3	57.1														

*All measures level   tbsp. = tablespoon   oz. = ounce   gm. = gram   mg. = milligram   I.U. = International Unit   —— = quantity insignificant

Table A.16 STRAINED DESSERTS
Average Nutrient Values per 100 Grams and per Jar

PRODUCT	MEASURE*	WEIGHT gm.	WEIGHT oz.	CALORIES	PROTEIN gm.	FAT gm.	CARBOHYDRATE gm.	CRUDE FIBER gm.	ASH gm.	TOTAL SOLIDS gm.	CALCIUM mg.	PHOSPHORUS mg.	IRON mg.	SODIUM mg.	POTASSIUM mg.	VITAMIN A I.U.	THIAMIN mg.	RIBOFLAVIN mg.	NIACIN mg.	VITAMIN B_6 mg.	ASCORBIC ACID mg.
BLUEBERRY BUCKLE	7 tbsp.	100	3.5	83	0.2	0.1	20.2	0.2	0.1	20.8	4	3	0.37	44	18	6	0.004	0.008	0.04	0.01	1.7
	1 jar	128	4.5	105	0.2	0.1	25.9	0.3	0.2	26.7	4	4	0.48	57	23	8	0.005	0.010	0.06	0.01	2.2
BUTTERSCOTCH PUDDING	7 tbsp.	100	3.5	100	1.7	2.4	18.0	0.2	0.7	23.0	48	52	0.31	123	62	4	0.013	0.202	0.04	0.02	2.0
	1 jar	128	4.5	129	2.1	3.1	23.1	0.2	0.9	29.4	62	67	0.40	157	79	5	0.017	0.259	0.06	0.03	2.6
CHERRY VANILLA PUDDING	7 tbsp.	100	3.5	86	0.3	1.0	18.9	0.3	0.2	20.7	7	7	0.40	51	42	144	0.007	0.049	0.05	—	2.3
	1 jar	134	4.7	115	0.4	1.3	25.4	0.4	0.3	27.8	9	9	0.54	69	56	193	0.009	0.065	0.06	—	3.1
CHOCOLATE CUSTARD PUDDING	7 tbsp.	100	3.5	94	1.9	1.6	18.1	0.9	0.8	23.3	58	62	0.69	101	80	226	0.021	0.145	0.06	0.03	2.4
	1 jar	128	4.5	122	2.4	2.1	23.3	1.1	1.0	29.9	74	80	0.88	129	103	289	0.026	0.186	0.07	0.04	3.0
COTTAGE CHEESE DESSERT WITH PINEAPPLE	7 tbsp.	100	3.5	91	3.1	1.2	16.9	0.1	0.3	21.6	22	27	0.10	137	21	41	0.020	0.030	0.04	0.02	13.7
	1 jar	128	4.5	116	4.0	1.5	21.6	0.1	0.4	27.6	28	35	0.13	175	27	52	0.026	0.038	0.05	0.03	17.5
DUTCH APPLE DESSERT	7 tbsp.	100	3.5	93	0.1	1.0	20.9	0.4	0.1	22.5	4	4	0.25	27	54	8	0.007	0.007	0.03	0.03	7.5
	1 jar	134	4.7	124	0.1	1.3	27.9	0.6	0.2	30.1	5	5	0.34	36	73	11	0.009	0.010	0.04	0.04	10.1
FRUIT DESSERT WITH TAPIOCA	7 tbsp.	100	3.5	90	0.3	0.3	21.5	0.2	0.3	22.6	7	7	0.43	38	91	152	0.021	0.011	0.14	0.04	3.4
	1 jar	134	4.7	120	0.4	0.4	28.7	0.3	0.4	30.2	10	10	0.58	51	122	203	0.029	0.015	0.19	0.05	4.5
ORANGE PUDDING	7 tbsp.	100	3.5	99	1.1	0.9	21.7	0.3	0.6	24.6	29	30	0.49	96	66	67	0.049	0.081	0.08	0.03	5.3
	1 jar	134	4.7	133	1.5	1.2	29.0	0.4	0.8	32.9	39	41	0.65	129	89	89	0.066	0.108	0.11	0.04	7.1
PEACH COBBLER	7 tbsp.	100	3.5	86	0.4	0.2	20.7	0.5	0.2	22.0	4	8	0.27	17	68	98	0.007	0.014	0.34	0.02	7.5
	1 jar	134	4.7	116	0.5	0.3	27.8	0.7	0.2	29.5	5	11	0.37	23	92	131	0.009	0.018	0.45	0.03	10.1
RASPBERRY COBBLER	7 tbsp.	100	3.5	79	0.2	0.1	19.4	0.2	0.2	20.1	5	4	0.27	49	27	12	0.004	0.006	0.06	0.01	1.3
	1 jar	128	4.5	102	0.3	0.1	24.9	0.3	0.2	25.8	6	5	0.35	62	35	15	0.005	0.008	0.08	0.01	1.7
VANILLA CUSTARD PUDDING	7 tbsp.	100	3.5	88	1.7	1.2	17.5	0.9	0.7	22.0	55	55	0.51	101	64	228	0.014	0.137	0.05	0.03	2.4
	1 jar	128	4.5	112	2.2	1.6	22.3	1.1	0.9	28.1	71	70	0.65	129	82	292	0.018	0.176	0.06	0.04	3.0
SUMMARY OF STRAINED DESSERTS	Average Values per Jar			118	1.3	1.2	25.4	0.5	0.5	28.9	28	31	0.49	92	71	117	0.020	0.081	0.11	0.03	5.9
	% RDA (2-6 mos. infant)			15.3	6.5						5.6	7.7	4.9			7.8	5.0	16.2	1.6	10.0	16.9
	% RDA (6-12 mo. infant)			13.1	5.7						4.7	6.2	3.3			7.8	4.0	13.5	1.4	7.5	16.9
	% Calories				4.4	9.2	86.4														

Table A.17   *BAKED GOODS*
Average Nutrient Content per 100 Grams and per Unit

PRODUCT	MEASURE *	WEIGHT gm. oz.	CALO-RIES	PRO-TEIN gm.	FAT gm.	CARBO-HYDRATE gm.	CRUDE FIBER gm.	ASH gm.	TOTAL SOLIDS gm.	CAL-CIUM mg.	PHOS-PHORUS mg.	IRON mg.	SODIUM mg.	POTAS-SIUM mg.	THIA-MIN mg.	RIBO-FLAVIN mg.	NIACIN mg.	VITAMIN B₆ mg.
COOKIES (Animal Shaped)	15.4 cookies	100 3.5	439	11.6	14.7	65.0	0.9	2.4	94.6	127	181	2.00	432	372	1.23	2.00	12.31	4.046
	1 cookie	6.5	29	0.8	1.0	4.2	0.1	0.2	6.1	8	12	0.13	28	24	0.08	0.13	0.80	0.263
PRETZELS	1 pretzel	100 3.5	382	13.9	2.3	76.3	0.5	1.9	94.9	30	131	1.91	597	54	0.19	0.07	1.15	0.800
		5.0	19	0.7	0.1	3.9	—	0.1	4.8	2	7	0.10	30	3	0.01	—	0.06	0.040
TEETHING BISCUITS	1 biscuit	100 3.5	382	11.3	5.2	72.6	0.7	3.3	93.1	466	438	2.01	532	298	0.40	0.39	2.47	0.200
		11.0	43	1.3	0.6	8.1	0.1	0.4	10.5	53	49	0.23	60	34	0.05	0.04	0.28	0.022
SUMMARY OF BAKED GOODS	Average Values per Unit		30	0.9	0.6	5.4	0.1	0.2	7.1	21	23	0.15	39	20	0.05	0.06	0.38	0.108
	% RDA (6-12 mos. infant)		3.3	3.9						3.5	4.6	1.0			10.0	10.0	4.7	27.0
	% RDA (1-2 year child)		2.7	3.6						3.0	3.3	1.0			8.3	10.0	4.7	21.6
	% Calories			11.8	17.7	70.6												

Table A.18 *JUNIOR FRUITS*
Average Nutrient Values per 100 Grams and per Jar

PRODUCT	MEASURE*	WEIGHT gm	WEIGHT oz	CALORIES	PROTEIN gm	FAT gm	CARBOHYDRATE gm	CRUDE FIBER gm	ASH gm	TOTAL SOLIDS gm	CALCIUM mg	PHOSPHORUS mg	IRON mg	SODIUM mg	POTASSIUM mg	VITAMIN A I.U.	THIAMIN mg	RIBOFLAVIN mg	NIACIN mg	VITAMIN B6 mg	ASCORBIC ACID† mg
APPLESAUCE	7 tbsp.	100	3.5	81	0.2	0.2	19.6	0.7	0.2	20.9	3	6	0.22	2	61	2	0.013	0.022	0.07	0.03	30.0
	1 jar	220	7.8	179	0.4	0.5	43.1	1.5	0.5	46.0	7	12	0.48	4	135	4	0.029	0.048	0.15	0.07	66.0
APPLESAUCE AND APRICOTS	7 tbsp.	100	3.5	87	0.3	0.3	20.8	0.6	0.7	22.7	4	6	0.35	2	82	244	0.014	0.020	0.18	0.03	9.1
	1 jar	220	7.8	192	0.7	0.7	45.7	1.3	1.6	50.0	9	14	0.78	3	180	537	0.030	0.045	0.39	0.07	20.0
APPLESAUCE WITH PINEAPPLE	7 tbsp.	100	3.5	74	0.2	0.1	18.0	1.0	0.2	19.5	4	6	0.31	2	70	15	0.027	0.017	0.08	0.04	9.1
	1 jar	220	7.8	162	0.5	0.3	39.4	2.3	0.4	42.9	9	13	0.68	4	153	33	0.059	0.038	0.17	0.09	20.0
APRICOTS WITH TAPIOCA	7 tbsp.	100	3.5	81	0.4	0.1	19.6	0.3	0.3	20.7	7	8	0.30	32	110	291	0.008	0.011	0.25	0.03	9.1
	1 jar	220	7.8	178	0.8	0.1	43.4	0.7	0.6	45.6	14	19	0.66	70	243	641	0.018	0.025	0.55	0.07	20.0
BANANAS WITH PINEAPPLE AND TAPIOCA	7 tbsp.	100	3.5	82	0.3	0.1	20.0	0.3	0.2	20.9	4	5	0.21	97	70	31	0.013	0.019	0.13	0.08	9.1
	1 jar	220	7.8	181	0.6	0.3	44.0	0.6	0.5	46.0	10	11	0.46	214	153	67	0.029	0.043	0.29	0.18	20.0
PEACHES	7 tbsp.	100	3.5	82	0.6	0.3	19.3	0.9	1.1	22.2	4	10	0.21	5	121	151	0.009	0.032	0.67	0.03	9.1
	1 jar	220	7.8	181	1.3	0.7	42.4	2.0	2.5	48.9	8	21	0.47	12	266	332	0.021	0.071	1.48	0.07	20.0
PEARS	7 tbsp.	100	3.5	69	0.3	0.2	16.6	1.3	0.3	18.7	8	9	0.23	2	91	3	0.013	0.022	0.19	0.02	9.1
	1 jar	220	7.8	152	0.7	0.4	36.4	3.0	0.6	41.1	18	20	0.51	4	199	7	0.029	0.048	0.41	0.04	20.0
PEARS AND PINEAPPLE	7 tbsp.	100	3.5	71	0.4	0.3	16.7	1.2	0.2	18.8	9	8	0.24	2	94	9	0.024	0.022	0.17	0.03	9.1
	1 jar	220	7.8	156	0.8	0.6	36.8	2.7	0.5	41.4	20	17	0.53	4	206	21	0.054	0.048	0.38	0.07	20.0
PLUMS WITH TAPIOCA	7 tbsp.	100	3.5	99	0.3	0.2	24.1	0.4	0.2	25.2	6	7	0.45	5	73	78	0.012	0.020	0.24	0.05	1.8
	1 jar	220	7.8	218	0.7	0.4	53.0	0.8	0.5	55.4	13	15	0.98	12	160	171	0.026	0.043	0.53	0.11	3.9
PRUNES WITH TAPIOCA	7 tbsp.	100	3.5	91	0.6	0.2	21.8	0.7	0.4	23.7	14	16	0.52	20	158	190	0.015	0.067	0.43	0.07	3.4
	1 jar	220	7.8	201	1.3	0.5	47.9	1.5	1.0	52.2	32	34	1.15	44	348	418	0.032	0.147	0.94	0.16	7.4
SUMMARY OF JUNIOR FRUITS	Average Values per Jar			180	0.8	0.4	47.2	1.6	0.9	47.0	14	18	0.67	37	204	223	0.033	0.056	0.53	0.09	21.7
	% RDA (6-12 mos. infant)			20.0	3.5						2.3	3.6	4.5			14.9	6.6	9.3	6.6	22.5	62.0
	% RDA (1-2 year child)			16.4	3.2						2.0	2.6	4.5			11.1	5.5	9.3	6.6	18.0	54.3
	% Calories				1.8	2.0	96.2														

Table A.19   *JUNIOR VEGETABLES*
Average Nutrient Values per 100 Grams and per Jar

PRODUCT	MEASURE*	WEIGHT gm.	WEIGHT oz.	CALORIES	PROTEIN gm.	FAT gm.	CARBOHYDRATE gm.	CRUDE FIBER gm.	ASH gm.	TOTAL SOLIDS gm.	CALCIUM mg.	PHOSPHORUS mg.	IRON mg.	SODIUM mg.	POTASSIUM mg.	VITAMIN A I.U.	THIAMIN mg.	RIBOFLAVIN mg.	NIACIN mg.	VITAMIN B6 mg.	ASCORBIC ACID mg.
CARROTS	7 tbsp.	100	3.5	30	0.7	0.2	6.3	0.7	1.0	8.9	22	21	0.34	122	204	13061	0.024	0.035	0.39	0.09	5.3
	1 jar	212	7.5	63	1.5	0.4	13.4	1.5	2.1	18.9	46	45	0.73	259	432	27690	0.052	0.075	0.84	0.19	11.3
CARROTS & PEAS	7 tbsp.	100	3.5	38	2.3	0.3	6.4	1.3	0.9	11.2	20	42	0.85	100	138	6253	0.077	0.055	0.94	0.07	4.9
	1 jar	212	7.5	79	4.9	0.7	13.3	2.8	2.0	23.7	42	89	1.81	213	293	13256	0.163	0.116	1.99	0.15	10.4
CREAMED CORN	7 tbsp.	100	3.5	62	1.5	0.2	13.6	0.3	0.9	16.5	31	38	0.24	101	68	21	0.013	0.073	0.31	0.04	2.1
	1 jar	212	7.5	133	3.2	0.5	28.8	0.6	1.8	34.9	66	81	0.51	214	145	44	0.029	0.155	0.67	0.08	4.5
CREAMED GREEN BEANS WITH BACON	7 tbsp.	100	3.5	67	1.8	2.8	8.6	0.4	0.9	14.5	30	32	0.47	308	89	106	0.029	0.050	0.30	0.13	3.7
	1 jar	212	7.5	141	3.9	5.9	18.1	0.9	1.9	30.7	64	68	1.00	652	188	224	0.061	0.107	0.64	0.28	7.8
CREAMED SPINACH	7 tbsp.	100	3.5	45	2.7	1.0	6.2	0.5	1.5	11.9	86	57	0.80	151	244	2281	0.031	0.100	0.25	0.07	12.3
	1 jar	212	7.5	95	5.8	2.2	13.1	1.0	3.1	25.2	182	121	1.70	320	517	4835	0.065	0.211	0.53	0.15	26.0
MIXED VEGETABLES	7 tbsp.	100	3.5	40	1.5	0.1	8.2	0.5	1.2	11.5	13	33	0.57	135	142	3944	0.039	0.026	0.69	0.07	3.6
	1 jar	212	7.5	85	3.2	0.3	17.3	1.1	2.5	24.4	28	69	1.22	286	302	8362	0.083	0.055	1.47	0.15	7.6
SQUASH	7 tbsp.	100	3.5	27	0.8	0.2	5.6	0.9	0.8	8.3	24	19	0.35	101	170	1239	0.021	0.041	0.45	0.06	9.6
	1 jar	212	7.5	57	1.8	0.5	11.4	2.0	1.8	17.5	52	41	0.74	214	360	2626	0.045	0.087	0.95	0.13	20.3
SWEET POTATOES	7 tbsp.	100	3.5	69	1.4	0.1	15.7	0.6	1.0	18.8	16	32	0.57	101	219	5344	0.036	0.035	0.44	0.11	12.4
	1 jar	220	7.8	153	3.1	0.2	34.6	1.3	2.2	41.4	35	71	1.25	222	483	11758	0.080	0.078	0.96	0.24	27.2
SUMMARY OF JUNIOR VEGETABLES	Average Values per Jar			101	3.4	1.3	18.8	1.4	2.2	27.1	64	73	1.12	298	340	8599	0.072	0.110	1.01	0.17	14.4
	% RDA (6-12 mos. infant)			11.0	14.8						10.7	14.6	7.5			573.3	14.4	18.3	12.6	42.5	41.1
	% RDA (1-2 year child)			9.0	13.6						9.1	10.4	7.5			430.0	12.0	18.3	12.6	34.0	36.0
	% Calories				13.5	11.6	74.8														

Table A 20 *JUNIOR CEREALS WITH FRUIT*
Average Nutrient Values per 100 Grams and per Jar

PRODUCT	MEASURE*	WEIGHT gm.	WEIGHT oz.	CAL-ORIES	PRO-TEIN gm.	FAT gm.	CARBO-HY-DRATE gm.	CRUDE FIBER gm.	ASH gm.	TOTAL SOLIDS gm.	CAL-CIUM mg.	PHOS-PHORUS mg.	IRON mg.	SODIUM mg.	POTAS-SIUM mg.	VITA-MIN A I.U.	THIA-MIN mg.	RIBO-FLAVIN mg.	NIACIN mg.	VITA-MIN B₆ mg.	ASCOR-BIC ACID mg.
HIGH PROTEIN CEREAL WITH APPLESAUCE AND BANANAS	7 tbsp.	100	3.5	93	4.6	0.5	17.6	0.3	0.8	23.8	30	83	7.77	121	181	—	0.195	0.469	3.12	0.20	20.0
	1 jar	220	7.8	205	10.1	1.1	38.7	0.7	1.8	52.4	66	183	17.10	266	398	—	0.429	1.032	6.86	0.44	44.0
MIXED CEREAL WITH APPLESAUCE AND BANANAS	7 tbsp	100	3.5	81	1.4	0.3	18.2	0.2	0.4	20.5	4	46	3.91	89	41	2	0.195	0.469	3.12	0.20	1.2
	1 jar	220	7.8	178	3.0	0.6	40.1	0.5	0.8	45.0	9	102	8.60	196	91	4	0.429	1.032	6.86	0.44	2.7
OATMEAL WITH APPLESAUCE AND BANANAS	7 tbsp.	100	3.5	76	1.6	0.7	15.8	0.3	0.5	18.9	8	62	3.91	139	48	13	0.195	0.469	3.12	0.22	2.4
	1 jar	220	7.8	167	3.5	1.5	34.8	0.6	1.1	41.5	18	135	8.60	306	105	29	0.429	1.032	6.86	0.44	5.4
RICE CEREAL WITH APPLESAUCE AND PINEAPPLE	7 tbsp.	100	3.5	87	1.2	0.1	20.3	0.2	0.4	22.2	20	27	7.50	85	45	—	0.195	0.469	3.12	0.20	20.0
	1 jar	220	7.8	191	2.6	0.2	44.7	0.4	0.9	48.8	44	59	16.50	187	99	—	0.429	1.032	6.86	0.44	44.0
SUMMARY OF JUNIOR CEREALS WITH FRUIT	Average Values per Jar			185	4.8	0.9	39.6	0.6	1.2	46.9	34	120	12.7	239	173	8	0.429	1.032	6.86	0.44	24.0
	% RDA (6-12 mos. infant)			20.6	20.8						5.7	24.0	84.7			0.5	85.8	172.0	85.7	110.0	68.6
	% RDA (1 - 2 year child)			16.8	19.2						4.9	17.1	84.7			0.4	71.5	172.0	85.7	88.0	60.1
	% Calories				10.3	4.3	85.5														

*All measures level   tbsp. = tablespoon   oz. = ounce   gm. = gram   mg. = milligram   I.U. = International Unit

Table A.21 *JUNIOR VEGETABLES AND MEATS*
Average Nutrient Values per 100 Grams and per Jar

PRODUCT	MEASURE*	WEIGHT gm.	WEIGHT oz.	CAL-ORIES	PRO-TEIN gm.	FAT gm.	CARBO-HY-DRATE gm.	CRUDE FIBER gm.	ASH gm.	TOTAL SOLIDS gm.	CAL-CIUM mg.	PHOS-PHORUS mg.	IRON mg.	SO-DIUM mg.	POTAS-SIUM mg.	VITA-MIN A I.U.	THIA-MIN mg.	RIBO-FLAVIN mg.	NIACIN mg.	VITA-MIN B₆ mg.	ASCOR-BIC ACID mg.
BEEF AND EGG NOODLES	7 tbsp.	100	3.5	51	2.7	1.0	7.7	0.2	1.0	12.6	6	30	0.62	105	64	286	0.025	0.049	0.70	0.08	2.4
	1 jar	212	7.5	107	5.8	2.1	16.3	0.4	2.1	26.7	13	64	1.32	222	137	607	0.054	0.103	1.48	0.17	5.2
CEREAL, EGG YOLKS AND BACON	7 tbsp.	100	3.5	75	2.2	4.2	7.0	0.1	0.8	14.3	26	46	0.44	134	35	7	0.033	0.078	0.17	0.10	1.4
	1 jar	212	7.5	158	4.7	8.8	14.9	0.2	1.7	30.3	56	97	0.94	284	75	16	0.070	0.165	0.35	0.21	3.0
CHICKEN NOODLE DINNER	7 tbsp.	100	3.5	44	2.0	0.5	7.8	0.2	0.8	11.3	11	24	0.45	151	26	481	0.027	0.030	0.45	0.05	2.1
	1 jar	212	7.5	93	4.3	1.0	16.6	0.4	1.7	24.0	24	51	0.95	320	55	1019	0.057	0.063	0.96	0.11	4.4
CREAM OF CHICKEN SOUP	7 tbsp.	100	3.5	55	2.5	1.0	8.9	0.2	1.0	13.6	33	39	0.42	138	70	352	0.014	0.062	0.36	0.05	1.9
	1 jar	212	7.5	116	5.2	2.1	19.1	0.5	2.0	28.9	70	82	0.90	293	148	746	0.031	0.131	0.75	0.11	4.0
MACARONI, TOMATO, BEEF AND BACON	7 tbsp.	100	3.5	62	2.3	1.4	10.1	0.3	0.8	14.9	15	29	0.49	125	82	306	0.045	0.056	0.72	0.04	2.3
	1 jar	212	7.5	132	5.0	3.0	21.3	0.6	1.7	31.6	33	61	1.03	265	173	648	0.096	0.119	1.53	0.08	4.9
SPAGHETTI, TOMATO SAUCE AND BEEF	7 tbsp.	100	3.5	68	2.9	0.8	12.4	0.4	1.4	17.9	16	37	0.65	220	118	339	0.094	0.085	1.17	0.08	3.1
	1 jar	212	7.5	145	6.2	1.6	26.4	0.8	3.0	38.0	33	78	1.39	483	249	718	0.199	0.180	2.48	0.17	6.5
SPLIT PEAS WITH BACON	7 tbsp.	100	3.5	85	3.1	2.6	12.3	0.3	1.1	19.4	20	49	0.53	126	88	564	0.054	0.045	0.46	0.05	2.3
	1 jar	212	7.5	179	6.6	5.4	26.0	0.6	2.4	41.0	41	104	1.12	267	186	1195	0.114	0.095	0.99	0.11	4.8
TURKEY RICE DINNER	7 tbsp.	100	3.5	44	2.0	0.7	7.3	0.2	0.9	11.1	10	17	0.41	149	36	594	0.008	0.032	0.34	0.04	2.3
	1 jar	212	7.5	92	4.3	1.5	15.4	0.5	1.9	23.6	20	36	0.87	316	77	1260	0.018	0.067	0.73	0.08	4.9
VEGETABLES & BACON	7 tbsp.	100	3.5	64	2.0	2.4	8.7	0.2	1.0	14.3	22	38	0.50	171	88	833	0.045	0.037	0.39	0.06	2.5
	1 jar	212	7.5	137	4.3	5.2	18.2	0.5	2.2	30.4	46	82	1.07	362	187	1767	0.096	0.079	0.83	0.13	5.2
VEGETABLES & BEEF	7 tbsp.	100	3.5	51	2.5	1.6	6.6	0.2	1.1	12.0	7	32	0.54	146	84	544	0.039	0.041	0.72	0.08	2.1
	1 jar	212	7.5	108	5.2	3.3	14.3	0.4	2.3	25.5	15	68	1.14	310	179	1154	0.083	0.088	1.53	0.17	4.5
VEGETABLES & CHICKEN	7 tbsp.	100	3.5	50	1.9	0.3	9.8	0.2	0.9	13.1	10	27	0.82	107	61	725	0.017	0.028	0.46	0.08	1.9
	1 jar	212	7.5	105	4.1	0.6	20.7	0.5	1.9	27.8	21	57	1.73	227	130	1537	0.035	0.059	0.97	0.17	4.1
VEGETABLES & HAM WITH BACON	7 tbsp.	100	3.5	58	1.7	1.9	8.5	0.2	0.9	13.2	6	26	0.39	210	43	260	0.045	0.025	0.39	0.07	1.9
	1 jar	212	7.5	122	3.6	4.0	18.0	0.5	1.9	28.0	12	55	0.84	445	91	551	0.096	0.054	0.82	0.15	4.0

Table A.21 (Continued)

	Measure																			
VEGETABLES & LAMB	7 tbsp	100	3.5	49	2.0	1.3	7.4	0.2	1.1	12.0	6	23	0.45	129	86	606	0.018	0.025	0.47	0.07	2.3
	1 jar	212	7.5	106	4.2	2.9	15.7	0.5	2.2	25.5	13	49	0.96	273	182	1284	0.038	0.054	0.99	0.15	4.8
VEGETABLES & LIVER WITH BACON	7 tbsp	100	3.5	49	2.0	1.0	8.1	0.3	1.0	12.4	9	38	1.66	235	100	2022	0.031	0.220	1.06	0.10	2.6
	1 jar	212	7.5	104	4.2	2.0	17.2	0.7	2.2	26.3	19	81	3.52	498	213	4287	0.066	0.467	2.26	0.21	5.6
VEGETABLES & TURKEY	7 tbsp	100	3.5	42	1.7	0.3	8.2	0.2	0.9	11.3	7	19	0.56	106	25	337	0.014	0.022	0.28	0.05	2.1
	1 jar	212	7.5	89	3.6	0.6	17.3	0.4	2.0	23.9	15	41	1.18	224	53	714	0.030	0.046	0.59	0.11	4.6
SUMMARY OF JR. VEGETABLES & MEAT COMBINATIONS	Average Values per Jar			120	4.8	2.9	18.5	0.5	2.1	28.8	29	67	1.26	319	142	1167	0.072	0.118	1.15	0.14	4.7
	% RDA (6-12 mo. infant)			13.3	20.9						4.8	13.4	8.4			77.8	14.4	19.7	14.4	35.0	13.4
	% RDA (1-2 year child)			10.9	19.2						4.1	9.6	8.4			58.3	12.0	19.7	14.4	28.0	11.7
	% Calories				16.1	21.9	62.0														

*All measures level   tbsp. = tablespoon   oz. = ounce   gm. = gram   mg. = milligram   I.U. = International Unit

Table A.22   JUNIOR MEATS
Average Nutrient Values per 100 Grams and per Jar

PRODUCT	MEASURE*	WEIGHT gm.	oz.	CAL-ORIES	PRO-TEIN gm.	FAT gm.	CARBO-HY-DRATE gm.	CRUDE FIBER gm.	ASH gm.	TOTAL SOLIDS gm.	CAL-CIUM mg.	PHOS-PHORUS mg.	IRON mg.	SODIUM mg.	POTAS-SIUM mg.	VITA-MIN A I.U.	THIA-MIN mg.	RIBO-FLAVIN mg.	NIACIN mg.	VITA-MIN B₆ mg.	ASCOR-BIC ACID mg.
BEEF	7 tbsp.	100	3.5	96	15.1	4.0	—	—	1.1	20.2	8	111	1.97	155	191	—	0.009	0.171	3.44	0.25	4.2
	1 jar	99	3.5	95	14.9	4.0	—	—	1.1	20.0	8	110	1.96	154	190	—	0.009	0.170	3.42	0.25	4.1
CHICKEN	7 tbsp.	100	3.5	135	14.6	8.3	0.5	—	1.0	24.4	28	122	1.61	208	123	—	0.016	0.215	3.79	0.32	3.0
	1 jar	99	3.5	133	14.4	8.2	0.5	—	1.0	24.1	27	121	1.60	206	122	—	0.016	0.213	3.75	0.32	3.0
CHICKEN STICKS	10 sticks	100	3.5	191	15.9	13.7	1.0	0.2	1.5	32.3	73	121	1.97	429	106	—	0.025	0.236	2.10	0.37	3.8
	1 jar*	70	2.5	134	11.1	9.6	0.7	0.1	1.0	22.5	51	84	1.38	300	74	—	0.018	0.179	1.47	0.26	2.7
HAM	7 tbsp.	100	3.5	117	14.9	6.1	0.6	—	1.2	22.8	6	128	1.36	206	222	—	0.165	0.175	2.83	0.39	3.6
	1 jar	99	3.5	116	14.8	6.0	0.6	—	1.2	22.6	6	127	1.35	204	219	—	0.164	0.174	2.80	0.39	3.6
LAMB	7 tbsp.	100	3.5	97	15.4	3.9	—	—	1.1	20.4	6	112	1.68	203	182	—	0.026	0.219	3.35	0.43	2.6
	1 jar	99	3.5	96	15.3	3.9	—	—	1.1	20.3	6	111	1.67	201	180	—	0.025	0.217	3.31	0.43	2.5
MEAT STICKS	10 sticks	100	3.5	164	15.7	10.7	1.1	0.2	1.4	29.1	35	103	2.00	465	114	—	0.149	0.217	1.53	0.17	2.9
	1 jar*	70	2.5	115	11.0	7.5	0.8	0.2	1.0	20.5	25	72	1.40	326	80	—	0.104	0.152	1.07	0.12	2.0
PORK	7 tbsp.	100	3.5	114	14.6	6.2	—	—	1.2	22.0	6	119	1.08	243	193	—	0.193	0.197	2.87	0.49	4.3
	1 jar	99	3.5	113	14.5	6.1	—	—	1.2	21.8	6	118	1.07	241	191	—	0.191	0.195	2.84	0.49	4.2
TURKEY	7 tbsp.	100	3.5	106	15.7	4.7	0.1	—	1.1	21.6	27	115	1.65	168	140	—	0.021	0.213	3.59	0.32	3.5
	1 jar	99	3.5	105	15.5	4.7	0.1	—	1.1	21.4	26	114	1.63	166	139	—	0.021	0.211	3.55	0.32	3.5
VEAL	7 tbsp.	100	3.5	100	15.6	4.2	—	—	1.1	20.9	6	120	1.27	168	204	—	0.019	0.191	3.86	0.30	4.2
	1 jar	99	3.5	99	15.4	4.2	—	—	1.1	20.7	6	119	1.26	166	202	—	0.019	0.190	3.83	0.30	4.2
SUMMARY OF JUNIOR MEATS	Average Values per Jar			112	14.1	6.0	0.3		1.1	21.5	18	108	1.48	220	155	—	0.063	0.189	2.89	0.32	3.3
	% RDA (6-12 mos. infant)			12.4	61.3						3.0	21.6	9.9				12.6	31.5	36.1	80.0	9.4
	% RDA (1-2 year child)			10.2	56.4						2.6	15.4	9.9				10.5	31.5	36.1	64.0	8.3
	% Calories				50.5	48.4	1.1														

*All measures level   tbsp. = tablespoon   oz. = ounce   gm. = gram   mg. = milligram   I.U. = International Unit   —— = quantity insignificant   * = 7 sticks per jar

Table A.23 *JUNIOR HIGH MEAT DINNERS*
Average Nutrient Values per 100 Grams and per Jar

PRODUCT	MEASURE*	WEIGHT gm.	oz.	CAL-ORIES	PRO-TEIN gm.	FAT gm.	CARBO-HY-DRATE gm.	CRUDE FIBER gm.	ASH gm.	TOTAL SOLIDS gm.	CAL-CIUM mg.	PHOS-PHORUS mg.	IRON mg.	SODIUM mg.	POTAS-SIUM mg.	VITA-MIN A I.U.	THIA-MIN mg.	RIBO-FLAVIN mg.	NIACIN mg.	VITA-MIN B_1 mg.	ASCOR-BIC ACID mg.
BEEF WITH VEGETABLES	7 tbsp.	100	3.5	82	6.5	3.6	6.0	0.3	1.1	17.5	8	60	0.99	218	108	369	0.026	0.078	1.45	0.20	2.5
	1 jar	128	4.5	105	8.4	4.6	7.6	0.3	1.5	22.4	10	77	1.27	279	138	473	0.033	0.099	1.86	0.26	3.1
CHICKEN WITH VEGETABLES	7 tbsp.	100	3.5	87	6.3	4.4	5.6	0.2	1.0	17.5	32	63	0.94	205	55	444	0.014	0.077	0.97	0.12	2.1
	1 jar	128	4.5	113	8.1	5.7	7.2	0.2	1.3	22.5	41	81	1.20	262	71	569	0.017	0.098	1.24	0.15	2.7
HAM WITH VEGETABLES	7 tbsp.	100	3.5	78	6.9	2.8	6.3	0.2	1.1	17.3	8	78	0.69	205	130	56	0.115	0.091	1.50	0.60	2.3
	1 jar	128	4.5	100	8.8	3.6	8.0	0.3	1.5	22.2	10	100	0.88	263	166	71	0.148	0.116	1.92	0.77	3.0
TURKEY WITH VEGETABLES	7 tbsp.	100	3.5	79	5.6	3.5	6.3	0.2	1.0	16.6	14	50	0.80	252	57	283	0.011	0.071	1.03	0.23	2.1
	1 jar	128	4.5	101	7.2	4.5	8.0	0.3	1.3	21.3	18	64	1.03	322	73	363	0.015	0.090	1.32	0.29	2.7
VEAL WITH VEGETABLES	7 tbsp.	100	3.5	64	6.3	1.2	7.1	0.3	1.2	16.1	8	68	0.76	226	128	239	0.031	0.093	1.78	0.13	2.8
	1 jar	128	4.5	83	8.1	1.6	9.0	0.4	1.5	20.6	10	87	0.97	289	164	306	0.040	0.119	2.27	0.17	3.6
SUMMARY OF JUNIOR HIGH MEAT DINNERS	Average Values per Jar			100	8.1	4.0	8.0	0.3	1.4	21.8	18	82	1.07	283	122	356	0.051	0.104	1.72	0.33	3.0
	% RDA (6-12 mos. infant)			11.1	35.2						3.0	16.4	7.1			23.7	10.2	17.3	21.5	82.5	8.6
	% RDA (1-2 year child)			9.1	32.4						2.6	11.7	7.1			17.8	8.5	17.3	21.5	66.0	7.5
	% Calories				32.3	35.9	31.9														

*All measures level   tbsp. = tablespoon   oz. = ounce   gm. = gram   mg. = milligram   I.U. = International Unit

Table A.24 *JUNIOR DESSERTS*
Average Nutrient Values per 100 Grams and per Jar

PRODUCT	MEASURE*	WEIGHT gm.	WEIGHT oz.	CAL-ORIES	PRO-TEIN gm.	FAT gm.	CARBO-HY-DRATE gm.	CRUDE FIBER gm.	ASH gm.	TOTAL SOLIDS gm.	CAL-CIUM mg.	PHOS-PHORUS mg.	IRON mg.	SO-DIUM mg.	POTAS-SIUM mg.	VITA-MIN A I.U.	THIA-MIN mg.	RIBO-FLAVIN mg.	NIACIN mg.	VITA-MIN B₆ mg.	ASCOR-BIC ACID mg.
BANANA PUDDING	7 tbsp.	100	3.5	96	0.9	0.7	21.4	0.6	0.5	24.1	8	24	0.51	124	52	24	0.019	0.052	0.10	0.09	1.5
	1 jar	220	7.8	210	2.1	1.6	46.9	1.3	1.1	53.0	18	52	1.11	273	114	53	0.043	0.114	0.22	0.20	3.4
BLUEBERRY BUCKLE	7 tbsp.	100	3.5	84	0.2	0.1	20.6	0.2	0.1	21.2	4	4	0.29	46	11	3	0.006	0.008	0.05	0.01	1.6
	1 jar	220	7.8	185	0.5	0.2	45.2	0.5	0.3	46.7	9	8	0.65	101	24	6	0.014	0.017	0.10	0.02	3.6
BUTTERSCOTCH PUDDING	7 tbsp.	100	3.5	92	1.7	1.3	18.3	0.4	0.7	22.4	50	53	0.35	120	52	2	0.014	0.195	0.04	0.02	2.4
	1 jar	212	7.5	195	3.6	2.8	38.9	0.8	1.4	47.5	105	112	0.75	254	110	4	0.029	0.413	0.09	0.04	5.0
CHERRY VANILLA PUDDING	7 tbsp.	100	3.5	86	0.3	0.7	19.7	0.1	0.2	21.0	7	7	0.27	50	36	129	0.009	0.036	0.04	—	2.1
	1 jar	220	7.8	190	0.8	1.6	43.0	0.3	0.5	46.2	16	16	0.59	110	78	284	0.020	0.080	0.10	—	4.6
CHOCOLATE CUSTARD PUDDING	7 tbsp.	100	3.5	95	2.1	1.5	18.2	0.5	0.7	23.0	57	61	0.42	100	70	226	0.014	0.143	0.05	0.03	2.2
	1 jar	220	7.8	208	4.5	3.3	40.1	1.0	1.6	50.5	125	135	0.93	221	153	479	0.031	0.314	0.12	0.07	4.7
COTTAGE CHEESE DESSERT WITH PINEAPPLE	7 tbsp.	100	3.5	91	3.1	1.2	16.9	0.1	0.3	21.6	22	27	0.10	137	21	41	0.020	0.030	0.04	0.02	9.1
	1 jar	220	7.8	199	6.8	2.6	37.2	0.2	0.7	47.5	48	59	0.22	301	46	90	0.044	0.066	0.09	0.04	20.0
DUTCH APPLE DESSERT	7 tbsp.	100	3.5	92	0.1	0.7	21.4	0.4	0.1	22.7	4	4	0.23	28	34	8	0.008	0.008	0.03	0.03	9.1
	1 jar	220	7.8	204	0.3	1.6	47.0	0.8	0.3	50.0	9	9	0.52	61	74	18	0.017	0.017	0.07	0.07	20.0
FRUIT DESSERT WITH TAPIOCA	7 tbsp.	100	3.5	92	0.3	0.1	22.4	0.2	0.3	23.3	7	8	0.44	41	90	124	0.014	0.011	0.17	0.04	2.8
	1 jar	220	7.8	202	0.6	0.3	49.2	0.5	0.6	51.2	16	18	0.97	91	197	274	0.030	0.024	0.36	0.09	6.2
PEACH COBBLER	7 tbsp.	100	3.5	87	0.4	0.1	21.2	0.3	0.2	22.2	4	9	0.22	17	61	64	0.008	0.014	0.31	0.02	9.1
	1 jar	220	7.8	192	0.9	0.3	46.4	0.7	0.4	48.7	9	19	0.49	38	134	141	0.019	0.030	0.68	0.04	20.0
RASPBERRY COBBLER	7 tbsp.	100	3.5	82	0.3	0.1	19.9	0.2	0.2	20.7	6	4	0.38	46	21	3	0.004	0.008	0.07	0.01	1.8
	1 jar	220	7.8	180	0.6	0.2	44.0	0.4	0.4	45.6	12	9	0.84	101	45	7	0.008	0.017	0.14	0.02	4.0
VANILLA CUSTARD PUDDING	7 tbsp.	100	3.5	95	1.9	1.7	18.0	0.6	0.7	22.9	54	54	0.29	108	65	228	0.017	0.118	0.04	0.03	1.4
	1 jar	212	7.5	202	4.0	3.5	38.5	1.2	1.4	48.6	114	114	0.61	229	139	483	0.035	0.251	0.08	0.06	3.0
SUMMARY OF JUNIOR DESSERTS	Average Values per Jar			197	2.2	1.6	43.3	0.7	0.8	48.7	44	50	0.70	162	101	167	0.026	0.122	0.19	0.06	8.6
	% RDA (6-12 mo. infant)			21.9	9.6						7.3	10.0	4.7			11.1	5.2	20.3	2.4	15.0	24.6
	% RDA (1-2 year child)			17.9	8.8						6.3	7.1	4.7			8.4	4.3	20.3	2.4	12.0	21.5
	% Calories				4.5	7.3	88.2														

Table A.25 *TODDLER MEALS* —
Average Nutrient Values per 100 Grams and per Jar

PRODUCT	MEASURE*	WEIGHT gm.	WEIGHT oz.	CAL-ORIES	PRO-TEIN gm.	FAT gm.	CARBO-HY-DRATE gm.	CRUDE FIBER gm.	ASH gm.	TOTAL SOLIDS gm.	CAL-CIUM mg.	PHOS-PHORUS mg.	IRON mg.	SODIUM mg.	POTAS-SIUM mg.	VITA-MIN A I.U.	THIA-MIN mg.	RIBO-FLAVIN mg.	NIACIN mg.	VITA-MIN B6 mg.	ASCOR-BIC ACID mg.
BEEF LASAGNA	7 tbsp.	100	3.5	76	4.3	2.3	9.5	0.2	1.3	17.6	17	55	0.82	434	88	808	0.052	0.065	1.05	0.07	2.4
	1 jar	177	6.2	135	7.6	4.1	16.8	0.4	2.3	31.2	30	96	1.46	768	155	1431	0.092	0.115	1.86	0.12	4.3
BEEF STEW	7 tbsp.	100	3.5	68	5.8	1.3	8.3	0.3	1.4	17.1	8	63	0.87	492	122	825	0.020	0.069	1.35	0.10	3.0
	1 jar	177	6.2	120	10.2	2.3	14.6	0.6	2.5	30.2	14	111	1.54	871	216	1460	0.035	0.122	2.39	0.17	5.3
CHICKEN STEW	7 tbsp.	100	3.5	75	4.8	2.4	8.5	0.3	1.3	17.3	31	62	0.72	421	64	875	0.030	0.075	0.98	0.07	2.4
	1 jar	170	6.0	128	8.2	4.1	14.5	0.5	2.2	29.5	52	105	1.23	716	109	1487	0.051	0.127	1.67	0.12	4.1
CREAMED POTATOES AND HAM	7 tbsp.	100	3.5	106	3.7	5.5	10.5	0.2	1.3	21.2	10	60	0.67	441	85	—	0.050	0.052	0.97	0.11	2.5
	1 jar	170	6.0	181	6.2	9.3	18.0	0.4	2.1	36.0	18	101	1.14	750	144	—	0.085	0.088	1.65	0.19	4.2
GREEN BEANS, POTATOES AND HAM CASSEROLE	7 tbsp.	100	3.5	79	2.3	3.4	9.7	0.4	1.2	17.0	13	44	0.53	419	84	96	0.044	0.046	0.69	0.09	4.2
	1 jar	177	6.2	139	4.2	6.0	17.1	0.7	2.1	30.1	22	77	0.94	742	148	170	0.078	0.082	1.22	0.16	7.5
MACARONI ALPHABETS AND BEEF CASSEROLE	7 tbsp.	100	3.5	83	6.5	1.8	10.1	0.3	1.6	20.3	43	95	1.02	497	103	200	0.037	0.105	1.18	0.06	3.0
	1 jar	177	6.2	146	11.5	3.1	18.0	0.6	2.8	36.0	76	168	1.81	881	182	354	0.066	0.186	2.09	0.11	5.3
SPAGHETTI AND MEAT BALLS	7 tbsp.	100	3.5	76	5.8	0.7	11.7	0.4	1.5	20.0	19	67	0.89	459	138	367	0.062	0.106	1.50	0.09	4.8
	1 jar	177	6.2	135	10.2	1.2	20.9	0.6	2.6	35.5	34	119	1.58	813	244	649	0.111	0.189	2.66	0.16	8.5
VEGETABLE AND TURKEY CASSEROLE	7 tbsp.	100	3.5	89	5.5	3.2	9.6	0.5	1.6	20.4	46	80	0.70	560	96	1692	0.027	0.107	0.74	0.08	5.1
	1 jar	177	6.2	158	9.7	5.6	17.2	0.8	2.9	36.2	82	142	1.25	991	170	2994	0.048	0.189	1.32	0.14	9.0
SUMMARY OF TODDLER MEALS	Average Values per Jar			143	8.5	4.5	17.1	0.6	2.4	33.1	41	115	1.37	816	171	1068	0.071	0.137	1.86	0.15	6.0
	% RDA (1-2 year child)			13.0	34.0						5.9	16.4	9.1			53.4	11.8	22.8	23.3	30.0	15.0
	% RDA (2-3 year child)			11.4	34.0						5.1	14.4	9.1			53.4	11.8	19.6	23.3	25.0	15.0
	% Calories				23.8	28.3	47.9														

*All measures level   tbsp. = tablespoon   oz. = ounce   gm. = gram   mg. = milligram   I.U. = International Unit   —— = quantity insignificant

NUTRITIVE VALUES OF THE EDIBLE PART OF FOODS (TABLE A.26)

The source of the data in Table A.26 is *Nutritive Value of Foods,* Home and Garden Bulletin 72, revised, U. S. Department of Agriculture, Washington, D. C. Data for some cooked and prepared foods are taken from Church and Church, *Food Values of Portions Commonly Used—Bowes and Church,* 9th ed., Lippincott, Philadelphia.

The abbreviation for trace (tr) is used to indicate fatty acid and vitamin values that would round to zero with the number of decimal places carried in these tables. For other components that would round to zero, a zero is used.

Dashes show that no basis could be found for imputing a value although there was some reason to believe that a measurable amount of the constituent might be present.

Other abbreviations used in Table A.26 are:

av—average	oz—ounce
c—cup	%—per cent
diam—diameter	pc—piece
hp—heaping	qt—quart
jc—juice	sc—section
lb—pound	serv—serving
lg—large	sl—slice
lv—leaves	sm—small
med—medium	sq—square
tbsp—tablespoon	

Table A.26   *Nutritive Values of the Edible Part of Foods*

Food	Weight, gm	Approximate Measure	Food Energy, Cal.	Pro-tein, gm	Fat (total lipid), gm
Almonds, shelled	142	1 c	850	26	77
Apple, raw	150	1 med	70	tr	tr
Apple brown betty	230	1 c	345	4	8
Apple butter	20	1 tbsp	37	tr	tr
Apple juice, bottled or canned	249	1 c	120	tr	tr
Applesauce, sweetened	254	1 c	230	1	tr
Apricots:					
raw	114	3 apricots	55	1	tr
sirup pack	259	1 c	220	2	tr
dried, uncooked	150	1 c	390	8	1
dried, cooked	285	1 c	240	5	1
Asparagus:					
fresh, cooked	175	1 c	35	4	tr
canned, green	96	6 spears	20	2	tr
Bacon:					
broiled or fried	16	2 sl	100	5	8
Canadian, cooked	21	1 sl	65	6	4
Banana, raw	150	1 med	85	1	tr
Beans:					
baked, with tomato sauce, with pork	261	1 c	320	16	7
baked, with tomato sauce, without pork	261	1 c	310	16	1
green snap, fresh cooked	125	1 c	30	2	tr
green snap, canned	239	1 c	45	2	tr
Lima, fresh, cooked	160	1 c	180	12	1
red kidney, canned	256	1 c	230	15	1
wax, canned	125	1 c	27	2	tr
Beef, cooked:					
cuts, braised, simmered, pot-roasted	72	2.5 oz, lean	140	22	5
cuts, braised, simmered, pot-roasted	85	3 oz, lean and fat	245	23	16
hamburger, ground lean	85	3 oz	185	23	10
hamburger, regular	85	3 oz	245	21	17
rib roast	51	1.8 oz, lean	125	14	7
rib roast	85	3 oz, lean and fat	375	17	34
round	78	2.7 oz, lean	125	24	3
round	85	3 oz, lean and fat	165	25	7
steak, sirloin	56	2 oz, lean	115	18	4
steak, sirloin	85	3 oz, lean and fat	330	20	27
Beef, canned:					
corned beef	85	3 oz	185	22	10
corned beef hash	85	3 oz	155	7	10

Table A.26 *(Continued)*

| | Fatty Acids | | | | | | | | | |
| Satur-ated (total), gm | Unsaturated | | Carbo-hydrate, gm | Cal-cium, mg | Iron, mg | Vitamin A Value, IU | Thia-min mg | Ribo-flavin, mg | Niacin, mg | Ascorbic Acid, mg |
	Oleic, gm	Lino-leic, gm								
6	52	15	28	332	6.7	0	0.34	1.31	5.0	tr
—	—	—	18	8	0.4	50	0.04	0.02	0.1	3
4	3	tr	68	41	1.4	230	0.13	0.10	0.9	3
—	—	—	9	3	0.1	0	tr	tr	tr	tr
—	—	—	30	15	1.5	—	0.01	0.04	0.2	2
—	—	—	60	10	1.3	100	0.05	0.03	0.1	3
—	—	—	14	18	0.5	2890	0.03	0.04	0.7	10
—	—	—	57	28	0.8	4510	0.05	0.06	0.9	10
—	—	—	100	100	8.2	16350	0.02	0.23	4.9	19
—	—	—	62	63	5.1	8550	0.01	0.13	2.8	8
—	—	—	6	37	1.0	1580	0.27	0.32	2.4	46
—	—	—	3	18	1.8	770	0.06	0.10	0.8	14
3	4	1	1	2	0.5	0	0.08	0.05	0.8	—
—	—	—	3	4	—	0	0.18	0.03	1.1	0
—	—	—	23	8	0.7	190	0.05	0.06	0.7	10
3	3	1	50	141	4.7	340	0.20	0.08	1.5	5
—	—	—	60	177	5.2	160	0.18	0.09	1.5	5
—	—	—	7	62	0.8	680	0.08	0.11	0.6	16
—	—	—	10	81	2.9	690	0.08	0.10	0.7	9
—	—	—	32	75	4.0	450	0.29	0.16	2.0	28
—	—	—	42	74	4.6	tr	0.13	0.10	1.5	—
—	—	—	6	45	2.1	150	0.05	0.06	0.5	6
2	2	tr	0	10	2.7	10	0.04	0.16	3.3	—
8	7	tr	0	10	2.9	30	0.04	0.18	3.5	—
5	4	tr	0	10	3.0	20	0.08	0.20	5.1	—
8	8	tr	0	9	2.7	30	0.07	0.18	4.6	—
3	3	tr	0	6	1.8	10	0.04	0.11	2.6	—
16	15	1	0	8	2.2	70	0.05	0.13	3.1	—
1	1	tr	0	10	3.0	tr	0.06	0.18	4.3	—
3	3	tr	0	11	3.2	10	0.06	0.19	4.5	—
2	2	tr	0	7	2.2	10	0.05	0.14	3.6	—
13	12	1	0	9	2.5	50	0.05	0.16	4.0	—
5	4	tr	0	17	3.7	20	0.01	0.20	2.9	—
5	4	tr	9	11	1.7	—	0.01	0.08	1.8	—

Table A.26   *(Continued)*

Food	Weight, gm	Approximate Measure	Food Energy, Cal.	Pro- tein, gm	Fat (total lipid), gm
Beef, dried or chipped	57	2 oz	115	19	4
Beef and vegetable stew	235	1 c	210	15	10
Beef potpie	227	1 pie, 4¼″ diam	560	23	33
Beer, av 3.6% alcohol	240	1 c	100	1	0
Beets, cooked, diced	165	1 c	50	2	tr
Beet greens, cooked	100	½ c	27	2	tr
Beverages, carbonated:					
cola type	240	1 c	95	0	0
gingerale	230	1 c	70	0	0
Biscuit, enriched flour	38	1, 2½″ diam	140	3	6
Blackberries, raw	144	1 c	85	2	1
Blueberries, raw	140	1 c	85	1	1
Bluefish, baked or broiled	85	3 oz	135	22	4
Bouillon cubes	4	1 cube	5	1	tr
Brains, all kinds, raw	85	3 oz	106	9	7
Bran, raisin	28	⅔ c	99	2	tr
Bran flakes, 40%	28	1 oz	85	3	1
Brazilnuts, shelled	140	1 c	915	20	94
Bread:					
Boston, enriched	48	1 sl	100	3	1
cracked-wheat	23	1 sl	60	2	1
French or Vienna, enriched	454	1 lb	1315	41	14
Italian, enriched	454	1 lb	1250	41	4
raisin, enriched	23	1 sl	60	2	1
rye, American	23	1 sl	55	2	tr
rye, pumpernickle	454	1 lb	1115	41	5
white, enriched	23	1 sl	60	2	1
white, unenriched	23	1 sl	60	2	1
whole wheat	23	1 sl	55	2	1
Breadcrumbs, dry	88	1 c	345	11	4
Broccoli, cooked	150	1 c	40	5	tr
Brussels sprouts, cooked	130	1 c	45	5	1
Buckwheat flour, light	98	1 c	342	6	1
Butter:					
stick, ⅛	14	1 tbsp	100	tr	11
pat or square	7	1 pat	50	tr	6
Buttermilk, cultured, skim	246	1 c	90	9	tr
Cabbage:					
raw	100	1 c	25	1	tr
cooked	170	1 c	35	2	tr
Chinese, raw	100	1 c	15	1	tr

[1] Calcium may not be usable because of presence of oxalic acid.
[2] Year-round average.

Table A.26 *(Continued)*

Fatty Acids

Saturated (total), gm	Unsaturated Oleic, gm	Linoleic, gm	Carbohydrate, gm	Calcium, mg	Iron, mg	Vitamin A Value, IU	Thiamin, mg	Riboflavin, mg	Niacin, mg	Ascorbic Acid, mg
2	2	tr	0	11	2.9	—	0.04	0.18	2.2	—
5	4	tr	15	28	2.8	2310	0.13	0.17	4.4	15
9	20	2	43	32	4.1	1860	0.25	0.27	4.5	7
—	—	—	9	12	tr	—	0.01	0.07	1.6	—
—	—	—	12	23	0.8	40	0.04	0.07	0.5	11
—	—	—	6	118[1]	3.2	6700	0.08	0.18	0.4	34
—	—	—	24	—	—	0	0	0	0	0
—	—	—	18	—	—	0	0	0	0	0
2	3	1	17	46	0.6	tr	0.08	0.08	0.7	tr
—	—	—	19	46	1.3	290	0.05	0.06	0.5	30
—	—	—	21	21	1.4	140	0.04	0.08	0.6	20
—	—	—	0	25	0.6	40	0.09	0.08	1.6	—
—	—	—	tr	—	—	—	—	—	—	—
—	—	—	1	14	3.1	0	0.20	0.22	3.7	15
—	—	—	22	0	1.0	0	0.10	—	1.1	0
—	—	—	23	20	1.2	0	0.11	0.05	1.7	0
19	45	24	15	260	4.8	tr	1.34	0.17	2.2	—
—	—	—	22	43	0.9	0	0.05	0.03	0.6	0
—	—	—	12	20	0.3	tr	0.03	0.02	0.3	tr
3	8	2	251	195	10.0	tr	1.26	0.98	11.3	tr
tr	1	2	256	77	10.0	0	1.31	0.93	11.7	0
—	—	—	12	16	0.3	tr	0.01	0.02	0.2	tr
—	—	—	12	17	0.4	0	0.04	0.02	0.3	0
—	—	—	241	381	10.9	0	1.05	0.63	5.4	0
tr	tr	tr	12	16	0.6	tr	0.06	0.04	0.5	tr
tr	tr	tr	12	16	0.2	tr	0.02	0.02	0.3	tr
tr	tr	tr	11	23	0.5	tr	0.06	0.03	0.7	tr
1	2	1	65	107	3.2	tr	0.19	0.26	3.1	tr
—	—	—	7	132	1.2	3750	0.14	0.29	1.2	135
—	—	—	8	42	1.4	680	0.10	0.18	1.1	113
—	—	—	78	11	1.0	0	0.08	0.04	0.4	0
6	4	tr	tr	3	0	460[2]	—	—	—	0
3	2	tr	tr	1	0	230[2]	—	—	—	0
—	—	—	13	298	0.1	10	0.09	0.44	0.2	2
—	—	—	5	49	0.4	130	0.05	0.05	0.3	47
—	—	—	7	75	0.5	220	0.07	0.07	0.5	56
—	—	—	3	43	0.6	150	0.05	0.04	0.6	25

Table A.26 *(Continued)*

Food	Weight, gm	Approximate Measure	Food Energy, Cal.	Pro- tein, gm	Fat (total lipid), gm
Cakes:					
angelfood	40	2″ sc, ⅟₁₂ of 8″ diam	110	3	tr
chocolate, chocolate icing	120	2″ sc, ⅟₁₆ of 10″ diam	445	5	20
cupcake, with chocolate icing	50	1, 2¾″ diam	185	2	7
cupcake, without icing	40	1, 2¾″ diam	145	2	6
fruitcake, dark	30	1 pc, 2″ x 2″ x ½″	115	1	5
plain, with chocolate icing	100	2″ sc, ⅟₁₆ of 10″ diam	370	4	14
plain, without icing	55	1 pc, 3″ x 2″ x 1½″	200	2	8
pound	30	1 sl, 2¾″ x 3″ x ⅝″	140	2	9
sponge	40	2″ sc, ⅟₁₂ of 8″ diam	120	3	2
Candy:					
butterscotch	5	1 pc	21	0	tr
caramels	28	1 oz	115	1	3
chocolate almond bar	32	1 bar	176	3	12
chocolate, milk	28	1 oz	150	2	9
chocolate cream	13	1 pc	51	1	2
fondant	11	1 av	4	—	—
fudge, plain	28	1 oz	115	1	3
hard	28	1 oz	110	0	tr
marshmallow	28	1 oz	90	1	tr
peanut brittle	25	1 pc	110	2	4
Cantaloupe, raw	385	½ of 5″ melon	60	1	tr
Carrots:					
raw	110	1 c, grated	45	1	tr
cooked	145	1 c, diced	45	1	tr
Cashew nuts	135	1 c	760	23	62
Cauliflower:					
raw	100	1 c	25	2	tr
cooked	120	1 c	25	3	tr
Celery:					
raw	100	1 c, diced	15	1	tr
cooked	65	½ c, diced	12	1	tr
Cheese:					
blue or Roquefort type	28	1 oz	105	6	9
Camembert	28	1 oz	84	5	7
Cheddar or American	17	1″ cube	70	4	5
Cheddar or American	112	1 c, grated	445	28	36
Cheddar, process	28	1 oz	105	7	9

[3] If the fat used in the recipe is butter or fortified margarine, the vitamin A value for chocolate cake with fudge icing will be 490 IU; 100 IU for fruit cake; 300 IU for plain cake without icing; 220 IU per cupcake; 400 IU for plain cake with icing; 220 IU per cupcake with icing; and 300 IU for pound cake.

Table A.26   *(Continued)*

Fatty Acids										
Satur-	Unsaturated					Vitamin				
ated		Lino-	Carbo-	Cal-		A	Thia-	Ribo-		Ascorbic
(total),	Oleic,	leic,	hydrate,	cium,	Iron,	Value,	min	flavin,	Niacin,	Acid,
gm	gm	gm	gm	mg	mg	IU	mg	mg	mg	mg
—	—	—	24	4	0.1	0	tr	0.06	0.1	0
8	10	1	67	84	1.2	190[3]	0.03	0.12	0.3	tr
2	4	tr	30	32	0.3	90[3]	0.01	0.04	0.1	tr
1	3	tr	22	26	0.2	70[3]	0.01	0.03	0.1	tr
1	3	1	18	22	0.8	40[3]	0.04	0.04	0.2	tr
5	7	1	59	63	0.6	180[3]	0.02	0.09	0.2	tr
2	5	1	31	35	0.2	90[3]	0.01	0.05	0.1	tr
2	5	1	14	6	0.2	80[3]	0.01	0.03	0.1	0
1	1	tr	22	12	0.5	180[3]	0.02	0.06	0.1	tr
—	—	—	4	1	0.1	0	0	tr	tr	0
2	1	tr	22	42	0.4	tr	0.01	0.05	tr	tr
—	—	—	16	68	0.9	40	0.03	0.16	0.3	tr
5	3	tr	16	65	0.3	80	0.02	0.09	0.1	tr
—	—	—	9	—	—	—	—	—	—	—
—	—	—	10	—	—	—	—	—	—	—
2	1	tr	21	22	0.3	tr	0.01	0.03	0.1	tr
—	—	—	28	6	0.5	0	0	0	0	0
—	—	—	23	5	0.5	0	0	tr	tr	0
—	—	—	18	10	0.5	7	0.02	0.12	1.2	0
—	—	—	14	27	0.8	6540[4]	0.08	0.06	1.2	63
—	—	—	11	41	0.8	12100	0.06	0.06	0.7	9
—	—	—	10	48	0.9	15220	0.08	0.07	0.7	9
10	43	4	40	51	5.1	140	0.58	0.33	2.4	—
—	—	—	5	22	1.1	90	0.11	0.10	0.6	69
—	—	—	5	25	0.8	70	0.11	0.10	0.7	66
—	—	—	4	39	0.3	240	0.03	0.03	0.3	9
—	—	—	2	33	0.3	0	0.03	0.02	0.2	3
5	3	tr	1	89	0.1	350	0.01	0.17	0.1	0
—	—	—	1	29	0.1	286	0.01	0.21	0.3	0
3	2	tr	tr	128	0.2	220	tr	0.08	tr	0
20	12	1	2	840	1.1	1470	0.03	0.51	0.1	0
5	3	tr	1	219	0.3	350	tr	0.12	tr	0

[4] Value based on varieties with orange-colored flesh, for green-fleshed varieties value is about 540 IU per ½ melon.

Table A.26 *(Continued)*

Food	Weight, gm	Approximate Measure	Food Energy, Cal.	Pro-tein, gm	Fat (total lipid), gm
foods, Cheddar	28	1 oz	90	6	7
cottage, creamed	225	1 c	240	31	9
cream	15	1 tbsp	55	1	6
Limburger	28	1 oz	97	6	8
Parmesan	28	1 oz	110	10	7
Swiss	28	1 oz	105	8	8
Cherries:					
raw, sweet, with stems[5]	130	1 c	80	2	tr
canned, red, sour, pitted,					
heavy sirup	260	1 c	230	2	1
Chicken:					
broiled	85	3 oz, flesh only	115	20	3
canned, boneless	85	3 oz	170	18	10
creamed	118	½ c, sm serv	208	18	12
fryer, breast, fried	94	½ breast, with bone	155	25	5
fryer, leg, fried	59	with bone	90	12	4
potpie	227	1 pie, 4¼″ diam	535	23	31
roasted	80	2 sl, 3″ x 3″ x ¼″	158	23	7
Chili con carne (no beans)	255	1 c	510	26	38
Chili sauce	17	1 tbsp	20	tr	tr
Chocolate:					
bitter or baking	28	1 oz	145	3	15
sweet	28	1 oz	150	1	10
Chocolate-flavored milk drink	250	1 c	190	8	6
Chocolate sirup	20	1 tbsp	50	tr	tr
Clams:					
raw	85	3 oz	65	11	1
canned, solids and liquid	85	3 oz	45	7	1
Cocoa beverage with milk	242	1 c	235	9	11
Coconut:					
dried, sweetened	62	1 c, shredded	340	2	24
fresh	97	1 c, shredded	335	3	34
Coleslaw	120	1 c	120	1	9
Cookies:					
plain and assorted	25	1 cooky, 3″ diam	120	1	5
wafers	10	2 wafers, 2⅛″ diam	49	1	2
Corn:					
fresh, cooked	140	1 ear, 5″ long	70	3	1
canned	256	1 c	170	5	2
Corn flakes	28	1 oz	110	2	tr

[5] Measure and weight apply to entire vegetable or fruit including parts not usually eaten.

Table A.26 *(Continued)*

Fatty Acids										
Satur-ated (total), gm	Unsaturated		Carbo-hydrate, gm	Cal-cium, mg	Iron, mg	Vitamin A Value, IU	Thia-min mg	Ribo-flavin, mg	Niacin, mg	Ascorbic Acid, mg
	Oleic, gm	Lino-leic, gm								
4	2	tr	2	162	0.2	280	0.01	0.16	tr	0
5	3	tr	7	212	0.7	380	0.07	0.56	0.2	0
3	2	tr	tr	9	tr	230	tr	0.04	tr	0
—	—	—	1	165	0.2	358	0.02	0.14	0.1	0
—	—	—	1	325	0.1	297	tr	0.20	0.1	0
4	3	tr	1	262	0.3	320	tr	0.11	tr	0
—	—	—	20	26	0.5	130	0.06	0.07	0.5	12
—	—	—	59	36	0.8	1680	0.07	0.06	0.4	13
1	1	1	0	8	1.4	80	0.05	0.16	7.4	—
3	4	2	0	18	1.3	200	0.03	0.11	3.7	3
—	—	—	7	83	1.1	328	0.04	0.18	3.8	tr
1	2	1	1	9	1.3	70	0.04	0.17	11.2	—
1	2	1	tr	6	0.9	50	0.03	0.15	2.7	—
10	15	3	42	68	3.0	3020	0.25	0.26	4.1	5
—	—	—	0	16	1.7	0	0.06	0.14	7.2	0
18	17	1	15	97	3.6	380	0.05	0.31	5.6	—
—	—	—	4	3	0.1	240	0.02	0.01	0.3	3
8	6	tr	8	22	1.9	20	0.01	0.07	0.4	0
6	4	tr	16	27	0.4	tr	0.01	0.04	0.1	tr
3	2	tr	27	270	0.4	210	0.09	0.41	0.2	2
tr	tr	tr	13	3	0.3	—	tr	0.01	0.1	0
—	—	—	2	59	5.2	90	0.08	0.15	1.1	8
—	—	—	2	47	3.5	—	0.01	0.09	0.9	—
6	4	tr	26	286	0.9	390	0.09	0.45	0.4	2
21	2	tr	33	10	1.2	0	0.02	0.02	0.2	0
29	2	tr	9	13	1.6	0	0.05	0.02	0.5	3
2	2	5	9	52	0.5	180	0.06	0.06	0.3	35
—	—	—	18	9	0.2	20	0.01	0.01	0.1	tr
—	—	—	7	—	—	—	—	—	—	—
—	—	—	16	2	0.5	310[6]	0.09	0.08	1.0	7
—	—	—	40	10	1.0	690[6]	0.07	0.12	2.3	13
—	—	—	24	5	0.4	0	0.12	0.02	0.6	0

[6] Based on yellow varieties; white varieties contain only a trace of cryptoxanthin and carotenes, the pigments in corn that have biological activity.

Table A.26 *(Continued)*

Food	Weight, gm	Approximate Measure	Food Energy, Cal.	Pro-tein, gm	Fat (total lipid), gm
Corn grits:					
enriched, cooked	242	1 c	120	3	tr
unenriched, cooked	242	1 c	120	3	tr
Corn muffin, enriched	48	1 med, 2¾" diam	150	3	5
Cornmeal, white or yellow, dry:					
enriched	145	1 c	525	11	2
unenriched	118	1 c	420	11	5
Crabmeat, canned	85	3 oz	85	15	2
Crackers:					
Graham	14	2 med	55	1	1
saltines	8	2 crackers	35	1	1
soda, plain	11	2 crackers	50	1	1
Cranberry sauce, sweetened	277	1 c	405	tr	1
Cream:					
half-and-half	15	1 tbsp	20	tr	2
heavy or whipping	15	1 tbsp	55	tr	6
light or coffee	15	1 tbsp	30	tr	3
Cucumber, raw	50	6 sl	5	tr	tr
Custard, baked	248	1 c	285	13	14
Dandelion greens, cooked	180	1 c	60	4	1
Dates, fresh and dried	178	1 c	490	4	1
Doughnut, cake type	32	1 doughnut	125	1	6
Eggs:					
raw, whole	50	1 med	80	6	6
boiled	100	2 med	160	13	12
scrambled	64	1 med	110	7	8
Farina, enriched, cooked	238	1 c	100	3	tr
Fats, cooking, vegetable	12.5	1 tbsp	110	0	12
Figs, dried	21	1 fig	60	1	tr
Fig bars	16	1 sm	55	1	1
Fishsticks, breaded, cooked	227	10 sticks	400	38	20
Fruit cocktail, canned	256	1 c	195	1	1
Gelatin, dry, plain	10	1 tbsp	35	9	tr
Gelatin dessert:					
plain	239	1 c	140	4	0
with fruit	241	1 c	160	3	tr
Gingerbread	55	1 pc, 2" x 2" x 2"	175	2	6

[7] Vitamin A value based on yellow product; white product contains only a trace.

[8] Iron, thiamine, riboflavin, and niacin are based on the minimal level of enrichment specified in standards of identity promulgated under the Federal Food, Drug, and Cosmetic Act.

[9] Based on recipe using white cornmeal; if yellow cornmeal is used, the vitamin A value is 140 IU per muffin.

Table A.26 *(Continued)*

Fatty Acids										
Satur-ated (total), gm	Unsaturated		Carbo-hydrate, gm	Cal-cium, mg	Iron, mg	Vitamin A Value, IU	Thia-min mg	Ribo-flavin, mg	Niacin, mg	Ascorbic Acid, mg
	Oleic, gm	Lino-leic, gm								
—	—	—	27	2	0.7[8]	150[7]	0.10[8]	0.07[8]	1.0[8]	0
—	—	—	27	2	0.2	150[7]	0.05	0.02	0.5	0
2	2	tr	23	50	0.8	80[9]	0.09	0.11	0.8	tr
tr	1	1	114	9	4.2[8]	640[7]	0.64[8]	0.38[8]	5.1[8]	0
1	2	2	87	24	2.8	600[7]	0.45	0.13	2.4	0
—	—	—	1	38	0.7	—	0.07	0.07	1.6	—
—	—	—	10	6	0.2	0	0.01	0.03	0.2	0
—	—	—	6	2	0.1	0	tr	tr	0.1	0
tr	1	tr	8	2	0.2	0	tr	tr	0.1	0
—	—	—	104	17	0.6	40	0.03	0.03	0.1	5
1	1	tr	1	16	tr	70	tr	0.02	tr	tr
3	2	tr	tr	11	tr	230	tr	0.02	tr	tr
2	1	tr	1	15	tr	130	tr	0.02	tr	tr
—	—	—	2	8	0.2	tr	0.02	0.02	0.1	6
6	5	1	28	278	1.0	870	0.10	0.47	0.2	1
—	—	—	12	252	3.2	21060	0.24	0.29	—	32
—	—	—	130	105	5.3	90	0.16	0.17	3.9	0
1	4	tr	16	13	0.4[10]	30	0.05[10]	0.05[10]	0.4[10]	tr
2	3	tr	tr	27	1.1	590	0.05	0.15	tr	0
4	5	1	1	54	2.3	1180	0.09	0.28	0.1	0
3	3	tr	1	51	1.1	690	0.05	0.18	tr	0
—	—	—	21	10	0.7[11]	0	0.11[11]	0.07[11]	1.0[11]	0
3	8	1	0	0	0	—	0	0	0	0
—	—	—	15	26	0.6	20	0.02	0.02	0.1	0
—	—	—	12	12	0.2	20	0.01	0.01	0.1	tr
5	4	10	15	25	0.9	—	0.09	0.16	3.6	—
—	—	—	50	23	1.0	360	0.04	0.03	1.1	5
—	—	—	—	—	—	—	—	—	—	—
—	—	—	34	—	—	—	—	—	—	—
—	—	—	40	—	—	—	—	—	—	—
1	4	tr	29	37	1.3	50	0.06	0.06	0.5	0

[10] Based on product made with enriched flour. With unenriched flour, approximate values per doughnut are: iron, 0.2 mg; thiamine, 0.01 mg; riboflavin, 0.03 mg; niacin, 0.2 mg.
[11] Iron, thiamine, riboflavin, and niacin are based on the minimum levels of enrichment specified in standards of identity promulgated under the Federal Food, Drug, and Cosmetic Act.

Table A.26　*(Continued)*

Food	Weight, gm	Approximate Measure	Food Energy, Cal.	Pro-tein, gm	Fat (total lipid), gm
Grapefruit:					
raw, white	285	½ med, 4¼″ diam	55	1	tr
raw, white	194	1 c, sc	75	1	tr
juice, canned	247	1 c, unsweetened	100	1	tr
juice, dehydrated,					
water added	247	1 c	100	1	tr
Grapes:					
Concord, Niagara	153	1 c	65	1	1
Muscat, Thompson, Tokay	160	1 c	95	1	tr
Grape juice, bottled	254	1 c	165	1	tr
Grapenut flakes	28	1 oz	110	3	tr
Gravy, meat, brown	18	1 tbsp	41	tr	4
Haddock, fried	85	3 oz	140	17	5
Heart, beef, lean, braised	85	3 oz	160	27	5
Herring:					
Atlantic, broiled	85	1 med	217	21	14
smoked, kippered	100	½ fish	211	22	13
Honey, strained or extracted	21	1 tbsp	65	tr	0
Honeydew melon	150	1 wedge, 2″ x 6½″	48	1	0
Ice cream, plain	71	1 sl, or ⅛ qt brick	145	3	9
Ice milk	187	1 c	285	9	10
Jams and preserves	20	1 tbsp	55	tr	tr
Jellies	20	1 tbsp	55	tr	tr
Kale, cooked	110	1 c	30	4	1
Kohlrabi, cooked	75	½ c	23	2	tr
Lamb:					
chop, cooked	137	1 chop, 4.8 oz	400	25	33
leg, roasted	71	2.5 oz, lean	130	20	5
shoulder, roasted	64	2.3 oz, lean	130	17	6
Lard	14	1 tbsp	125	0	14
Lemon	106	1 med	20	1	tr
Lemon juice, fresh	15	1 tbsp	5	tr	tr
Lettuce:					
head, Iceberg	454	1 head, 4¼″ diam	60	4	tr
leaves	50	2 lg	10	1	tr
Lime juice, fresh	246	1 c	65	1	tr
Liver:					
beef, fried	57	2 oz	130	15	6
calf, cooked	72	2 sl, 3″ x 2¼″ x ⅜″	147	16	7
pork, fried	74	2 sl, 3″ x 2¼″ x ⅜″	170	18	7
Lobster:					
boiled or broiled	334	1 (¾ lb) + 2 tbsp butter	308	20	25
canned	85	½ c	75	15	1

Table A.26   *(Continued)*

Fatty Acids										
Satur-	Unsaturated					Vitamin				
ated (total), gm	Oleic, gm	Lino- leic, gm	Carbo- hydrate, gm	Cal- cium, mg	Iron, mg	A Value, IU	Thia- min mg	Ribo- flavin, mg	Niacin, mg	Ascorbic Acid, mg
—	—	—	14	22	0.6	10	0.05	0.02	0.2	52
—	—	—	20	31	0.8	20	0.07	0.03	0.3	72
—	—	—	24	20	1.0	20	0.07	0.04	0.4	84
—	—	—	24	22	0.2	20	0.10	0.05	0.5	92
—	—	—	15	15	0.4	100	0.05	0.03	0.2	3
—	—	—	25	17	0.6	140	0.07	0.04	0.4	6
—	—	—	42	28	0.8	—	0.10	0.05	0.6	tr
—	—	—	23	—	1.2	0	0.13	—	1.6	0
—	—	—	2	—	0.2	0	0.15	0.01	tr	—
1	3	tr	5	34	1.0	—	0.03	0.06	2.7	2
—	—	—	1	5	5.0	20	0.21	1.04	6.5	1
—	—	—	0	—	1.2	130	0.01	0.15	3.3	0
—	—	—	0	66	1.4	0	tr	0.28	2.9	0
—	—	—	17	1	0.1	0	tr	0.01	0.1	tr
—	—	—	13	26	0.6	60	0.08	0.05	0.3	34
5	3	tr	15	87	0.1	370	0.03	0.13	0.1	1
6	3	tr	42	292	0.2	390	0.09	0.41	0.2	2
—	—	—	14	4	0.2	tr	tr	0.01	tr	tr
—	—	—	14	4	0.3	tr	tr	0.01	tr	1
—	—	—	4	147	1.3	8140	—	—	—	68
—	—	—	5	35	0.5	tr	0.03	0.03	0.2	28
18	12	1	0	10	1.5	—	0.14	0.25	5.6	—
3	2	tr	0	9	1.4	—	0.12	0.21	4.4	—
3	2	tr	0	8	1.0	—	0.10	0.18	3.7	—
5	6	1	0	0	0	0	0	0	0	0
—	—	—	6	18	0.4	10	0.03	0.01	0.1	38
—	—	—	1	1	tr	tr	tr	tr	tr	7
—	—	—	13	91	2.3	1500	0.29	0.27	1.3	29
—	—	—	2	34	0.7	950	0.03	0.04	0.2	9
—	—	—	22	22	0.5	30	0.05	0.03	0.3	80
—	—	—	3	6	5.0	30280	0.15	2.37	9.4	15
—	—	—	3	5	9.0	19130	0.13	2.39	11.7	15
—	—	—	8	10	15.6	12070	0.25	2.30	12.4	10
—	—	—	1	80	0.7	920	0.11	0.06	2.3	0
—	—	—	0	55	0.7	—	0.03	0.06	1.9	

Table A.26 *(Continued)*

Food	Weight, gm	Approximate Measure	Food Energy, Cal.	Pro- tein, gm	Fat (total lipid), gm
Macaroni:					
enriched, cooked	130	1 c	190	6	1
unenriched, cooked	130	1 c	190	6	1
Macaroni & cheese, baked	220	1 c	470	18	24
Mackerel, canned	85	3 oz	155	18	9
Malted milk beverage	270	1 c	280	13	12
Mangos	100	1 sm	66	1	tr
Margarine:					
stick, ⅛	14	1 tbsp	100	tr	11
pat or sq	7	1 pat	50	tr	6
Metrecal	237	8 oz	225	18	5
Milk:					
whole	244	1 c	160	9	9
nonfat, skim	246	1 c	90	9	tr
dry, nonfat, instant	70	1 c	250	25	tr
condensed	306	1 c	980	25	27
evaporated	252	1 c	345	18	20
Molasses:					
light	20	1 tbsp	50	—	—
blackstrap	20	1 tbsp	45	—	—
Muffins, white, enriched	48	1 med, 2¾" diam	140	4	5
Mushrooms, canned	244	1 c	40	5	tr
Mustard greens, cooked	140	1 c	35	3	1
Noodles:					
enriched, cooked	160	1 c	200	7	2
unenriched, cooked	160	1 c	200	7	2
Oats, puffed	28	1 oz	115	3	2
Oatmeal, cooked	236	1 c	130	5	2
Oils, salad, corn	14	1 tbsp	125	0	14
Okra, cooked	85	8 pods	25	2	tr
Olives:					
green, pickled	16	4 med	15	tr	2
ripe, pickled	10	3 sm	15	tr	2
Onions:					
raw	110	1 onion, 2½" diam	40	2	tr
cooked	210	1 c	60	3	tr
young green	50	6 onions	20	1	tr
Orange:					
navel	180	1 med	60	2	tr

[12] Iron, thiamine, riboflavin, and niacin are based on the minimum levels of enrichment specified in standards of identity promulgated under the Federal Food, Drug, and Cosmetic Act.

[13] Based on the average vitamin A content of fortified margarine. Federal specifications for

Table A.26 *(Continued)*

Fatty Acids

Saturated (total), gm	Unsaturated Oleic, gm	Unsaturated Linoleic, gm	Carbohydrate, gm	Calcium, mg	Iron, mg	Vitamin A Value, IU	Thiamin, mg	Riboflavin, mg	Niacin, mg	Ascorbic Acid, mg
—	—	—	39	14	1.4[12]	0	0.23[12]	0.14[12]	1.9[12]	0
—	—	—	39	14	0.6	0	0.02	0.02	0.5	0
11	10	1	44	398	2.0	950	0.22	0.44	2.0	tr
—	—	—	0	221	1.9	20	0.02	0.28	7.4	—
—	—	—	32	364	0.8	670	0.17	0.56	0.2	2
—	—	—	17	9	0.2	6350	0.06	0.06	0.9	41
2	6	2	tr	3	0	460[13]	—	—	—	0
1	3	1	tr	1	0	230[13]	—	—	—	0
—	—	—	28	500	3.8	1250	0.50	0.75	3.8	25
5	3	tr	12	288	0.1	350	0.08	0.42	0.1	2
—	—	—	13	298	0.1	10	0.10	0.44	0.2	2
—	—	—	36	905	0.4	20	0.24	1.25	0.6	5
15	9	1	166	802	0.3	1090	0.23	1.17	0.5	3
11	7	1	24	635	0.3	820	0.10	0.84	0.5	3
—	—	—	13	33	0.9	—	0.01	0.01	tr	—
—	—	—	11	137	3.2	—	0.02	0.04	0.4	—
1	3	tr	20	50	0.8	50	0.08	0.11	0.7	tr
—	—	—	6	15	1.2	tr	0.04	0.60	4.8	4
—	—	—	6	193	2.5	8120	0.11	0.19	0.9	68
1	1	tr	37	16	1.4[14]	110	0.23[14]	0.14[14]	1.8[14]	0
1	1	tr	37	16	1.0	110	0.04	0.03	0.7	0
tr	1	1	21	50	1.3	0	0.28	0.05	0.5	0
tr	1	1	23	21	1.4	0	0.19	0.05	0.3	0
1	4	7	0	0	0	—	0	0	0	0
—	—	—	5	78	0.4	420	0.11	0.15	0.8	17
tr	2	tr	tr	8	0.2	40	—	—	—	—
tr	2	tr	tr	9	0.1	10	tr	tr	—	—
—	—	—	10	30	0.6	40	0.04	0.04	0.2	11
—	—	—	14	50	0.8	80	0.06	0.06	0.4	14
—	—	—	5	20	0.3	tr	0.02	0.02	0.2	12
—	—	—	16	49	0.5	240	0.12	0.05	0.5	75

fortified margarine require a minimum of 15000 IU of vitamin A per pound.

[14] Iron, thiamine, riboflavin, and niacin are based on the minimum levels of enrichment specified in standards of identity promulgated under the Federal Food, Drug, and Cosmetic Act.

Table A.26   *(Continued)*

Food	Weight, gm	Approximate Measure	Food Energy, Cal.	Protein, gm	Fat (total lipid), gm
other varieties	210	1 med	75	1	tr
sections	97	½ c	44	1	tr
juice, fresh	247	1 c	100	1	tr
juice, frozen	248	1 c	110	2	tr
juice, dehydrated, water added	248	1 c	115	1	tr
Orange and grapefruit juice, frozen	248	1 c	110	1	tr
Ocean perch, breaded, fried	85	3 oz	195	16	11
Oyster meat, raw	240	1 c	160	20	4
Oyster stew	230	1 c with 3–4 oysters	200	11	12
Pancakes:					
white, enriched	27	1 cake, 4″ diam	60	2	2
buckwheat	27	1 cake, 4″ diam	55	2	2
Papayas, raw	182	1 c	70	1	tr
Parsley, raw, chopped	3.5	1 tbsp	1	tr	tr
Parsnips, cooked	155	1 c	100	2	1
Peaches:					
raw	114	1 med	35	1	tr
raw	168	1 c, sliced	65	1	tr
canned, sirup pack	257	1 c	200	1	tr
dried, cooked	270	1 c	220	3	1
frozen	340	12-oz carton	300	1	tr
Peanuts, roasted	9	1 tbsp	55	2	4
Peanut butter	16	1 tbsp	95	4	8
Pears:					
raw	182	1 med	100	1	1
canned, sirup pack	255	1 c	195	1	1
Peas, green:					
fresh, cooked	160	1 c	115	9	1
canned	249	1 c	165	9	1
Pecans, chopped	7.5	1 tbsp	50	1	5
Peppers, green, raw	62	1 med	15	1	tr
Pickles:					
dill	135	1 pickle, 4″ long	15	1	tr
relish	13	1 tbsp	14	tr	tr
sour	30	1 sl, 1½″ diam x 1″	3	tr	tr
sweet	20	1 pickle, 2¾″ long	30	tr	tr
Pies:					
apple	135	⅐ of 9″ pie	345	3	15

[15] Based on yellow-fleshed varieties; for white-fleshed varieties value is about 50 IU per 114-gm peach and 80 IU per cup of sliced peaches.
[16] Average weight in accordance with commercial freezing practices. For products without

Table A.26 *(Continued)*

Fatty Acids										
Satur-ated (total), gm	Unsaturated		Carbo-hydrate, gm	Cal-cium, mg	Iron, mg	Vitamin A Value, IU	Thia-min mg	Ribo-flavin, mg	Niacin, mg	Ascorbic Acid, mg
	Oleic, gm	Lino-leic, gm								
—	—	—	19	67	0.3	310	0.16	0.06	0.6	70
—	—	—	11	32	0.4	180	0.08	0.03	0.3	48
—	—	—	23	25	0.5	490	0.22	0.06	0.9	127
—	—	—	27	22	0.2	500	0.21	0.03	0.8	112
—	—	—	27	25	0.5	500	0.20	0.06	0.9	108
—	—	—	26	20	0.2	270	0.16	0.02	0.8	102
—	—	—	6	28	1.1	—	0.08	0.09	1.5	—
—	—	—	8	226	13.2	740	0.33	0.43	6.0	—
—	—	—	11	269	3.3	640	0.13	0.41	1.6	—
tr	1	tr	9	27	0.4	30	0.05	0.06	0.3	tr
1	1	tr	6	59	0.4	60	0.03	0.04	0.2	tr
—	—	—	18	36	0.5	3190	0.07	0.08	0.5	102
—	—	—	tr	7	0.2	300	tr	0.01	tr	6
—	—	—	23	70	0.9	50	0.11	0.13	0.2	16
—	—	—	10	9	0.5	1320[15]	0.02	0.05	1.0	7
—	—	—	16	15	0.8	2230[15]	0.03	0.08	1.6	12
—	—	—	52	10	0.8	1100	0.02	0.06	1.4	7
—	—	—	58	41	5.1	3290	0.01	0.15	4.2	6
—	—	—	77	14	1.7	2210	0.03	0.14	2.4	135[16]
1	2	1	2	7	0.2	—	0.03	0.01	1.5	0
2	4	2	3	9	0.3	—	0.02	0.02	2.4	0
—	—	—	25	13	0.5	30	0.04	0.07	0.2	7
—	—	—	50	13	0.5	tr	0.03	0.05	0.3	4
—	—	—	19	37	2.9	860	0.44	0.17	3.7	33
—	—	—	31	50	4.2	1120	0.23	0.13	2.2	22
tr	3	1	1	5	0.2	10	0.06	0.01	0.1	tr
—	—	—	3	6	0.4	260	0.05	0.05	0.3	79
—	—	—	3	35	1.4	140	tr	0.03	tr	8
—	—	—	3	2	0.2	14	0	tr	tr	1
—	—	—	1	8	0.4	93	tr	0.02	tr	2
—	—	—	7	2	0.2	20	tr	tr	tr	1
4	9	1	51	11	0.4	40	0.03	0.02	0.5	1

added ascorbic acid, value is about 37 mg per 12-oz carton and 50 mg per 16-oz carton; for those with added ascorbic acid, 139 mg per 12-oz carton and 186 mg per 16-oz carton.

Table A.26 *(Continued)*

Food	Weight, gm	Approximate Measure	Food Energy, Cal.	Pro-tein, gm	Fat (total lipid), gm
cherry	135	⅐ of 9″ pie	355	4	15
custard	130	⅐ of 9″ pie	280	8	14
lemon meringue	120	⅐ of 9″ pie	305	4	12
mince	135	⅐ of 9″ pie	365	3	16
pumpkin	130	⅐ of 9″ pie	275	5	15
Piecrust, plain, baked	135	1, 9″ crust	675	8	45
Pimentos, canned	38	1 med	10	tr	tr
Pineapple:					
raw	140	1 c, diced	75	1	tr
canned, sirup pack	260	1 c, crushed	195	1	tr
canned, sirup pack	122	2 sm sl + 2 tbsp jc	90	tr	tr
juice, canned	249	1 c	135	1	tr
Pizza, cheese	75	5½″ sector	185	7	6
Plums:					
raw	60	1 plum, 2″ diam	25	tr	tr
canned, sirup pack	122	3 plums + 2 tbsp jc	100	tr	tr
Popcorn, popped	14	1 c	65	1	3
Pork:					
chop, cooked	98	1 chop, 3.5 oz	260	16	21
ham, cured	85	3 oz	245	18	19
ham, fresh, lean	107	2 sl, 2″ x 1½″ x 1″	254	40	9
boiled ham	57	2 oz	135	11	10
Potatoes:					
baked	99	1 med	90	3	tr
French fried	57	10 pc	155	2	7
hash-browned	100	½ c	241	3	12
mashed	195	1 c with milk	125	4	1
mashed	195	1 c with milk & butter	185	4	8
Potato chips	20	10 chips	115	1	8
Pretzels	5	5 sm sticks	20	tr	tr
Prunes:					
dried, uncooked	32	4 prunes	70	1	tr
dried, cooked, sirup	270	1 c (17–18 prunes)	295	2	1
juice, canned	256	1 c	200	1	tr
Puddings:					
chocolate	144	½ c	219	5	7
lemon snow	130	1 serv	114	3	tr
tapioca	132	½ c	181	5	5
vanilla	248	1 c	275	9	10
Pumpkin, canned	228	1 c	75	2	1
Radishes, raw	40	4 sm	5	tr	tr
Raisins, dried	160	1 c	460	4	tr
Raspberries, red, raw	123	1 c	70	1	1
Rhubarb, cooked, sugar added	272	1 c	385	1	tr

Table A.26 *(Continued)*

Saturated (total), gm	Unsaturated Oleic, gm	Unsaturated Linoleic, gm	Carbohydrate, gm	Calcium, mg	Iron, mg	Vitamin A Value, IU	Thiamin, mg	Riboflavin, mg	Niacin, mg	Ascorbic Acid, mg
4	10	1	52	19	0.4	590	0.03	0.23	0.6	1
5	8	1	30	125	0.8	300	0.07	0.21	0.4	0
4	7	1	45	17	0.6	200	0.04	0.10	0.2	4
4	10	1	56	38	1.4	tr	0.09	0.05	0.5	1
5	7	1	32	66	0.6	3210	0.04	0.15	0.6	tr
10	29	3	59	19	2.3	0	0.27	0.19	2.4	0
—	—	—	2	3	0.6	870	0.01	0.02	0.1	36
—	—	—	19	24	0.7	100	0.12	0.04	0.3	24
—	—	—	50	29	0.8	120	0.20	0.06	0.5	17
—	—	—	24	13	0.4	50	0.09	0.03	0.2	8
—	—	—	34	37	0.7	120	0.12	0.04	0.5	22
2	3	tr	27	107	0.7	290	0.04	0.12	0.7	4
—	—	—	7	7	0.3	140	0.02	0.02	0.3	3
—	—	—	26	11	1.1	1470	0.03	0.02	0.5	2
2	tr	tr	8	1	0.3	—	—	0.01	0.2	0
8	9	2	0	8	2.2	0	0.63	0.18	3.8	—
7	8	2	0	8	2.2	0	0.40	0.16	3.1	—
—	—	—	0	7	2.5	0	0.69	0.33	5.4	0
4	4	1	0	6	1.6	0	0.25	0.09	1.5	—
—	—	—	21	9	0.7	tr	0.10	0.04	1.7	20
2	2	4	20	9	0.7	tr	0.07	0.04	1.8	12
—	—	—	32	18	1.2	30	0.08	0.06	1.7	7
—	—	—	25	47	0.8	50	0.16	0.10	2.0	19
4	3	tr	24	47	0.8	330	0.16	0.10	1.9	18
2	2	4	10	8	0.4	tr	0.04	0.01	1.0	3
—	—	—	4	1	0	0	tr	tr	tr	0
—	—	—	18	14	1.1	440	0.02	0.04	0.4	1
—	—	—	78	60	4.5	1860	0.08	0.18	1.7	2
—	—	—	49	36	10.5	—	0.02	0.03	1.1	4
—	—	—	37	147	0.2	196	0.05	0.22	0.2	0
—	—	—	27	4	0.1	0	tr	0.02	tr	10
—	—	—	28	151	0.6	195	0.05	0.21	0.6	0
5	3	tr	39	290	0.1	390	0.07	0.40	0.1	2
—	—	—	18	57	0.9	14590	0.07	0.12	1.3	12
—	—	—	1	12	0.4	tr	0.01	0.01	0.1	10
—	—	—	124	99	5.6	30	0.18	0.13	0.9	2
—	—	—	17	27	1.1	160	0.04	0.11	1.1	31
—	—	—	98	212	1.6	220	0.06	0.15	0.7	17

Table A.26 *(Continued)*

Food	Weight, gm	Approximate Measure	Food Energy, Cal.	Protein, gm	Fat (total lipid), gm
Rice:					
parboiled, cooked	176	1 c	185	4	tr
puffed	14	1 c	55	1	tr
white, cooked	168	1 c	185	3	tr
Rice flakes	30	1 c	115	2	tr
Rolls:					
plain, enriched	38	12 per lb	115	3	2
plain, unenriched	38	12 per lb	115	3	2
sweet	43	1 roll	135	4	4
Rutabagas, cooked	100	½ c	38	1	tr
Rye flour, light	80	1 c	285	8	1
Salads:					
apple, celery, walnut	154	3 hp tbsp, 2 lv lettuce	137	2	8
carrot & raisin	134	3 hp tbsp, 2 lv lettuce	153	2	6
fruit, fresh	195	3 hp tbsp, 2 lv lettuce	174	2	11
gelatin with fruit	188	1 sq, 2 lv lettuce	139	2	6
gelatin with vegetable	164	1 sq, 2 lv lettuce	115	2	6
lettuce, tomato, mayonnaise	115	4 lv lettuce, 3 sl tomato	80	2	6
potato	123	½ c, French dressing	184	2	11
Salad dressings:					
blue cheese	16	1 tbsp	80	1	8
commercial, plain	15	1 tbsp	65	tr	6
French	15	1 tbsp	60	tr	6
home cooked, boiled	17	1 tbsp	30	1	2
mayonnaise	15	1 tbsp	110	tr	12
Thousand Island	15	1 tbsp	75	tr	8
Salmon, pink, canned	85	3 oz	120	17	5
Sardines, Atlantic	85	3 oz	175	20	9
Sauerkraut, canned	235	1 c	45	2	tr
Sausage:					
bologna	227	8 sl	690	27	62
frankfurter, cooked	51	1 frankfurter	155	6	14
liverwurst	30	1 sl, 3″ diam x ¼″	79	5	6
pork, links or patty, cooked	113	4 oz	540	21	50
Vienna	18	1 av, 2″ x ¾″ diam	39	3	3
Scallops, fried	145	5–6 med pc	427	24	28
Shad, baked	85	3 oz	170	20	10
Sherbet, orange	193	1 c	260	2	2
Shortbread	16	2 pc, 58 per lb	78	1	3

[17] Iron, thiamine, and niacin are based on the minimum levels of enrichment specified in standards of identity promulgated under the Federal Food, Drug, and Cosmetic Act. Riboflavin based on unenriched rice. When the minimum level of enrichment for riboflavin speci-

Table A.26 *(Continued)*

Saturated (total), gm	Oleic, gm	Linoleic, gm	Carbohydrate, gm	Calcium, mg	Iron, mg	Vitamin A Value, IU	Thiamin, mg	Riboflavin, mg	Niacin, mg	Ascorbic Acid, mg
	Fatty Acids — Unsaturated									
—	—	—	41	33	1.4[17]	0	0.19[17]	0.02[17]	2.0[17]	0
—	—	—	13	3	0.3	0	0.06	0.01	0.6	0
—	—	—	41	17	1.5[17]	0	0.19[17]	0.01[17]	1.6[17]	0
—	—	—	26	9	0.5	0	0.10	0.02	1.6	0
tr	1	tr	20	28	0.7	tr	0.11	0.07	0.8	tr
tr	1	tr	20	28	0.3	tr	0.02	0.03	0.3	tr
1	2	tr	21	37	0.3	30	0.03	0.06	0.4	0
—	—	—	9	55	0.4	330	0.07	0.08	0.9	36
—	—	—	62	18	0.9	0	0.12	0.06	0.5	0
—	—	—	16	32	0.8	355	0.08	0.08	0.4	5
—	—	—	28	48	1.5	4708	0.08	0.08	0.5	6
—	—	—	21	45	0.8	685	0.08	0.09	0.4	32
—	—	—	22	23	0.5	391	0.04	0.05	0.3	16
—	—	—	15	24	0.5	1977	0.04	0.06	0.3	8
—	—	—	7	20	0.8	1115	0.06	0.07	0.5	19
—	—	—	21	21	0.8	243	0.07	0.04	0.8	16
2	2	4	1	13	tr	30	tr	0.02	tr	tr
1	1	3	2	2	tr	30	tr	tr	tr	—
1	1	3	3	2	0.1	—	—	—	—	—
1	1	tr	3	15	0.1	80	0.01	0.03	tr	tr
2	3	6	tr	3	0.1	40	tr	0.01	tr	—
1	2	4	2	2	0.1	50	tr	tr	tr	tr
1	1	tr	0	167[18]	0.7	60	0.03	0.16	6.8	—
1	—	—	0	372	2.5	190	0.02	0.17	4.6	—
—	—	—	9	85	1.2	120	0.07	0.09	0.4	33
—	—	—	2	16	4.1	—	0.36	0.49	6.0	—
—	—	—	1	3	0.8	—	0.08	0.10	1.3	—
—	—	—	1	3	1.6	1725	0.05	0.34	1.4	0
18	21	5	tr	8	2.7	0	0.89	0.39	4.2	—
—	—	—	0	2	0.4	0	0.02	0.02	0.6	0
—	—	—	19	41	3.1	0	0.09	0.17	2.3	0
—	—	—	0	20	0.5	20	0.11	0.22	7.3	—
—	—	—	59	31	tr	110	0.02	0.06	tr	4
—	—	—	11	2	tr	0	0.01	tr	tr	0

fied in the standards of identity becomes effective the value will be 0.12 mg per cup of parboiled rice and of white rice.

[18] Based on total contents of can. If bones are discarded, value will be greatly reduced.

Table A.26   *(Continued)*

Food	Weight, gm	Approximate Measure	Food Energy, Cal.	Pro-tein, gm	Fat (total lipid), gm
Shrimp, canned	85	3 oz	100	21	1
Sirups, table blends	20	1 tbsp	60	0	0
Soups:					
bean	250	1 c	170	8	6
beef	250	1 c	100	6	4
beef noodle	250	1 c	70	4	3
beef bouillon, broth, consomme	240	1 c	30	5	0
chicken	250	1 c	75	4	2
chicken noodle	250	1 c	65	4	2
clam chowder	255	1 c	85	2	3
cream, mushroom	240	1 c	135	2	10
pea, green	245	1 c	130	6	2
tomato	245	1 c	90	2	2
vegetable with beef broth	250	1 c	80	3	2
vegetable-beef	203	1 serv, 3 from can	64	6	2
Soy flour, medium fat	88	1 c	232	37	6
Spaghetti:					
enriched, cooked	140	1 c	155	5	1
unenriched, cooked	140	1 c	155	5	1
in tomato sauce	250	1 c with cheese	260	9	9
Italian style	292	1 serv, with meat sauce	396	13	21
Italian style	302	1 serv, as above with grated cheese	436	15	24
Spinach	180	1 c	40	5	1
Squash:					
summer, cooked	210	1 c	30	2	tr
winter, cooked	205	1 c	130	4	1
Strawberries:					
raw	149	1 c	55	1	1
frozen	284	10-oz carton	310	1	1
Sugar:					
brown	14	1 tbsp	50	0	0
maple	15	1 pc, 1¼″ x 1″ x ½″	52	—	—
white, granulated	12	1 tbsp	45	0	0
white, powdered	8	1 tbsp	30	0	0
Sweet potatoes:					
baked	110	1 med, 5″ x 2″	155	2	1
candied	175	1 sm, 3½″ x 2¼″	295	2	6
Tangerine	114	1 med	40	1	tr

[19] Iron, thiamine, riboflavin, and niacin are based on the minimum levels of enrichment specified in standards of identity promulgated under the Federal Food, Drug, and Cosmetic Act.

Table A.26   *(Continued)*

Satur-ated (total), gm	Unsaturated Oleic, gm	Unsaturated Lino-leic, gm	Carbo-hydrate, gm	Cal-cium, mg	Iron, mg	Vitamin A Value, IU	Thia-min mg	Ribo-flavin, mg	Niacin, mg	Ascorbic Acid, mg
—	—	—	1	98	2.6	50	0.01	0.03	1.5	—
—	—	—	15	9	0.8	0	0	0	0	0
1	2	2	22	62	2.2	650	0.14	0.07	1.0	2
2	2	tr	11	15	0.5	—	—	—	—	—
1	1	1	7	8	1.0	50	0.05	0.06	1.1	tr
0	0	0	3	tr	0.5	tr	tr	0.02	1.2	—
1	1	tr	10	20	0.5	—	0.02	0.12	1.5	—
tr	1	1	8	10	0.5	50	0.02	0.02	0.8	tr
—	—	—	13	36	1.0	920	0.03	0.03	1.0	—
1	3	5	10	41	0.5	70	0.02	0.12	0.7	tr
1	1	tr	23	44	1.0	340	0.05	0.05	1.0	7
tr	1	1	16	15	0.7	1000	0.06	0.05	1.1	12
—	—	—	14	20	0.8	3250	0.05	0.02	1.2	—
—	—	—	6	5	0.5	2340	0.03	0.04	0.8	—
—	—	—	33	215	11.4	100	0.72	0.30	2.3	0
—	—	—	32	11	1.3[19]	0	0.19[19]	0.11[19]	1.5[19]	0
—	—	—	32	11	0.6	0	0.02	0.02	0.4	0
2	5	1	37	80	2.2	1080	0.24	0.18	2.4	14
—	—	—	39	27	2.1	901	0.12	0.12	3.0	24
—	—	—	40	99	2.2	1041	0.12	0.16	3.0	24
—	—	—	6	167	4.0	14580	0.13	0.25	1.0	50
—	—	—	7	52	0.8	820	0.10	0.16	1.6	21
—	—	—	32	57	1.6	8610	0.10	0.27	1.4	27
—	—	—	13	31	1.5	90	0.04	0.10	0.9	88
—	—	—	79	40	2.0	90	0.06	0.17	1.5	150
—	—	—	13	12	0.5	0	tr	tr	tr	0
—	—	—	14	27	0.5	—	—	—	—	—
—	—	—	12	0	tr	0	0	0	0	0
—	—	—	8	0	tr	0	0	0	0	0
—	—	—	36	44	1.0	8910	0.10	0.07	0.7	24
2	3	1	60	65	1.6	11030	0.10	0.08	0.8	17
—	—	—	10	34	0.3	350	0.05	0.02	0.1	26

Table A.26 *(Continued)*

Food	Weight, gm	Approximate Measure	Food Energy, Cal.	Protein, gm	Fat (total lipid), gm
Tomatoes:					
raw	150	1 med	35	2	tr
canned	242	1 c	50	2	tr
Tomato juice, canned	242	1 c	45	2	tr
Tomato catsup	17	1 tbsp	15	tr	tr
Tongue, beef, simmered	85	3 oz	210	18	14
Tuna, canned, drained	85	3 oz	170	24	7
Turkey, roasted	100	3 sl, 3″ x 2½″ x ¼″	200	31	8
Turnips, cooked, diced	155	1 c	35	1	tr
Turnip greens, cooked	145	1 c	30	3	tr
Veal:					
chop, loin, cooked	122	1 med	514	28	44
cutlet, broiled	85	3 oz	185	23	9
roast	85	3 oz	230	23	14
Vinegar	15	1 tbsp	2	0	—
Waffles, baked	75	1 waffle, ½″ x 4½″ x 5½″	210	7	7
Walnuts, English	8	1 tbsp, chopped	50	1	5
Watermelon:					
raw	100	½ c cubes	28	1	tr
raw	925	1 wedge, 4″ x 8″	115	2	1
Wheat:					
puffed	28	1 oz	105	4	tr
shredded	28	1 oz	100	3	1
Wheat flakes	28	1 oz	100	3	tr
Wheat flours:					
all-purpose or family, enriched	110	1 c, sifted	400	12	1
all-purpose or family, unenriched	110	1 c, sifted	400	12	1
cake or pastry flour	110	1 c, sifted	365	8	1
self-rising, enriched	110	1 c	385	10	1
whole wheat	120	1 c	400	16	2
Wheat germ	68	1 c	245	18	7
White sauce, medium	265	1 c	430	10	33
Yeast, brewer's, dry	8	1 tbsp	25	3	tr
Yoghurt	246	1 c	120	8	4

Table A.26 *(Continued)*

Fatty Acids

Saturated (total), gm	Unsaturated Oleic, gm	Unsaturated Linoleic, gm	Carbohydrate, gm	Calcium, mg	Iron, mg	Vitamin A Value, IU	Thiamin, mg	Riboflavin, mg	Niacin, mg	Ascorbic Acid, mg
—	—	—	7	20	0.8	1350	0.10	0.06	1.0	34[20]
—	—	—	10	15	1.2	2180	0.13	0.07	1.7	40
—	—	—	10	17	2.2	1940	0.13	0.07	1.8	39
—	—	—	4	4	0.1	240	0.02	0.01	0.3	3
—	—	—	tr	6	1.9	—	0.04	0.25	3.0	—
—	—	—	0	7	1.6	70	0.04	0.10	10.1	—
—	—	—	0	30	5.1	tr	0.08	0.17	9.8	0
—	—	—	8	54	0.6	tr	0.06	0.08	0.5	33
—	—	—	5	267	1.6	9140	0.21	0.36	0.8	100
—	—	—	0	7	3.5	0	0.17	0.26	5.8	0
5	4	tr	—	9	2.7	—	0.06	0.21	4.6	—
7	6	tr	0	10	2.9	—	0.11	0.26	6.6	—
—	—	—	1	1	0.1	—	—	—	—	—
2	4	1	28	85	1.3	250	0.13	0.19	1.0	tr
tr	1	3	1	8	0.2	tr	0.03	0.01	0.1	tr
—	—	—	7	7	0.2	590	0.05	0.05	0.2	6
—	—	—	27	30	2.1	2510	0.13	0.13	0.7	30
—	—	—	22	8	1.2	0	0.15	0.07	2.2	0
—	—	—	23	12	1.0	0	0.06	0.03	1.3	0
—	—	—	23	12	1.2	0	0.18	0.04	1.4	0
tr	tr	tr	84	18	3.2[21]	0	0.48[21]	0.29[21]	3.8[21]	0
tr	tr	tr	84	18	0.9	0	0.07	0.05	1.0	0
tr	tr	tr	79	17	0.5	0	0.03	0.03	0.7	0
tr	tr	tr	82	292	3.2[21]	0	0.49[21]	0.29[21]	3.9[21]	0
tr	1	1	85	49	4.0	0	0.66	0.14	5.2	0
1	2	4	32	49	6.4	0	1.36	0.46	2.9	0
18	11	1	23	305	0.5	1220	0.12	0.44	0.6	tr
—	—	—	3	17	1.4	tr	1.25	0.34	3.0	tr
2	1	tr	13	295	0.1	170	0.09	0.43	0.2	2

[20] Year-round average. Samples marketed from November through May average around 15 mg per 150-gm tomato; from June through October, around 39 mg.

[21] Iron, thiamine, riboflavin, and niacin are based on the minimum level of enrichment specified in the standards of identity promulgated under the Federal Food, Drug, and Cosmetic Act.

Glossary

Amino acids — The basic building blocks of protein; contain an organic acid radical and an amino radical.

Amylase — Enzyme that breaks down starch into smaller molecules.

Amylose — The fraction of starch that is in a straight chain.

Anabolism — Synthesis of new compounds in the body.

Anemia — A condition in which the red blood cells are abnormal either in number, shape, or size. Iron deficiency anemia is characterized by a low hemoglobin count; large red blood cells (immature) may be the result of folacin or vitamin B_{12} deficiency.

Apatite — Crystalline masses that form the structure of bones and teeth, and contain a variety of chemical substances such as calcium, phosphate, fluoride, and hydroxyl ions.

Arteriosclerosis — Disease in which the walls of the arteries become hardened and thickened.

Ascorbic acid — A synonym for vitamin C.

Atherosclerosis — Type of arteriosclerosis; fatty substances such as cholesterol form mushy deposits in the arteries and partially obstruct blood flow.

Basal metabolic rate — Rate at which energy is used in the body to maintain vital body functions; measured in a resting, post-absorptive state.

Beriberi — Condition characterized by disturbances of nerve function; caused by a deficiency of thiamin.

Biotin — A water soluble vitamin in the B complex.

Blastogenesis — Transmission of inherited characteristics via germ plasm; trophoblastic (external) cells and internal cells are formed and separated by fluid.

Blastocyst – Embryonic cell of a mammal.

Blood serum – Fluid, colorless plasma remaining when the cells, clotting factor, and fibrin have been removed from the blood.

Calciferol – Synonym for vitamin D.

calorie – Heat required to raise the temperature of a gram of water at an atmosphere of pressure a degree Celsius.

Calorie – Heat required to raise the temperature of a kilogram of water at an atmosphere of pressure a degree Celsius. This unit is synonymous with kilocalorie and is a thousand times larger than a calorie.

Carbohydrates – Organic compounds containing carbon, hydrogen, and oxygen, with the ratio of hydrogen to oxygen being two to one. Starch and sugar are examples.

Carotenes – Yellow pigments that can be converted into vitamin A in the body; sometimes called provitamin A.

Catabolism – Process of breaking down complex compounds in the body.

Catalyst – Compound capable of altering the speed of a chemical reaction without being changed during the reaction.

Cellulose – Complex carbohydrate (polysaccharide) found in plants and important as roughage in man's diet.

Cheilosis – Lesions on the lips and cracks at corners of mouth; condition caused by riboflavin deficiency.

Cholesterol – Steroid alcohol found in some foods and also manufactured in the body; occurs in mushy deposits in arteries in cases of atherosclerosis.

Chorionic villi – Villi (small convolutions) in the outer membrane of the placenta; contain capillaries which transport the nutrients absorbed through these villi to the fetus.

Cobalamin – Synonym for vitamin B_{12}; indicates the cobalt atom found in the vitamin molecule.

Coenzyme A – Compound containing pantothenic acid; required for metabolism of fats.

Collagen – Type of connective tissue in the body.

Colostrum – Thin, somewhat yellow fluid secreted during the first few days of lactation prior to the development of mature human milk.

Cytochrome system – Iron-containing enzymes functioning in the release of energy in the body.

Deamination – Removal of the amino (nitrogen-containing) group from an amino acid.

Decalcification – Loss of calcium from bones and/or teeth.

Dermatitis – Inflammation of the skin.

Diglyceride – Fat molecule containing two fatty acids.

Disaccharide – Sugars that are composed of two monosaccharides united into a single molecule by the loss of a molecule of water. Lactose is a disaccharide found in milk.

DNA – Deoxyribonucleic acid.

Eclampsia – Severe toxemia in pregnancy; convulsions are symptomatic.

Ectoderm – Outer germinal layer formed during the embryonic period; brain, nervous system, outer skin, hair, and nails develop from this layer.

Edema – Accumulation of fluid in the tissues.

Embryo – The developing being, from implantation to the end of the second month of pregnancy (in humans).

Emulsify – To form an emulsion.

Emulsion – Colloidal dispersion of two immiscible liquids; suspension of small droplets of a liquid (such as an oil) in another liquid (such as water).

Endemic – Occurring with some constancy in a geographic region.

Endocrine gland – Any of the glands comprising the endocrine system; a gland that secretes hormones in the body.

Endoderm – Inner germinal layer formed during the embryonic period; inner linings of the digestive and respiratory tracts and the glands (including liver and pancreas) develop from this layer.

Enzymes – Proteins that catalyze reactions in the body.

Epiphysis – The bony formation that gradually replaces cartilage at the ends of bones.

Epithelium – Outer layer of skin and mucous membranes.

Essential fatty acid – Linoleic acid; fatty acid needed by the body and which must be supplied by the diet because the body cannot synthesize this specific unsaturated fatty acid.

FAD – Flavin-adenine dinucleotide.

Fatty acid – Organic acid which can combine with glycerol to form a fat.

Fetus – Developing, unborn being; fetal period for humans is from third month to birth.

Flavin-adenine dinucleotide – Coenzyme required for normal cellular respiration; contains riboflavin. Synonym is FAD.

Flavoprotein – Protein containing riboflavin; functions in release of energy in the body.

Fluorapatite – Fluoride-containing compound which gives strength to bones and teeth.

Fluoridation – Process of regulating fluoride level in water at a desirable level, normally at 1 part fluoride per million parts of water.

Fluorosis – Condition characterized by a mottled appearance of the teeth caused by a very high intake of fluoride over an extended period of time.

Folacin – Also termed folic acid; one of the water soluble B vitamins.

Fructose – A simple sugar or monosaccharide; a specific carbohydrate.

Galactose – A simple sugar resulting from the breakdown of lactose in milk; a specific carbohydrate.

Gestation – Pregnancy.

Gastrulation – Formation of the three germinal layers during the embryonic period.

Glucagon – Pancreatic hormone that releases glucose from storage in the liver.

Glucose – A simple sugar or monosaccharide; a specific carbohydrate. The type of sugar found in the blood; the most common of the monosaccharides.

Glyceride – Fatty compound formed when glycerol and fatty acids are combined.

Glycogen – Polysaccharide; form in which carbohydrate is stored in man and animals. Starch is the counterpart in plants.

Goiter – Enlargement of the thyroid gland in the throat; caused by lack of iodine.

Hemoglobin – Iron-containing protein in red blood cells.

Hemosiderosis – Condition caused by toxic levels of iron in the diet.

Hormone – Compound secreted by an endocrine gland that influences the functioning of an organ in another part of the body.

Hydrogenation – Addition of hydrogen to an unsaturated fatty acid; process raises the melting point and increases the firmness of the fatty acid.

Hydrolysis – Chemical splitting of a compound by the addition of a water molecule.

Hydroxyapatite – Structural compound of bones and teeth; can be replaced by fluorapatite, a harder compound, when fluoride is available.

Hypercalcemia – Excessive calcium in the blood.

Hypervitaminosis – Condition caused by an excessive intake of a vitamin; vitamin A and vitamin D excesses have been found to lead to this condition.

Keratin – Insoluble structural protein in epidermis, hair, and nails.

Ketone bodies – Compounds (acetone, acetoacetic acid, and beta-hydroxybutyric acid) which cause ketosis when they accumulate in the body; can lead to coma and even death.

Ketosis – Condition caused by the accumulation of ketone bodies; occurs when insufficient carbohydrate derivatives are available for normal metabolism of fats in the body.

Kilocalorie – Amount of heat required to raise a kilogram of water at an atmosphere of pressure a degree Celsius; synonymous with Calorie.

Kwashiorkor – Condition in children caused by inadequate intake of protein.

Lactase – Enzyme required for digestion of lactose, the sugar in milk.

Lactation – Production of milk by the mammary glands.

Lacunae – Intervillous spaces in the placenta containing the maternal blood supply to the placenta.

Linoleic acid – Essential fatty acid; contains 18 carbons and 3 double bonds.

Lipase – Enzyme that digests fats.

Lipids – Organic compounds composed of carbon, hydrogen, and oxygen; fat or fatlike substances.

Lipoprotein – Compound containing a lipid and a protein.

Macrocytic anemia – Condition in which the red blood cells fail to mature, hence the cells remain large.

Marasmus – Condition caused by a severely restricted caloric (and usually protein) intake; starvation.

Megaloblastic anemia – Blood condition in which the red blood cells do not mature.

Melanin – Dark pigments in skin and hair.

Mesoderm – Middle germinal layer formed during the embryonic period; voluntary muscles, excretory system, the covering of internal organs, inner skin layer, circulatory system (including heart), and bones and cartilage develop from this layer.

Metabolism – Chemical changes involved in utilizing nutrients for the functioning of the body; general term covering both anabolism and catabolism.

Mitochondria – Rod-shaped organelles in cells where energy-releasing reactions take place.

Monoglyceride – Compound composed of a fatty acid attached to glycerol.

Monosaccharide – Carbohydrate in its simplest form; common examples are galactose, fructose, and glucose.

Myelin – Protective, sheath-like coating around nerves.

NAD – Nicotinamide adenine dinucleotide.

Niacin – One of the water soluble B vitamins.

Nicotinamide adenine dinucleotide – Coenzyme containing niacin which is needed in the release of energy; also called NAD.

Night blindness – Limited ability to adapt to changes in light intensity; occurs in deficiency of vitamin A.

Obesity – Condition of being 20 percent or more above desirable weight.

Osmotic pressure – The force which enables a solvent to pass through a semipermeable membrane when the concentrations of solutes on both sides of the membrane are different.

Ossification – Formation of bone.

Ovum – Egg.

Pancreatic amylase – Starch-digesting enzyme formed in the pancreas and acting in the small intestine.

Pantothenic acid – A water soluble B vitamin; component of coenzyme A.

Pectin – Carbohydrate composed of methylated galacturonic acid units.

Pellagra – Deficiency condition due to insufficient niacin.

Pernicious anemia – Condition in which nerve function and red blood cell development are modified; caused by inadequate vitamin B_{12} in the body.

Phenylalanine – An essential amino acid.

Phenyketonuria – Condition caused by an inborn metabolic error which causes phenylalanine to accumulate in the blood, resulting in permanent brain damage; also called PKU.

Phospholipid – Fat in which phosphate and a nitrogenous substance have replaced one of the fatty acids.

Placenta – The organ of reproduction responsible for the nourishment and excretory functions of the developing being.

Polysaccharide – Carbohydrate of very large molecular size; examples include starch, cellulose, glycogen, and pectin.

Polyunsaturated fatty acid – Fatty acid with more than one (commonly two or three) double bond.

Protease – Enzyme that digests protein.

Protein – Organic compound composed of amino acids; contains carbon, hydrogen, oxygen and nitrogen.

Protein-calorie malnutrition – Condition caused by inadequate intake of protein and calories; also called PCM.

Ptyalin – Enzyme in the mouth that initiates the digestion of starch; also called salivary amylase.

Pyridoxine – A water soluble B vitamin.

Renal solute load – Level of ions in the kidney.

Reticulum – Network in the placenta.

Riboflavin – A water soluble B vitamin.

Ribosome – Organelle in which protein is synthesized in the cell.

Ribonucleic acid – Compound playing a prominent role in protein synthesis in the cell; also called RNA.

Rickets – Deficiency condition in which insufficient vitamin D is available to promote adequate absorption of calcium.

Rhodopsin – Compound formed in the rods of the retina of the eye and which is required for vision in dim light; also called visual purple. Vitamin A is needed for formation of rhodopsin.

Salivary amylase – Starch splitting enzyme in mouth; also called ptyalin.

Saturated fatty acid – Fatty acid containing as much hydrogen as it is capable of holding.

Scurvy – Deficiency condition caused by inadequate intake of ascorbic acid.

Starch – Carbohydrate composed of many glucose units linked together into very large molecules.

Sterile field sterilization – Method of formula preparation in which the bottles and other equipment are sterilized separately before sterilized formula is poured into the bottles.

Terminal sterilization – Preparation of formula by sterilizing the formula in the bottles.

Thiamin – A water soluble B vitamin; occasionally called vitamin B_1.

Thiamin pyrophosphate – Thiamin-containing coenzyme utilized in releasing energy in the body; also called TPP.

Thyroxine – Hormone containing iodine and secreted by the thyroid gland to regulate basal metabolic rate.

Tocopherol – Compound with vitamin E activity.

Transamination – Transfer of an amino group from an amino acid to another compound to form a new, nonessential amino acid in the body.

Trophoblastic cells – Cells formed during blastogenesis and which form the external cover of the embryo.

Vitamin A – Fat soluble vitamin.

Vitamin B_6 – Water soluble B vitamin; also called pyridoxine.

Vitamin B_{12} – Water soluble B vitamin; also called cobalamin.

Vitamin C – Water soluble vitamin; also called ascorbic acid.

Vitamin D – Fat soluble vitamin.

Vitamin E – Fat soluble vitamin.

Xerophthalmia – Disease of the eye which can result in blindness; caused by a vitamin A deficiency.

Photo Credits

Index

G

Galactosemia, 347
Gallbladder, 66, 68
Gastric lipase, 6
Gastrulation, 50
Gelatin, 8
Genital system, 65
Germinal layers, 50
Gestagens, 56
Giantism, 67
Glucose, 2, 56
Glycerol, 5
Glycogen, 4, 37, 38
Goiter, 25, 357
Gonadotropic hormones, 56, 67
Gonads, 68
Granulated sugar, 3
Growth, 22, 28, 47 – 70
  antenatal, 47 – 56
  height, 56 – 58
  hormone, 67
  human vs. cow's milk, 128
  Negro, 57
  placental, 54 – 56
  postnatal, 56 – 70
  predictions, 63
  pregnancy, 48 – 51
  preschool, 188
  rate, 56 – 58
  sex, 57 – 60
  skeletal, 61 – 63
  teeth, 19, 21, 22, 49, 52
  weight, 58 – 61
Growth hormone, 67

H

Hair, 48 – 50
Hair proteins, 18
Hallucinogens, 131
Handicapped children, 347 – 350
Head, 61
Head Start, 252
Health, 288
Health foods, 374
Heart, 48 – 49, 51, 53, 65
  abnormalities, 109
  in pregnancy, 103
Heartburn, 103
Heavy metals, 26
Height, 56 – 58
Hemoglobin, 18, 20, 23, 38, 66, 172, 287
  in adolescents, 189 – 290
  in pregnancy, 102   103

  levels, 297
  race, 289
  sex, 289
Hemorrhages, 33, 34
Hemosiderosis, 23
High meat dinners, 172 – 175
Histamine, 11
Histidine, 8, 11, 126
Homogenization, 121
Hormones, 11, 18
Hospital feeding, 344 – 346
  premature infant, 344 – 345
  older child, 345 – 346
Human milk
  carbohydrate in, 126 – 127
  composition of, 120
  fat in, 120 – 123
  linoleic acid in, 122
  medications, 131 – 132
  minerals in, 127 – 128
  protein, 123 – 125
  safety of, 131
  vitamins in, 128 – 129
Hydrochloric acid, 18, 19
Hydrogenation, 5
Hydroxyapatite, 24
Hyperparathyroidism, 69
Hyperplasia, 74
Hyperthyroidism, 14
Hypervitaminosis A, 30
Hypervitaminosis D, 32
Hypothyroidism, 114

I

Immunities, 137
Implantation, 48
Inborn errors of metabolism, 11
INCAP, 13
Incaparina, 13
Incomplete protein, 8 – 9, 12 – 13
Incremental lines, 64
Infant feeding, 159 – 183
  breads, 173
  cereals, 165 – 168
  desserts, 173
  eggs, 171 – 172
  family participation, 161
  fruits, 168 – 171
  junior foods, 178 – 179
  meats, 171 – 174
  menus, 176 – 179
  minerals, 164 – 165
  overfeeding, 175
  pastas, 173
  RDA for, 163

schedule, 159—161, 173—174
serving size, 178
setting, 179—181
solid foods, 165—174
vegetables, 168—171
vitamins, 161—164
Influenza, 137
Inner skin, 48
Insulin, 18, 21
Internal cells, 48
International Unit
vitamin A, 32
vitamin D, 32
vitamin E, 33
Intestinal lipase, 6
Intestinal tract, 48, 52, 66
Intestinal wall, 4, 49
Iodide, 17, 18, 20, 24—26
in infancy, 128
in pregnancy, 108
Iodized salt, 25—26, 111, 357
Iron, 17, 18, 20, 22—23, 192
in adolescence, 289—290
in cereals, 167—168
in infancy, 28, 164
in lactation, 112
in pregnancy, 107—108
supplement, 108
Isoleucine, 8, 125, 126

J

Junior foods, 178—179

K

Keratin, 30
Ketone bodies, 7
Ketosis, 2
Kidney, 48, 67
Kidney disease, 135
Kilocalorie, 15
Kwashiorkor, 13, 77—78

L

Lactase, 4, 90, 147
Lactation, 12, 111—113
drugs, 131—132
nutritional needs, 111—112
ovulation, 137
Lactose, 3, 22, 127
Lactose intolerance, 90—91, 147
Lacto-ovo-vegetarian diets, 294

Lacto-vegetarians, 295
Lacunae, 54
LaLeche League, 138
Larynx, 66
Lead, 26—27
Legs, 48, 52, 61
Legumes, 9
Leucine, 8, 11, 125, 126
Linoleic acid, 7, 122
Lipase, 6
gastric, 6
intestinal, 6
Lipids, 5—8
absorption, 6
classification, 5
compound, 5
derived, 5
digestion, 6
functions, 7
metabolism, 6—7
simple, 3
sources, 5—6
Liver, 48, 51, 66
Long bones, 52, 62, 63
Lungs, 48—50, 51, 65, 66
Lysine, 8, 125, 126

M

Macrocytic anemia, 39
Macronutrient minerals, 17
Magnesium, 17, 18, 20
Maltase, 4
Maltose, 3
Manganese, 17, 18, 20, 26
Marasmus, 13, 76
Margarine, 362—363
Marijuana, 132
Meat-based formula, 148
Meat group, 91—94, 188—189
preparation, 198
Meats, strained, 172
Medications
in lactation, 131—132
Megaloblastic anemia, 108
Melanin, 19, 24
Menarche, 288
Mental development, 73—80
birth weight, 75
brain weight, 75
postnatal, 75—80
premature, 75
prenatal, 73—75
social class, 75
Mental retardation, 11, 108—109